A PRACTICAL MANUAL OF
RENAL MEDICINE
Nephrology, Dialysis and Transplantation

A PRACTICAL MANUAL OF
RENAL MEDICINE
Nephrology, Dialysis and Transplantation

edited by

Kar Neng Lai
The University of Hong Kong, Hong Kong

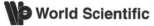

World Scientific

NEW JERSEY · LONDON · SINGAPORE · BEIJING · SHANGHAI · HONG KONG · TAIPEI · CHENNAI

Published by

World Scientific Publishing Co. Pte. Ltd.

5 Toh Tuck Link, Singapore 596224

USA office: 27 Warren Street, Suite 401-402, Hackensack, NJ 07601

UK office: 57 Shelton Street, Covent Garden, London WC2H 9HE

British Library Cataloguing-in-Publication Data
A catalogue record for this book is available from the British Library.

Disclaimer:
Every effort has been made to ensure that drug doses and other information are accurately portrayed in this book. However, the responsibility for all prescriptions rests with the physician. Neither the publisher nor the editor/authors can be held responsible for errors or any consequences arising from the information contained herein. Please consult the standard prescribing information and instructions on use that are issued by the manufacturers and available in each country.

ISBN-13 978-981-283-871-1 (pbk)
ISBN-10 981-283-871-6 (pbk)

Typeset by Stallion Press
Email: enquiries@stallionpress.com

Printed in Singapore.

This book is dedicated to my parents
and
my brother, Ka Siu LAI, MD

Preface

Most textbooks of kidney diseases provide comprehensive information on etiology, epidemiology, physiology, pathology, pathogenetic mechanisms, symptomatology, investigation and management. While the importance of an understanding of the pathophysiology of disease is pivotal in our clinical practice, most physicians, fellows and medical residents value handy, updated, instructive, and evidence-based practical manual during their bedside duty. *A Practical Manual of Renal Medicine: Nephrology, Dialysis and Transplantation* is written explicitly for practising clinicians with primary emphasis on therapeutic approach.

The objective of this *Manual* is to provide a set of updated and well-accepted information to guide those who provide acute and long-term management to patients with kidney diseases. The topics covered include common problems in clinical nephrology such as electrolyte and fluid disturbance, acute renal failure, hypertension, urinary tract infection, glomerular diseases, pregnancy-related renal dysfunction and renal imaging. The sections on dialysis and transplantation place major emphasis on making correct clinical decision, appropriate therapeutic approach and step-by-step treatment protocols. With expert contributors from different countries, the recommended therapeutic approach will be gauged at an international standard applicable to most regional referral centers. These treatment protocols are by no means exhaustive but serve as an effective and accountable guide for patient management worldwide.

The absence of discussions of pathophysiology in most chapters is not meant to diminish its critical role in the understanding and practice of renal medicine. I feel that it is more important to conserve space for management thrust of this *Manual* while keeping down the size for this *Manual* to be carried in the pocket conveniently. For easy reading and rapid reference, bullet points, short notes, tables and diagrams are used throughout the *Manual* instead of lengthy texts.

My sincere thanks to all contributing authors of this *Manual* not only because of their expertise in the science of medicine, but because they are physicians who are able to translate and apply their scientific knowledge in a practical way to allow for a systematic and evidence-based plan of therapy and treatment in the best interests of our patients.

Kar Neng LAI
MD, DSc, FRCPath, FRCP, FRACP
Yu Chiu Kwong Chair of Medicine and
University Chair of Nephrology
University of Hong Kong
February 2009

Contents

List of Contributors

Daniel T. M. CHAN, MD, FRCP
Professor of Medicine
Department of Medicine
University of Hong Kong
Queen Mary Hospital
Hong Kong

James C. M. CHAN, MD
Professor of Pediatrics
University of Vermont College of Medicine
Burlington, VT 05405
USA

Director of Research
The Barbara Bush Children's Hospital
Maine Medical Center
22 Bramhall Street
Portland, ME 04102-3175
USA

Laurence K. CHAN, MD, PhD, FRCP
Professor, Department of Renal Medicine
University of Colorado Health Sciences Center
4200 East Ninth Avenue, C281
Denver, CO 80262
USA

Siu-Kim CHAN, MBBS, MRCP
Fellow, Division of Nephrology
Department of Renal Medicine
University of Colorado Health Sciences Center
4200 East Ninth Avenue, C281
Denver, CO 80262
USA

Present Address:
Renal Division
Department of Medicine
Pamela Youde Nethersole Eastern Hospital
Chai Wan
Hong Kong

Jeremy R. CHAPMAN, MD, FRCP, FRACP
Clinical Professor, Renal Medicine
Westmead Hospital
University of Sydney
Westmead, NSW 2145
Australia

Alfred K. H. CHEUNG, MD
Professor of Medicine
Division of Nephrology & Hypertension
University of Utah
85 North Medical Drive East
Salt Lake City, UT 84112
USA

Kai-Ming CHOW, MBChB, MRCP
Associate Consultant, Renal Unit
Chinese University of Hong Kong
Prince of Wales Hospital
Hong Kong

Bo-Ying CHOY, MBBS, FRCP
Consultant
Department of Medicine
University of Hong Kong
Queen Mary Hospital
Hong Kong

Ferdinand S. K. CHU, MBBS, FRCR, FACLM
Consultant
Department of Radiology
Queen Mary Hospital
Hong Kong

Simon J. DAVIS, MD, FRCP
Professor of Nephrology and Dialysis Medicine
Institute for Science and Technology in Medicine
Keele University
UK

Consultant Nephrologist
Department of Nephrology
University Hospital of North Staffordshire
Stoke-on-Trent, ST4 7LN
UK

Mohsen EL KOSSI, MD, MRCP
Consultant Renal Physician
Doncaster Royal Infirmary
Armthorpe Road
Doncaster, DN2 5LT
UK

Meguid EL NAHAS, PhD, FRCP
Professor of Nephrology
Sheffield Kidney Institute
Northern General Hospital (Sorby Wing)
Herries Road, Sheffield S5 7AU
UK

Barbara ENGEL, BSc, RD, PhD
Tutor in Nutrition and Dietetics
Faculty of Health & Medical Sciences
University of Surrey
Guildford, Surrey GU2 7XH
UK

Dae-Suk HAN, MD
Professor of Medicine
Department of Internal Medicine
Yonsei University College of Medicine
134 Shinchon-dong, Seodaemoon-gu
Seoul, 120-752
Korea

Susan HOU, MD
Professor of Medicine
Department of Medicine
Loyola University
Stritch School of Medicine
2160 South First Avenue
Maywood, IL 60153
USA

Todd S. ING, MBBS, FACP, FRCP
Emeritus Professor
Department of Medicine
Loyola University Chicago
Veterans Affairs Hospital
Hines, IL
USA

Peter G. KERR, MBBS, PhD, FRACP
Professor and Director of Nephrology
Department of Nephrology
Monash Medical Centre
Clayton, Victoria 3168
Australia

Orly F. KOHN, MD, FACP
Associate Professor of Medicine
Department of Medicine
University of Chicago Medical Center
5841 S. Maryland Avenue, MC 5100
Chicago, IL 60637
USA

Andrew S. H. LAI, MBBS
Registrar
Department of Radiology
Queen Mary Hospital
Hong Kong

Kar Neng LAI, MD, DSc, FRCPath, FRCP, FRACP
Professor of Medicine
Department of Medicine
University of Hong Kong
Queen Mary Hospital
Hong Kong

David B. N. LEE, MBBS, FRCP, FACP
Nephrology Consultant
VA Greater Los Angeles Healthcare System
16111 Plummer Street (111), North Hills
Los Angeles, CA 91343
USA

Professor of Medicine
David Geffen School of Medicine
University of California, Los Angeles
Los Angeles, CA
USA

Evan J. C. LEE, MD, FRCP
Associate Professor of Medicine
Department of Medicine
Yong Loo Lin School of Medicine
National University of Singapore
Main Building Level 3
5 Lower Kent Ridge Road
Singapore 119074

Philip K. T. LI, MD, FRCP, FACP
Chief of Nephrology and Honorary Professor of Medicine
Chinese University of Hong Kong
Prince of Wales Hospital
Hong Kong

Wai-Kei LO, MBBS, FRCP
Consultant, Renal Unit
Department of Medicine
University of Hong Kong
Tung Wah Hospital
Hong Kong

Sing-Leung LUI, MD, PhD, FRCP
Consultant, Renal Unit
Department of Medicine
University of Hong Kong
Tung Wah Hospital
Hong Kong

Bruce A. PUSSELL, MBBS, PhD, FRACP
Professor of Medicine
Department of Nephrology
Prince of Wales Hospital
Barker Street
Randwick, Sydney, New South Wales 2031
Australia

Bharathi REDDY, MD
Assistant Professor of Medicine
University of Chicago Medical Center
5841 S. Maryland Avenue, MC 5100
Chicago, IL 60637
USA

Ramin SAM, MD, FACP
Associate Professor of Medicine
Division of Nephrology
Department of Medicine
University of California, San Francisco
San Francisco General Hospital
Building 100, Room 342
1001 Potrero Avenue
San Francisco, CA 94110
USA

Sydney C. W. TANG, MD, PhD, FRCP
Associate Professor of Medicine
Department of Medicine
University of Hong Kong
Queen Mary Hospital
Hong Kong

Matthew K. L. TONG, MBBS, FRCP
Consultant
Department of Medicine and Geriatrics
Princess Margaret Hospital
Lai Chi Kok
Hong Kong

Rowan G. WALKER, MD, FRACP
Associate Professor of Medicine
Department of Nephrology
Royal Melbourne Hospital
Grattan Street
Melbourne, Victoria 3050
Australia

Part 1

General Management of Renal Patients

1

Assessment of Patients with Renal Diseases

Sydney C. W. Tang

1.1 Urinalysis

- It is a fundamental step in diagnosing renal disease.
- Freshly voided morning urine is preferred.
- Three characteristics should be observed: physical, biochemical, and microscopic.
- In clinical practice, direct examination and dipstick testing are usually sufficient.

1.1.1 *Physical Properties*

(i) Color
   The most important color change to observe is a red-through-brown discoloration, which occurs in:

   - hematuria
   - hemoglobinuria
   - myoglobinuria (Fig. 1.1)
   - bilirubinuria (increased urine urobilinogen)
   - ingestion of food dyes (beetroot, blackberries, vegetable dyes) or drugs (rifampicin, phenazopyridine, chloroquine, nitrofurantoin, doxorubicin)
   - presence of metabolites (porphyrin, melanin, homogentisic acid)

(ii) Turbidity

   - Pyuria
   - Chyluria
   - Excessive salt (urate, phosphate, oxalate)

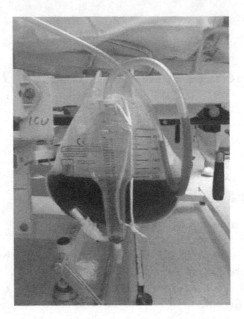

Fig. 1.1 Myoglobinuria in a patient with acute rhabdomyolysis.

(iii) Frothiness

- Proteinuria.

(iv) Specific gravity (SG)
Urine SG, defined as the weight of the urine compared with that of an equal volume of pure water, reflects solute load. Its clinical value is limited, as it depends on the hydration status and other factors. In general:

- SG > 1.030: proteinuria, glycosuria, radiocontrast
- 1.030 > SG > 1.020: volume depletion
- fixed SG = 1.010: chronic renal impairment
- fixed SG = 1.000–1.005: diabetes insipidus.

1.1.2 Biochemical Properties

Commercially available urine Multistix strips can yield semiquantitative detection of:

- albumin (but not Bence-Jones proteins)
- blood
- glucose
- nitrites
- leukocytes
- ketone
- pH

Microalbuminuria can be detected using a specialized dipstick, which usually yields a semiquantitative estimation of urine albumin-to-creatinine ratio.

1.1.3 Microscopy

- Microscopy allows identification of abnormal cells, casts, crystals, and even microorganisms. Phase-contrast microscopy is superior to conventional microscopy.
- Dysmorphic red blood cells (RBCs; Fig. 1.2) of glomerular origin can be distinguished from nonglomerular RBCs. The absence of RBCs together with dipstick-positive hematuria is classical of myoglobinuria in acute rhabdomyolysis.
- The presence of white blood cells (WBCs) may signify urinary tract infection. Sometimes, bacteria may be seen (Fig. 1.3).
- Epithelial cells lining the urinary tract at any level sloughing into the urine are generally of little diagnostic utility (Fig. 1.4).
- Urine crystals are present in minute quantities in normal urine, but should be absent in freshly voided urine. Commonly observed crystals (Fig. 1.5) in association with renal stones include calcium oxalate, uric acid, and magnesium ammonium phosphate.

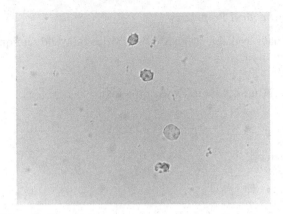

Fig. 1.2 Dysmorphic RBCs with varying sizes, shapes and hemoglobin contents, reflecting glomerular bleeding (courtesy of Dr Susanna Lau, Associate Professor, Department of Microbiology, The University of Hong Kong).

1.2 Interpretation of Laboratory Tests

1.2.1 *Assessment of Renal Function Using Plasma Creatinine*

- The standard measure of renal function is the glomerular filtration rate (GFR). In clinical practice, creatinine clearance (CrCl) is often used to reflect the GFR. CrCl is calculated using either a timed urine collection, given by $[U_{Cr} \times V]/P_{Cr}$, where U_{Cr} = urine creatinine concentration, V = urine volume, and P_{Cr} = plasma creatinine concentration, or accepted equations.
- For timed urine collection, a 24-hour urine sample is usually obtained, since shorter collections tend to yield less accurate results:

$$\text{CrCl (mL/min)} = [U_{Cr} \times V \times 1000]/[P_{Cr} \times 24 \times 60].$$

For patients with significant renal insufficiency, the average of creatinine and urea clearances is computed:

$$\text{UrCl (mL/min)} = [U_{Ur} \times V \times 1000]/[P_{Ur} \times 24 \times 60]$$
$$\text{Corrected GFR} = [\text{CrCl} + \text{UrCl}]/2.$$

- Commonly used estimation equations include:

  (i) the abbreviated 4-variable MDRD (Modification of Diet in Renal Disease study) equation

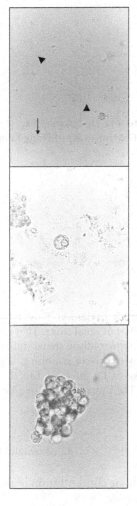

Fig. 1.3 WBCs and bacteria. *Left:* a clump of WBCs. *Middle:* WBCs and bacteria. *Right:* cocci in chains (arrow) and pairs (arrowheads) (courtesy of Dr Susanna Lau, Associate Professor, Department of Microbiology, The University of Hong Kong).

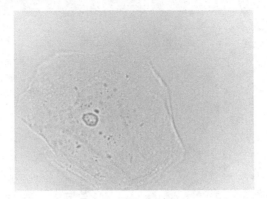

Fig. 1.4 Epithelial cell (courtesy of Dr Susanna Lau, Associate Professor, Department of Microbiology, The University of Hong Kong).

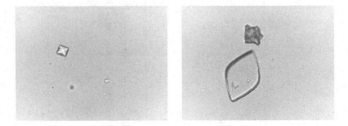

Fig. 1.5 Urine crystals. *Left*: Ca oxalate crystals, typically cuboidal in shape, are the most common type of renal stone. They are seen in patients with hypercalciuria, hyperparathyroidism, renal tubular acidosis, and hypocitraturia, and also in ethylene glycol poisoning. *Right*: Urate crystals are diamond-shaped (courtesy of Dr Susanna Lau, Associate Professor, Department of Microbiology, The University of Hong Kong).

GFR (mL/min/1.73 m^2)
$$= 186.3 \times (P_{Cr})^{-1.154} \times (\text{age})^{-0.203} \times 0.742 \text{ (if female)} \times 1.21 \text{ (if black)},$$

where P_{Cr} = plasma creatinine concentration in mg/dL (to convert from µmol/L to mg/dL, divide by 88.4).

— The equation was developed by regression analysis in 1628 patients with a lower range of GFR in the USA.

Table 1.1   K/DOQI classification for the 5 stages of CKD.

Stage	Description	GFR (mL/min/1.73 m²)
1	Kidney damage with normal or ↑ in GFR	≥90
2	Kidney damage with mild ↓ in GFR	60–89
3	Moderate ↓ in GFR	30–59
4	Severe ↓ in GFR	15–29
5	Kidney failure	<15 (or dialysis)

— Most of the study subjects were Caucasians without diabetes.
— The equation does not carry a body weight variable because it normalizes GFR to body surface area.
— It is most accurate in subjects with moderate chronic kidney disease (CKD) and less accurate at the extremes of GFR, underestimating at high GFR but overestimating with advanced CKD.
— It is increasingly utilized as recommended by the Kidney Disease Outcomes Quality Initiative (K/DOQI) guidelines, which define CKD (see Table 1.1) as structural or functional abnormalities of the kidney for ≥3 months, as manifested by either:

(a) kidney damage, with or without decreased GFR, as defined by:

— pathologic abnormalities
— markers of kidney damage (urinary abnormalities e.g. proteinuria), blood abnormalities, imaging abnormalities; or

(b) GFR <60 mL/min/1.73 m², with or without kidney damage. It has been validated in African-Americans, and has been modified using multiple regression methods for Chinese subjects as:

$$\text{GFR (mL/min/1.73 m}^2) = 175 \times (P_{Cr})^{-1.234} \times (\text{age})^{-0.179} \times 0.79 \text{ (if female).}$$

(ii) the Cockcroft–Gault equation

$$CrCl(mL/min) = \frac{(140 - age) \times lean\ body\ weight\ [kg]}{P_{Cr}[mg/dL] \times 72}$$
$$\times 0.85\ (if\ female).$$

(To convert P_{Cr} from mg/dL to μmol/L, multiply by 88.4.)

— The equation was developed in 1976 in 249 men with stable serum creatinine.
— It is suitable only for patients with stable renal function.
— The adjustment factor for women is based on the theoretical assumption of a 15% lower muscle mass than men.
— The weight element in the numerator overestimates GFR in edematous or obese subjects.
— This equation is being increasingly replaced by the MDRD formula.

- A potential error in using serum creatinine stems from its propensity to drug interaction. Medications that affect serum creatinine without actually altering renal function are listed as follows:

(i) Drugs that increase serum creatinine by inhibiting its tubular secretion

— Amiloride
— Cimetidine
— Probenecid
— Spironolactone
— Triamterene
— Trimethoprim

(ii) Drugs that increase serum creatinine due to interference with creatinine measurement

— Ascorbic acid
— Cephalosporins

1.2.2 Assessment of Renal Function Using Plasma Cystatin C

An inherent defect of P_{Cr}-based prediction equation is that different levels of P_{Cr} do not necessarily reflect the true variation of GFR. This is particularly true during the early stages of CKD because of tubular secretion of creatinine.

- Cystatin C is a small, 13-kDa basic protein produced by all nucleated cells at a constant rate and eliminated exclusively by glomerular filtration.
- Plasma cystatin C level increases earlier than P_{Cr} as GFR decreases, and hence is useful in detecting early renal function impairment.
- Plasma cystatin C level starts to rise at a GFR of around 90 mL/min/ 1.73 m^2.
- Renal plasma clearance correlates strongly with that of ^{51}Cr-EDTA, with a linear coefficient of 0.99.
- A uniformly agreed cystatin C-based GFR-estimating equation has yet to be proposed.
- Cystatin C measurement is more expensive that P_{Cr} assay.

1.3 Renal Biopsy

Percutaneous renal biopsy under real-time ultrasound guidance using spring-loaded automated 16G to 18G Tru-Cut needles is the favored approach.

1.3.1 *Indications*

- For diagnosis of renal parenchymal disease (proteinuria, abnormal sediments, or impaired function)
- For diagnosis of renal allograft rejection and recurrent or *de novo* disease
- As protocol biopsy for early detection of chronic allograft nephropathy

1.3.2 *Contraindications*

Absolute	*Relative*
Bleeding diathesis	Extreme obesity
Uncooperative patient	Contracted kidney
Uncontrolled hypertension	Hydronephrosis
Currently on antiplatelet agent,	Acute pyelonephritis
warfarin, or non-steroidal	Large cysts or tumor
anti-inflammatory drug	Solitary kidney (consider
(NSAID)	laparoscopic approach)
	Respiratory distress
	Pregnancy (second and third
	trimesters)

1.3.3 Preparation

- Ensure blood pressure (BP) < 150/95 mmHg.
- Stop aspirin/clopidogrel/warfarin/NSAID for at least 5 days before biopsy.
- Ensure platelet count ≥ 100 × 10⁹/L.
- Ensure normal coagulation times (except in lupus anticoagulant-positive patients).
- If serum urea > 20 mmol/L, consider DDAVP infusion at 0.3 µg/kg i.v. over 30 mins before biopsy.
- Type and screen.

1.3.4 Complications

- Microscopic hematuria   100%
- Macroscopic hematuria   3%–5%
- Perinephric hematoma   visible in computed tomography (CT) scan in 50%–90%, usually asymptomatic
- Arteriovenous fistula or aneurysm   rare
- Mortality   <0.1%

1.3.5 Post-Renal Biopsy Care

- Complete overnight bed rest.
- Regular blood pressure monitoring.

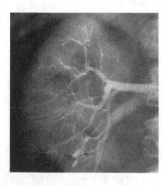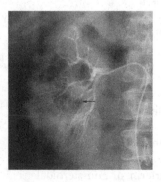

Fig. 1.6 Persistent post-renal biopsy bleeding and embolization. *Left*: Renal arteriography in a patient with persistent post-renal biopsy hematuria. Arrow shows bleeding vessel with extravasation of contrast. *Right*: After successful embolization, there is acute cut-off of the branch renal artery supplying the bleeder (arrow).

- Voided urine should be inspected.
- Anti-platelet agents or warfarin intake can be resumed after 2 days if there is no sign of bleeding.
- Excessive physical activities should be avoided for 1 week.

If gross hematuria occurs with stable hemodynamic status:

- Continue bed rest.
- Optimize blood pressure and monitor hemoglobin level.

If there is hemodynamic compromise:

- Consider renal angiography with embolization of bleeder, if necessary (Fig. 1.6).
- Blood transfusion may be required.

Suggested Reading

de Jong PE, Gansevoort RT. (2006) Prevention of chronic kidney disease: the next step forward! *Nephrology* 11:240–244.

Kidney Disease Outcome Quality Initiative. (2002) K/DOQI clinical practice guidelines for chronic kidney disease: evaluation, classification, and stratification. *Am J Kidney Dis* 39(Suppl 1):S1–S246.

Lane C, Brown M, Dunsmuir W, *et al.* (2006) Can spot urine protein/creatinine ratio replace 24 h urine protein in usual clinical nephrology? *Nephrology* 11:245–249.

Levey AS, Bosch JP, Lewis JB, *et al.* (1999) A more accurate method to estimate glomerular filtration rate from serum creatinine: a new prediction equation. Modification of Diet in Renal Disease Study Group. *Ann Intern Med* 130:461–470.

Lewis J, Agodoa L, Cheek D, *et al.*, African-American Study of Hypertension and Kidney Disease. (2001) Comparison of cross-sectional renal function measurements in African Americans with hypertensive nephrosclerosis and of primary formulas to estimate glomerular filtration rate. *Am J Kidney Dis* 38:744–753.

Ma YC, Zuo L, Chen JH, *et al.* (2006) Modified glomerular filtration rate estimating equation for Chinese patients with chronic kidney disease. *J Am Soc Nephrol* 17:2937–2944.

Ma YC, Zuo L, Chen JH, *et al.* (2007) Improved GFR estimation by combined creatinine and cystatin C measurements. *Kidney Int* 72:1535–1542.

Tang S, Li JH, Lui SL, *et al.* (2002) Free-hand, ultrasound-guided percutaneous renal biopsy: experience from a single operator. *Eur J Radiol* 41:65–69.

Tidman M, Sjostrom P, Jones I. (2008) A comparison of GFR estimating formulae based upon s-cystatin C and s-creatinine and a combination of the two. *Nephrol Dial Transplant* 23:1072–1073.

2

Acid-Base Disturbances

Orly F. Kohn and Todd S. Ing

2.1 Simple Acid-Base Disturbances

An acid is a proton or hydrogen donor; and a base, a proton or hydrogen acceptor. For example, lactic acid = lactate$^-$ + H$^+$. Lactic acid is an acid because it can donate H$^+$, whereas lactate is a base because it can accept H$^+$.

Normal arterial blood pH varies between 7.35 and 7.45. Normal arterial P_{CO_2} = 40 ± 4 (± 2 SD[a]) mmHg, and normal arterial serum [HCO$_3$$^-$] = 25 ± 1 (± 2 SD) mmol/L (Note: [...] refers to concentrations). Acidemia is defined by a blood pH of less than 7.35; alkalemia, when pH is higher than 7.45. Acidosis is a process generating excess acid, while alkalosis is a process generating excess base. Acidosis can occur without acidemia if blood pH is higher than 7.35, and alkalosis can take place without alkalemia if blood pH is less than 7.45. The pH range that is compatible with survival is estimated to be between 6.8 and 7.8 (16–160 nmol H$^+$/L). Acidosis and alkalosis can coexist, but acidemia and alkalemia cannot.

In the determination of acid-base changes in the blood, arterial blood pH and P_{CO_2} are measured while arterial serum [HCO$_3$$^-$] is derived by applying the Henderson–Hasselbalch equation. This calculated arterial serum [HCO$_3$$^-$] is as accurate as if it had actually been measured. Serum electrolytes in the form of [Na], [K], [Cl], and [T$_{CO_2}$] (also known as total CO$_2$ or carbon dioxide content) are ordinarily obtained from venous serum; note that [HCO$_3$$^-$] is often not part of the regular venous serum electrolyte panel. [T$_{CO_2}$] is the sum of serum [HCO$_3$$^-$] and [H$_2CO_3$] (the latter including dissolved CO$_2$ gas; see below for the calculation of [H$_2$CO$_3$]). Since venous

---

[a] SD: standard deviation.

P_{CO_2} is commonly in the neighborhood of 46 mmHg and the solubility coefficient of carbon dioxide in venous serum at 20°C is 0.046, the venous serum $[H_2CO_3]$ is (46 × 0.046) = 2.1 mmol/L. Since venous $[HCO_3^-]$, having a value of 25 mmol/L, is a little higher than its arterial counterpart, the normal value for venous serum $[T_{CO_2}]$ is (25 + 2.1) = 27.1 with a range of 25 to 29 mmol/L. When metabolic acidosis is the only disturbance, venous serum $[T_{CO_2}]$ is <25 mmol/L. If metabolic alkalosis is the sole disorder, venous serum $[T_{CO_2}]$ will be >29 mmol/L.

2.1.1 *Definition of pH*

$$pH = -\log[H^+ \text{ mol/L}]. \text{ For } H^+, g/L = \text{mol/L} = \text{Eq/L}.$$

For example:

$$pH\ 7 = -\log[10^{-7}\text{ mol } H^+/L]$$
$$[H^+] = [10^{-7}\text{ mol } H^+/L] = [100\text{ nmol } H^+/L].$$

Whenever the pH changes by 0.3, the H^+ concentration changes by a factor of 2, either multiplying or dividing by 2, depending on whether the H^+ concentration is increasing or decreasing. One can use this method to obtain any H^+ concentration from any pH value (only applicable to pH values with one or no decimal place). This is shown in Table 2.1.

The HCO_3/CO_2 system is the principal buffer in extracellular fluid (ECF). The relationship between pH and the ratio of HCO_3 to CO_2 is expressed by the Henderson–Hasselbalch equation:

$$pH = 6.1 + \log([HCO_3^-]/[H_2CO_3]) = 6.1 + \log([HCO_3^-]/0.03\ P_{CO_2}),$$

in which 6.1 is the pK_a of H_2CO_3 and $[H_2CO_3]$ is calculated as the product of P_{CO_2} and 0.03 (the latter being the solubility coefficient of carbon dioxide gas in serum at 37°C, the temperature at which arterial

Table 2.1 Relationship between pH and $[H^+]$ in nmol/L.

pH	$[H^+]$	pH	$[H^+]$	pH	$[H^+]$	pH	$[H^+]$	pH	$[H^+]$	pH	$[H^+]$	pH	$[H^+]$
8	10	7.7	20	7.4	40	7.1	80	6.8	160				
7	100	7.3	50	7.6	25								
6	1000	6.3	500	6.6	250	6.9	125	7.2	63	7.5	32	7.8	16

P_{CO_2} is obtained). [HCO_3^-] and [H_2CO_3] are expressed in mmol/L, and P_{CO_2} in mmHg (for a monovalent ion, mmol/L and mEq/L can be used interchangeably).

The Henderson–Hasselbalch equation is derived from the Henderson equation, namely (in arterial blood) [H^+] = K[H_2CO_3]/[HCO_3^-], with K being the dissociation constant for H_2CO_3 and having a value of 800. Therefore, [H^+] = 800(0.03 P_{CO_2})/[HCO_3^-]. After solving 800(0.03), the Henderson equation for clinical use becomes:

$$[H^+] \text{ nanomol/L} = 24 \, P_{CO_2} \text{ mmHg}/[HCO_3^-] \text{ mmol/L.}$$

Example

Arterial pH 7.1, P_{CO_2} = 40 mmHg. What is the [HCO_3^-]?

(1) By applying the Henderson equation:

   80 = 24(40)/[HCO_3^-].

Therefore, [HCO_3^-] is found to have a value of 12 mmol/L.

(2) By applying the Henderson–Hasselbalch equation:

   7.1 = 6.1 + log[HCO_3^-]/40(0.03) = 6.1 + log[HCO_3^-]/1.2.
   log[HCO_3^-]/1.2 = 1, so [HCO_3^-]/1.2 = 10.

Therefore, [HCO_3^-] = 10(1.2) = 12 mmol/L.

[HCO_3^-] is regulated by the kidneys (via HCO_3^- reclamation and H^+ secretion). P_{CO_2} is regulated by the lungs (alveolar ventilation). The lungs and kidneys adapt for metabolic and respiratory disturbances, respectively. As the body's adaptive mechanism is never complete, with a simple disturbance the pH is always abnormal. The expected respiratory or renal adaptations for a primary renal or respiratory disorder have been empirically derived from humans with those disorders. Whereas the expected respiratory adaptation to a metabolic disturbance has been thought to be of similar magnitude be it acute or chronic, renal adaptation is more complete if the respiratory disturbance is chronic than if it is acute (Table 2.2). Of note, mild acute metabolic acidosis brought on by NH_4Cl ingestion was recently shown to result in only 0.85 mmHg decline in P_{CO_2} per 1 mmol/L decline in [HCO_3^-], raising the possibility of some difference in respiratory adaptation between acute and chronic metabolic acidosis conditions as well.

Table 2.2 Expected adaptive response to a primary acid-base disturbance.

Disturbance	pH	[HCO$_3^-$]	P$_{CO_2}$
Metabolic acidosis	⇓	⇓ primary	Adaptive ⇓ in P$_{CO_2}$ of 1.2 (range, 1–1.5) mmHg per 1 mmol/L ⇓ in [HCO$_3^-$], i.e. ΔP$_{CO_2}$ = Δ[HCO$_3^-$] × 1.2
Metabolic alkalosis	⇑	⇑ primary	Adaptive ⇑ in P$_{CO_2}$ of 0.7 (range, 0.25–1) mmHg per 1 mmol/L ⇑ in [HCO$_3^-$], i.e. ΔP$_{CO_2}$ = Δ[HCO$_3^-$] × 0.7. An adaptive rise in P$_{CO_2}$ above 55 mmHg is unlikely because of the hypoventilation-induced hypoxia that stimulates respiration
Respiratory acidosis	⇓	Adaptive ⇑ in [HCO$_3^-$] of 1 mmol/L (acute) and 3.5 mmol/L (chronic) per 10 mmHg ⇑ in P$_{CO_2}$	⇑ primary
Respiratory alkalosis	⇑	Adaptive ⇓ in [HCO$_3^-$] of 2 mmol/L (acute) and 4 mmol/L (chronic) per 10 mmHg ⇓ in P$_{CO_2}$	⇓ primary

2.2 Mixed Acid-Base Disturbances

A mixed disorder is present when there is less than or more than the expected degree of adaptation.

Example

Arterial pH 7.23, $[HCO_3^-]$ = 15 mmol/L, P_{CO_2} = 37 mmHg (normal values, pH 7.4, $[HCO_3^-]$ 24 mmol/L, P_{CO_2} 40 mmHg).

- ⇓ pH, ⇓ $[HCO_3^-]$, therefore metabolic acidosis.
- Expect 1.2 mmHg ⇓ in P_{CO_2} for each 1 mmol/L ⇓ in $[HCO_3^-]$

(adaptation starts within 1 hour and complete by 12–24 hours).

Expected respiratory adaptation is calculated as follows:

$[HCO_3^-]$ drop = 24 – 15 = 9 mmol/L.

Expected drop in P_{CO_2} is 9 × (1.2) ≈ 11 mmHg; expected P_{CO_2} then is 40 – 11 = 29 mmHg. At 37 mmHg, the measured P_{CO_2} is higher than expected; therefore, a combination of metabolic acidosis and respiratory acidosis is present.

One of the classical mixed acid-base disorders is seen with salicylate overdose. Salicylates stimulate the respiratory center in the medulla, leading to hyperventilation and respiratory alkalosis. It also leads to an increased production of lactic acid and ketoacids, resulting in metabolic acidosis. Salicylic acid itself only accounts for a few mmol/L of the total acids present.

2.3 Metabolic Acidosis

2.3.1 *Normal Physiology*

Daily net acid (H^+) production = 0.3–1 mmol/kg/day. This is derived from:

- sulfuric acid resulting from the metabolism of sulfur-containing amino acids such as cysteine, cystine, and methionine
- phosphoric acid resulting from the metabolism of phosphoproteins and phosphoesters
- H^+ resulting from the metabolism of cationic amino acids such as lysine and arginine.

Daily renal net acid excretion (NAE, in mmol/day) = $V([NH_4^+] + [TA] - [HCO_3^-])$, where V is urine volume; and $[NH_4^+]$, $[TA]$ (titratable acid), and $[HCO_3^-]$ refer to their respective urine concentrations.

- TA is relatively fixed in quantity, consisting mostly of the acidic monosodium dihydrogen phosphate, generated as follows: $Na_2HPO_4 + H^+ \rightarrow NaH_2PO_4 + Na^+$.
- NH_4^+ production varies by need: with acidosis, more NH_4^+ is synthesized from glutamine, up to as high as 200 mmol/day.

The causes for metabolic acidosis can be classified in terms of: (a) a high H^+ production rate, (b) excessive loss of HCO_3^-, and (c) inability to excrete the amount of acids generated as a result of normal metabolism. In practical terms, differentiation among the various types of acidosis usually relies on the anion gap, as depicted in Fig. 2.1. A high anion gap acidosis is almost always due to increased acid generation (the only exception being that of advanced renal insufficiency), whereas excess urine HCO_3^- loss or stool HCO_3^- (and/or HCO_3^- precursor) loss and decreased renal acid excretion can lead to a normal anion gap acidosis.

2.3.2 *High Anion Gap (or Normochloremic) Metabolic Acidosis*

- Anion gap $[AG^-]$ in serum = measured cations minus measured anions = $[Na^+] - [Cl^-] - [T_{CO_2}]$. Sodium is the major cation in the

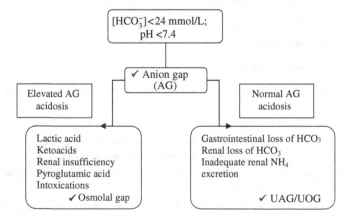

Fig. 2.1 Approach to differential diagnosis of metabolic acidosis. UAG: urine anion gap; UOG: urine osmolal gap.

serum; therefore, $[Na^+]$ is used here to represent measured cations. Measured anions are represented by $[Cl^-]$ and $[T_{CO_2}]$. $[T_{CO_2}]$ takes the place of $[HCO_3^-]$ here.

• $[AG^-]$ is the concentration of anions that are not ordinarily measured when serum electrolytes are estimated. These unmeasured anions include albumin (accounting for most of the $[AG^-]$), phosphates, sulfate, and certain organic anions. Normal $[AG^-] = 138 - 101 - 27 = 10$ mEq/L (mEq is a measure of charges).

• $[AG^-]$ decreases by ~2.5 mEq/L per 1 g/dL fall in serum $[albumin^-]$ below 4.4 g/dL.

• $[AG^-]$ is usually about 7–13 mEq/L.

With the generation of an acid (HX), bicarbonate is consumed:

$$HX + NaHCO_3 \rightarrow NaX + H_2CO_3 \rightarrow CO_2 + H_2O + NaX.$$

X is an unmeasured anion that increases the $[AG^-]$.

Example

In a patient with diabetic ketoacidosis, serum $[Na^+] = 138$, $[Cl^-] = 101$, $[T_{CO_2}] = 10$. $[AG^-] = 138 - 101 - 10 = 27$ mEq/L of unmeasured anions, 10 of which are due to albumin and other normally present but unmeasured anions, and 17 of which are due to ketoacid anions, (i.e. acetoacetate and β-hydroxybutyrate). Note the normochloremia.

2.3.2.1 *Causes*

⇑ acid generbation

(i) Lactic acidosis
  • L-lactic acidosis, type A: impaired tissue oxygenation, hypoperfusion.
  • L-lactic acidosis, type B: malignancy, metformin, drug-induced mitochondrial dysfunction (e.g. HIV nucleoside reverse transcriptase inhibitors, linezolid), inhibitors of mitochondrial ATP generation (e.g. cyanide toxicity from nitroprusside), thiamine deficiency, propofol. Also see under (iii) ingestions/intoxications below.

- D-lactic acidosis: jejunoileal bypass, short bowel syndrome. D-lactic acid is produced by an abnormal colonic bacterial flora. D-lactate is not detected by standard clinical laboratory assays, which only measure L-lactate using the enzyme L-lactic dehydrogenase.

(ii) Ketoacidosis
  - Due to acetoacetic and/or β-hydroxybutyric acids, e.g. in diabetes mellitus, ethanol ketoacidosis, and during fasting or on a low-carbohydrate, high-protein diet.

(iii) Ingestions/Intoxications
  - Formic acid from methanol (via alcohol dehydrogenase).[b]
  - Glycolic, glyoxylic, and oxalic acids from ethylene glycol (via alcohol dehydrogenase).[b]
  - Lactic acid from propylene glycol (a diluent for lorazepam, phenobarbital, diazepam, phenytoin, trimethoprim-sulfamethoxazole, and other medications) (via alcohol dehydrogenase).[b]
  - Acetoacetic, β-hydroxybutyric, and lactic acids from salicylates.
  - Pyroglutamic acid: from acquired glutathione depletion (due to acetaminophen/paracetamol, vigabatrin, flucloxacillin, netilmicin), or rarely due to inherited glutathione synthetase or 5-oxoprolinase deficiency.

A mnemonic for common causes of high anion gap metabolic acidosis is AKA MULE (AKA is typically the abbreviation for "also known as"):

- A = aspirin (salicylate, acetoacetate, β-hydroxybutyrate, lactate)
- K = ketoacidosis (acetoacetate, β-hydroxybutyrate)
- A = alcohol [ethanol] (β-hydroxybutyrate)
- M = methanol (formate)
- U = uremia (phosphate, sulfate)
- L = lactic acidosis (lactate)
- E = ethylene glycol (glycolate, glyoxylate, oxalate).

Anions within brackets refer to the involved unmeasured anions.

---

[b] Note the increased osmolal gap with methanol, ethylene glycol, and propylene glycol intoxication because these agents are particles that contribute to osmolality. Osmolal gap (normal values, 5–10 mmol/kg) is the difference between serum osmolality determined by freezing point depression and that calculated from: $2 \times$ [Na] (mmol/L) + glucose (mg/L)/180 + urea nitrogen (mg/L)/28.

If $[AG^-] > 25$ mEq/L, one of the above conditions is almost always present. If $[AG^-] < 20$ mEq/L, often one cannot find the involved anion (may be Krebs cycle intermediate(s) such as citrate, isocitrate, alpha-ketoglutarate, succinate, malate).

Decreased excretion of nonvolatile acids

High anion gap acidosis is often seen with end-stage renal failure not because of increased acid generation, but because of reduced excretion of the normally produced nonvolatile acids — such as phosphoric, sulfuric, and certain organic acids (see above) — along with retention of those acids' conjugate bases (such as phosphate, sulfate, urate, and hippurate anions) with a glomerular filtration rate (GFR) of <15 mL/min.

2.3.3 *Normal Anion Gap (or Hyperchloremic) Metabolic Acidosis*

> **Example**
>
> Bicarbonate consumption by HCl:
>
> $$HCl + NaHCO_3 \rightarrow NaCl + H_2CO_3 \rightarrow CO_2 + H_2O + NaCl.$$
>
> There are no new unmeasured anions here.

2.3.3.1 *Causes*

Renal

(i) Loss of HCO_3 (failure of reclamation): proximal renal tubular acidosis
- Proximal tubule dysfunction either as a part of a generalized proximal tubular dysfunction, known as Fanconi syndrome, or as an isolated bicarbonate reclamation defect.
  - (a) Acquired: monoclonal immunoglobulin light chain, ifosfamide.
  - (b) Genetic: inherited defects in sodium bicarbonate transporter, inherited defect in Na^+/H^+ exchanger, cystinosis.

- Carbonic anhydrase inhibition by drugs, e.g. acetazolamide, zonisamide, topiramate, topical mefanide acetate.

(ii) Decreased acid excretion
- Distal renal tubular acidosis
  (a) Genetic: gene mutations in the H^+ ATPase or Cl^-/HCO_3^- exchanger.
  (b) Acquired: often associated with hypergammaglobulinemia (Sjogren's syndrome, HIV, systemic lupus erythematosus), amphotericin B.
- Type 4 renal tubular acidosis (hyperkalemia with reduced NH_4^+ excretion).
- Hypoaldosteronism and aldosterone resistance: primary hypoaldosteronism, Addison's disease, hyporeninemic hypoaldosteronism (e.g. secondary to nonsteroidal anti-inflammatory agents), ACE inhibitors, HIV, spironolactone, heparin, cyclosporine or tacrolimus.
- Renal insufficiency (with GFR < 30 mL/min): decreased NH_4^+ excretion due to a reduced renal mass (the residual renal function is still capable of excreting the abnormal anions mentioned above).

Gastrointestinal loss of HCO_3

- Intestinal secretions at sites below the stomach have a bicarbonate or bicarbonate-precursor organic anion concentration of 50–70 mmol/L. Profound loss of intestinal fluids (via diarrhea, drainage tube, or fistula) will result in hyperchloremic metabolic acidosis, often with hypokalemia.
- Ureterosigmoidostomy results in hyperchloremic metabolic acidosis due to colonic absorption of chloride (in exchange for bicarbonate) and ammonium from urine. Ureteroileostomy may also bring about acidosis if there is a prolonged contact between the urine and the intestinal mucosa (e.g. as a result of intestinal obstruction).

Gain of HCl

- Administration of NH_4Cl, HCl, calcium chloride (oral), cholestyramine hydrochloride, sevelamer hydrochloride.
- Formation of hydrogen mainly from metabolism of cationic amino acids from total parenteral nutrition (TPN).

Example

A patient with ureterosigmoidostomy has serum $[Na^+] = 138$, $[Cl^-] = 118$, $[T_{CO_2}] = 10$. $[AG^-] = 138 - 118 - 10 = 10$ mEq/L, all of which are due to albumin and other normally present but unmeasured anions. There are no abnormal anions present.

The low $[T_{CO_2}]$ is due to loss of serum HCO_3^- in the feces as a result of exchange with urinary Cl^- in the colonic lumen. Note the hyperchloremia as a result of the increased colonic absorption of Cl^-.

Entry of intracellular H⁺ into ECF

- Hyperthyroidism: encountered at times among Asians especially after a high carbohydrate meal. Extracellular fluid (ECF) potassium enters cells in exchange for hydrogen.
- Hypokalemic periodic paralysis: ECF potassium enters cells in exchange for hydrogen as well.

A mnemonic for common causes of normal anion gap metabolic acidosis is USED CAR:

- U = ureteroenterostomy
- S = saline given intravenously in the face of renal dysfunction (serum $[HCO_3^-]$ diluted by saline)
- E = endocrine disturbances such as hypoaldosteronism, hyperthyroidism, antialdosterone agents
- D = diarrhea
- C = carbonic anhydrase inhibitors
- A = alimentation (TPN), various hydrochlorides
- R = renal tubular acidosis

Normal anion gap metabolic acidosis caused by excessive gastrointestinal loss of HCO_3^- or by gain of H^+ will result in an increased NH_4^+ excretion by the kidneys. Urinary $[NH_4^+]$ is not ordinarily determined by clinical laboratories, but can be estimated by either the urinary anion gap (UAG^-) or the urinary osmolal gap (UOG), with the latter being less prone to error.

2.3.4 *Urinary Anion Gap (UAG⁻)*

UAG^- measurement may be useful in the workup of a normal anion gap metabolic acidosis.

In urine: $[Na^+] + [K^+] + $ [unmeasured cations]
$= [Cl^-] + $ [unmeasured anions].
UAG^- in $mEq/L = [Na^+] + [K^+] - [Cl^-]$
$= $ [unmeasured anions] $- $ [unmeasured cations].

Normal UAG^- may be positive or near 0 (with urinary $[NH_4^+]$ of about 20–40 mEq/L). With non-renal metabolic acidosis, such as that due to diarrhea, UAG^- is expected to become more negative as NH_4^+ (an unmeasured cation) and Cl^- excretion increase (NH_4^+ excretion to as high as 200 mEq/day); in this case, $UAG^- = -20$ to -70 mEq/L.

With renal acidification defects (all types of renal tubular acidosis [RTA] and renal insufficiency), UAG^- will remain 0 to positive despite metabolic acidosis because NH_4^+ excretion is reduced. However, note that UAG^- does not accurately reflect NH_4^+ excretion in the urine in states of metabolic acidosis in which urinary unmeasured anion excretion is also increased. Examples of such unmeasured anions include hippurate (from metabolism of toluene to hippuric acid in glue sniffing), D-lactate (with inability of D-lactate to be reabsorbed by the renal tubules in the face of D-lactic acidosis), and ketoacid anions (in ketoacidosis). The acidosis-induced increase in NH_4^+ excretion is accompanied by an increase in excretion of those unmeasured organic anions rather than by that of chloride. Since urinary $[Cl^-]$ is low, urinary $[Na^+] + [K^+] - [Cl^-]$ will be positive even though NH_4^+ excretion is increased. Therefore, UAG^- is not a useful measure under such circumstances and will misleadingly suggest the presence of RTA. In such cases, measurement of the urinary osmolal gap will be helpful.

2.3.5 Urinary Osmolal Gap (UOG)

UOG is useful in estimating urinary NH_4^+ excretion if UAG^- is 0 or positive and there is a high suspicion of an increased excretion of urinary unmeasured anions.

$$UOG \ (mmol/kg) = \text{measured } U_{osm} - \text{calculated } U_{osm}$$
$$= \text{measured } U_{osm} - \{2 \times [Na \ mmol/L] + 2$$
$$\times [K \ mmol/L] + [\text{urea nitrogen, } mg/L]/28$$
$$+ [\text{glucose, } mg/L]/180\},$$

where U_{osm} is the urine osmolality. If the urine dipstick is negative for glucose, one can ignore urine glucose for the osmolality calculation.

Since UOG is mainly the sum of $[NH_4^+]$ and its accompanying anions, UOG/2 is an approximate estimation of urinary $[NH_4^+]$. A low UOG (e.g. <100 mmol/kg) suggests low NH_4^+ excretion, and thus renal disease such as RTA. The combination of a high UOG (because of high $[NH_4^+]$ and $[Cl^-]$) and a highly negative UAG⁻ (because of high $[NH_4^+]$ and $[Cl^-]$) suggests diarrhea or exogenous acid loading. The coupling of a high UOG (because of high $[NH_4^+]$ and high [unmeasured organic anions]) and a positive UAG⁻ (because of low $[Cl^-]$ and high [unmeasured organic anions]) suggests the presence of hippurate, D-lactate, and ketoacid anions in the urine (and their respective causative diseases).

A high anion gap acidosis and a normal anion gap acidosis can coexist in the same patient. $\Delta[\text{anion gap}^-]/\Delta[HCO_3^-]$ may be helpful in recognizing the coexistence of the two types of acidosis. With high anion gap acidosis, $\Delta[\text{anion gap}^-]$ and $\Delta[HCO_3^-]$ are not far apart. In the face of normal anion gap acidosis, $\Delta[\text{anion gap}^-]$ is normal while $\Delta[HCO_3^-]$ and $\Delta[Cl^-]$ are high.

Example

A patient with D-lactic acidosis (high anion gap acidosis) and proximal renal tubular acidosis (normal anion gap acidosis) has serum $[Na^+] = 138$, $[Cl^-] = 110$, $[T_{CO_2}] = 10$. $[AG^-] = 138 - 110 - 10 = 18$ mEq/L, 10 of which are due to albumin and other normally present but unmeasured anions while 8 (the Δ anion gap⁻) of which are due to D-lactate. However, $[T_{CO_2}]$ has decreased by a total of $27 - 10 = 17$. Original serum values $[Na^+] = 138$, $[Cl^-] = 101$, $[T_{CO_2}] = 27$.

Eight of the 17 $[T_{CO_2}]$ lost was due to titration with the 8 mmol/L of $[H^+]$ derived from the 8 mmol/L of D-lactic acid. The remaining nine of the 17 $[T_{CO_2}]$ lost was due to loss of HCO_3^- in the urine (filtered bicarbonate which was not reclaimed). $[Cl^-]$ increases by 9 in an attempt to balance the electrical charges as a result of increased absorption of chloride from the tubular fluid.

When considering $\Delta[\text{anion gap}^-]/\Delta[HCO_3^-]$ in high anion gap metabolic acidosis, one should be mindful that, in order for the ratio to be close to unity, the volume of distribution for H^+ and that for the abnormal anion need to be similar. If H^+ has a larger volume of distribution than the abnormal anion, the ratio will not be unity. For example, as more H^+ ions move into the intracellular compartment relative to the anion, there will be a smaller decline in the extracellular HCO_3^- as more buffering will be provided by intracellular buffers as opposed to extracellular HCO_3^-. If relatively more of the anion remains in the ECF, the increase in anion gap level will exceed the fall in extracellular HCO_3^-. Thus, $\Delta[\text{anion gap}^-]/\Delta[HCO_3^-]$ may be greater than 1, even in a pure high anion gap metabolic acidosis.

2.3.6 Clinical Consequences

Stimulation of the respiratory center in the brainstem by marked systemic metabolic acidosis (e.g. pH < 7.2) can lead to a deep and rapid breathing pattern called Kussmaul's respiration. Severe acidosis can bring about vasodilatation and myocardial depression with resultant hypotension, pulmonary edema, dysrhythmias, and death. Chronic acidosis, even if mild, can cause both hypercalciuria and osteopenia as a result of buffering of hydrogen by calcium salts. Chronic acidosis can lead to growth retardation in children. Acidosis has also been suggested to cause catabolism.

2.3.7 Treatment

- HCO_3^- replacement is particularly controversial for high anion gap acidosis such as diabetic ketoacidosis and type A lactic acidosis.
- The most critical actions under those conditions are correcting the underlying acidemia-causing process and thereby allow the body's homeostatic mechanisms to correct the acid-base abnormality.
- For severe high anion gap acidosis (pH < 7.1–7.2), $NaHCO_3$ may be administered with the aim of raising serum $[HCO_3^-]$ to 10–12 mmol/L and the pH to just over 7.2.

2.3.7.1 Estimation of HCO_3^- Deficit

- Target serum $[HCO_3^-]$ at 10–12 mmol/L (pH ≥ 7.2) and calculate the total HCO_3^- deficit up to this level.

- HCO_3^- space increases as serum $[HCO_3^-]$ declines:

$$HCO_3^- \text{ space} = V_{HCO_3} = \{0.4 + (2.6/[HCO_3^-])\}* \text{ lean BW (in kg)},$$

where V_{HCO_3} is the HCO_3^- volume and BW is the body weight.

Calculate HCO_3^- space (a) at the start of therapy ($V_{HCO_3^- ini}$) and (b) after the target serum $[HCO_3^-]$ of 12 mmol/L has been reached as a result of the proposed $NaHCO_3$ therapy ($V_{HCO_3^- fin}$). Then, average the two values so obtained ($V_{HCO_3^- ave}$).

Example

A patient with lactic acidosis has arterial serum $[HCO_3^-]$ of 5 mmol/L, lean BW of 60 kg, and target arterial serum $[HCO_3^-]$ of 12 mmol/L. What amount of HCO_3^- might be required to bring the patient to the target level?

$V_{HCO_3^- ini} = [0.4 + (2.6/[HCO_3^-])] \times \text{lean BW (kg)} = [0.4 + 2.6/5] \times 60 = (0.4 + 0.52) \times 60 = 55.2$ L.

$V_{HCO_3^- fin} = [0.4 + (2.6/[HCO_3^-])] \times \text{lean BW (kg)} = [0.4 + 2.6/12] \times 60 = (0.4 + 0.2) \times 60 = 36$ L.

$V_{HCO_3^- ave} = (55.2 + 36)/2 = 45.6$ L.

Since $\Delta[HCO_3^-] = 12 - 5 = 7$ mmol/L, the total amount of HCO_3^- (i.e. $NaHCO_3$) needed is estimated to be $7 \times 45.6 = 319$ mmol.

A simpler approach is to estimate the HCO_3^- space as half of the lean body weight. This will result in an underestimation of the amount of total HCO_3^- needed to reach the target. In the above example, the estimate by the simplified method is 210 mmol (0.5×60 kg $\times 7$ (7 being the $\Delta[HCO_3^-]$). Since periodic monitoring of the results of HCO_3^- administration with arterial acid-base and electrolyte measurements is required anyway, the simpler approach provides a good start and then further supplementation can be based on the rate of improvement in acidosis.

Other important considerations in the treatment of metabolic acidosis:

- Replace ongoing HCO_3^- losses.
- Avoid hypernatremia ($NaHCO_3$ ampoules have a sodium level of 44 mmol/50 mL or 50 mmol/50 mL, equivalent to 880 mmol/L or 1000 mmol/L).

- Avoid volume overload, especially in the face of compromised renal or cardiac function.
- Avoid hypocalcemia and hypokalemia. Excercise caution in patients with limited pulmonary function in whom bicarbonate therapy may result in elevation of P_{CO_2}.
- Follow acid-base changes during therapy, as formulas provide only estimates of HCO_3 deficit.

2.3.7.2 *Correction of Normal Anion Gap Metabolic Acidosis*

While there are no evidence-based recommendations for HCO_3^- replacement for normal anion gap acidosis, most recommend HCO_3^- therapy to raise $[HCO_3^-]$ initially to about 15 mmol/L. One can then gradually increase the serum bicarbonate level towards normal with sodium bicarbonate therapy over a number of days, if clinically indicated. For example, if the cause of the non-anion gap acidosis was severe diarrhea which has been resolved, with time the normal kidneys will correct the acidosis and no further bicarbonate therapy will be necessary. If, on the other hand, the hyperchloremic acidosis is due to a distal renal tubular acidosis, chronic bicarbonate therapy will be necessary to keep serum bicarbonate in the normal range.

> **Example**
>
> A patient with normal anion gap acidosis due to severe diarrhea has arterial serum $[HCO_3^-]$ of 10 mmol/L, lean BW of 60 kg.
>
> If target $[HCO_3^-]$ is 15 mmol/L, the HCO_3^- deficit is roughly estimated as follows:
>
> $$\text{Lean BW (kg)} * 0.5 * \Delta[HCO_3^-] = 60 * 0.5 * (15 - 10)$$
> $$= 150 \text{ mmol.}$$

2.3.7.3 *Metabolic Acidosis in Renal Patients*

- Reduction in renal mass compromises NH_4^+ excretion. Metabolic acidosis, however, does not develop in chronic kidney disease (CKD) patients until the GFR falls to ≤ 20–30 mL/min.
- If metabolic acidosis is present when GFR is >30 mL/min, consider another disorder such as hyporeninemic hypoaldosteronism, renal tubular defects, or gastrointestinal HCO_3^- loss (see "Gastrointestinal loss of HCO_3" in Sec. 2.3.3.1).

- With further decline in renal function, a high anion gap metabolic acidosis develops due to the retention of nonvolatile acids (see "Decreased excretion of nonvolatile acids" in Sec. 2.3.2.1). Titratable acid excretion decreases when GFR is <15 mL/min; this may occur earlier in CKD if protein intake is low or if hypophosphatemia is present (e.g. due to excessive intake of phosphate binders).
- Hemodialysis patients on conventional thrice-weekly dialysis with a dialysate [HCO_3^-] of 35 mmol/L are usually slightly acidotic, with an average predialysis serum [HCO_3^-] of 22 mmol/L. Raising dialysate [HCO_3^-] to 40 mmol/L normalizes predialysis serum [HCO_3^-] in the majority of patients. However, patients who consume a high protein diet may not normalize even with this higher dialysate [HCO_3^-]; under such circumstances, oral sodium bicarbonate therapy may be necessary. Another factor contributing to the acidosis is a large interdialytic fluid gain, which dilutes the total amount of HCO_3^- in the body, thus lowering the serum [HCO_3^-].
- The majority of peritoneal dialysis patients dialyzing with 35 mmol/L lactate-based dialysate have normal serum [HCO_3^-]. Only about 10% have a serum [HCO_3^-] of <22 mmol/L.
- Metabolic acidosis in dialysis patients has been associated with muscle wasting and hypoalbuminemia. Other negative effects include increased bone resorption, worsening hypertriglyceridemia, and stunted growth in children. The US National Kidney Foundation K/DOQI guidelines recommend maintaining a serum [HCO_3^-] of ≥22 mmol/L in end-stage renal disease (ESRD) and CKD patients.
- Sevelamer hydrochloride decreases serum [HCO_3^-] due to the provision of an increased acid load as HCl is released in exchange for bound phosphate and bile acids. Sevelamer carbonate eliminates this problem. Additionally, binding of short-chain fatty acid anions and their elimination in stool is thought to exacerbate the acidosis of sevelamer hydrochloride, as these anions are HCO_3^- precursors.

2.4 Metabolic Alkalosis

2.4.1 *Pathogenetic Mechanism*

This mechanism consists of two phases:

- Generation phase: addition of new HCO_3^- to the ECF, or loss of water in excess of HCO_3^- from the ECF.
- Maintenance phase: failure to excrete excess HCO_3^-.

2.4.1.1 *Generation Phase*

(i) Loss of hydrogen from the ECF (with resultant addition of new HCO_3^- to the ECF)
  • Via gastric juice: vomiting, nasogastric suction.
  • Via kidney: loop and thiazide diuretics; mineralocorticoid excess; Conn's Cushing's, Liddle's, Bartter's, and Gitelman's syndromes; licorice gluttony; nonabsorbable anions (by renal tubules) such as sodium penicillin and carbenicillin.
  • Into cells: hypokalemia.

(ii) Loss from ECF of fluid poor in HCO_3^- and rich in Cl^- (water loss in excess of HCO_3^- loss from the blood, hence serum [HCO_3^-] rises)
  • Sweat in cystic fibrosis.
  • Diarrheal fluid in congenital chloridorrhea or in villous adenoma of the colon.

(iii) Excessive intake of HCO_3^- or HCO_3^- precursors.
  • Baking soda (i.e. $NaHCO_3$): pica, treatment for dyspepsia.
  • Salts of citrate, lactate, acetate, malate.
  • Calcium carbonate: milk alkali syndrome.

2.4.1.2 *Maintenance Phase*

This phase is due to (a) enhanced renal HCO_3^- reclamation as a result of decreased effective circulating volume and Cl^- depletion and (b) ongoing generation of metabolic alkalosis.

2.4.2 *Assessment of Urinary Chloride*

Urinary [Cl^-] is valuable in the evaluation of metabolic alkalosis as a marker of volume depletion and as a means to help sort out the causes of metabolic alkalosis. When blood volume is high, urine [Cl^-] will be high (except in diuretic therapy; see below). In the face of a low blood volume, urine [Cl^-] will usually be low (less than 20 mmol/L).

Urinary [Na^+] may be misleading at certain time points in the evolution of metabolic alkalosis as a marker of volume depletion. For example, early in the course of alkalosis due to vomiting or extrarenal loss of HCO_3^- - poor and Cl^--rich fluid, the patient may have a high urinary [Na^+] despite volume depletion because the kidneys are attempting to correct the alkalosis by excreting excess HCO_3^- with a cation (Na^+ or K^+). When the bicarbonaturia is ongoing, the urine pH will also be elevated. As the patient becomes even more volume- and Cl^--depleted, the bicarbonaturia will stop and the urine will become paradoxically acidic.

A high urinary [Cl⁻] may be seen in a patient who recently consumed diuretics, reflecting the effect of the diuretic on the renal tubules. When the diuretic effect on the tubules wears off, urinary [Cl⁻] will decline, once again accurately reflecting volume status.

2.4.3 Clinical Consequences

Patients with mild or moderate metabolic alkalosis ([HCO$_3^-$] < 40 mmol/L) often have few symptoms, unless there is marked associated hypokalemia.

Patients with severe metabolic alkalosis ([HCO$_3^-$] > 40 mmol/L) can develop a number of nonspecific manifestations in the form of weakness, lethargy, headache, constipation, muscle cramps, tetany, delirium, seizures, and even stupor. Some of these symptoms may be related to a combination of metabolic alkalosis-induced/associated abnormalities such as hypokalemia, hypercapnea, hypoxemia, and reduction in serum ionized calcium levels. Severe metabolic alkalosis may be associated with malignant arrhythmias such as ventricular tachycardia and fibrillation in seriously ill patients. Hypokalemia, hypoxemia, as well as the use of digitalis preparations in cardiac failure and underlying heart disease settings may all contribute to the occurrence of the above-mentioned arrhythmias.

2.4.4 Treatment

When the blood volume is low as reflected by a low urine [Cl⁻], it is key to correct volume depletion and Cl⁻ depletion in order to allow the kidneys to excrete the excess HCO$_3^-$. This can be achieved with NaCl replacement orally or intravenously. Correction of alkalosis by NaCl (e.g. normal saline) in these chloride-responsive conditions is achieved by both decreased bicarbonate reclamation by the proximal tubules and enhanced bicarbonate secretion by the β-intercalated cells of the distal tubule. Potassium depletion is also common in metabolic alkalosis and mandates repletion.

In edematous disorders such as congestive heart failure, a different strategy is used as total body sodium content is increased and further volume overload must be avoided. In these conditions, it is imperative to replete KCl (for hypokalemia and alkalosis) and enhance bicarbonate excretion in the urine by the use of a carbonic anhydrase inhibitor, namely, acetazolamide. The effectiveness of acetazolamide therapy may be short-lived, but can be ascertained by monitoring the urine pH and the serum [HCO_3^-] serially. Acetazolamide will also increase urinary potassium loss, which has to be replaced. In cases where acetazolamide is ineffective or contraindicated, one can administer isotonic hydrochloric acid, preferably buffered in amino acid or fat emulsion via a large central vein. If the alkalosis is due to excessive gastric acid losses, then gastric H^+ secretion should be blocked with either a proton pump inhibitor or a H_2 blocker. Finally, hemodialysis, peritoneal dialysis, hemofiltration, or hemodiafiltration using chloride-rich and bicarbonate-poor or bicarbonate precursor-poor dialysate or replacement solutions can be effective in the treatment of metabolic alkalosis in patients with compromised renal function.

When the blood volume is high and the urine [Cl^-] is not low as in the case of mineralocorticoid excess states, NaCl administration will not be an effective therapy. Under such chloride-nonresponsive conditions, the cause of the particular metabolic alkalosis should be treated, e.g. resection of an adrenal adenoma that causes the mineralocorticoid excess.

2.4.5 *Metabolic Alkalosis in Renal Patients*

CKD and particularly ESRD patients have a limited ability to excrete excess HCO_3^-. Thus, a HCO_3^- load which would be excreted by normal kidneys may result in a metabolic alkalosis in those patients. Some of the unique causes reported in CKD/ESRD patients are:

- Heavy crack/freebase cocaine use in a dialysis patient can lead to severe metabolic alkalosis because of the high strong base content in the cocaine preparation. Cocaine base is prepared by dissolving cocaine HCl in water and adding sodium hydroxide. Furthermore, baking soda is often added to raise the weight of the mixture.
- Use of sodium citrate for regional anticoagulation for continuous renal replacement therapy (CRRT) or for plasmapheresis can lead to metabolic alkalosis, as the citrate is metabolized to HCO_3^-. The dialysate or replacement fluid used in CRRT must be adjusted to provide a lesser amount of HCO_3^- or HCO_3^- precursor in order to avoid the alkalosis caused by the citrate. Timely hemodialysis after a plasmapheresis procedure in a renal dysfunction patient can avert the alkalosis caused by citrate given during the plasmapheresis procedure.
- Intermittent hemodialysis with a high [HCO_3^-] dialysate (used to achieve a predialysis serum [HCO_3^-] > 22 mmol/L) often results in transient metabolic alkalosis post-dialysis.

- The ingestion of nonabsorbable antacids (magnesium hydroxide, aluminum hydroxide, or calcium carbonate), combined with a cation exchange resin (sodium polysterene sulfonate), by renal insufficiency patients may lead to metabolic alkalosis. This occurs because of the binding of some of the cations (magnesium, aluminum, or calcium) to the resin, leaving more pancreatic HCO_3^- to be absorbed from the intestinal lumen.

2.5 Combined Metabolic Acidosis and Metabolic Alkalosis

High anion gap metabolic acidosis and metabolic alkalosis can occur in the same patient.

Example

For a patient with metabolic alkalosis due to nasogastric suction followed by the development of diabetic ketoacidosis, serum $[Na^+] = 138$, $[Cl^-] = 87$, $[T_{CO_2}] = 32$. Original serum values: $[Na^+] = 138$, $[Cl^-] = 101$, $[T_{CO_2}] = 27$.

$[AG^-] = 138 - 87 - 32 = 19$ mEq/L of unmeasured anions, 10 of which are due to albumin and other normally present unmeasured anions while the remaining 9 (Δ anion gap$^-$ = 19 − 10 = 9) of which are due to other unmeasured anions in the form of acetoacetate and β-hydroxybutyrate.

The Δ anion gap of 9 means that the $[T_{CO_2}]$ has correspondingly decreased by 9 as a result of the presence of a high anion gap metabolic acidosis in the form of diabetic ketoacidosis. The $[T_{CO_2}]$ of 32 signifies the presence of a metabolic alkalosis as well. Had there not been the loss of 9 mmol/L of $[T_{CO_2}]$ due to titration with 9 mmol/L of $[H^+]$ derived from the 9 mmol/L of acetoacetic and β-hydroxybutyric acids (the presence of those acids is reflected by the Δ anion gap$^-$ of 9), the $[T_{CO_2}]$ would have had a value of 32 + 9 = 41 — evidence of the original greater degree of metabolic alkalosis.

$[Cl^-]$ falls by $(101 - 87) = 14$. This is because, prior to the onset of diabetic ketoacidosis, the original $[T_{CO_2}]$ was 41, an increase of $(41 - 27) = 14$ from the normal value of 27. The decrease in $[Cl^-]$ was an accompaniment of the increase in $[T_{CO_2}]$ that had occurred prior to the development of the diabetic ketoacidosis.

The combination of a normal anion gap metabolic acidosis and a metabolic alkalosis cannot be diagnosed by changes in serum electrolytes.

If, in addition, serum P_{CO2} is higher or lower than 40 mmHg, then a diagnosis of respiratory acidosis or respiratory alkalosis can be added to the clinical condition, fulfilling a picture commonly referred to as a "triple disturbance".

2.6 Respiratory Acid-Base Disturbances in Renal Patients

The lungs are often affected by the same specific diseases that lead to kidney failure (e.g. systemic lupus erythematosus, Wegener's granulomatosis) and also by long-standing uremia (pulmonary calcifications). Even more commonly seen are the effects of volume overload, such as pleural effusions and alveolar edema, resulting in a restrictive defect and increase in the work of spontaneous breathing. Consequently, the lungs' ability to compensate for metabolic acidosis is impaired. In addition, hypoxemia may lead to hyperventilation and respiratory alkalosis.

With HCO_3^--based dialysis, the dialysate compartment has a relatively high P_{CO_2} (as high as 130 mmHg), generated by the addition of a small amount of acetic acid into the HCO_3^- solution. Excess CO_2 diffuses through the dialysis membrane into the venous blood. With normal lungs, the excess CO_2 is rapidly disposed of via ventilation; when ventilation is severely compromised, however, P_{CO_2} may rise, leading to respiratory acidosis. Of historical interest, this situation is the reverse of what had been seen with acetate-based dialysis, where the dialysate had low P_{CO_2}, leading to a rapid loss of CO_2 into the bath, decreasing ventilatory drive, and contributing to the hypoxemia which was often seen during hemodialysis when using an acetate-based bath.

Metabolic acidosis needs to be corrected so as to allow permissive hypercapnea and also to tolerate weaning in mechanically ventilated renal failure patients.

Suggested Reading

Bushinsky DA, Coe FL, Katzenberg C, et al. (1982) Arterial P_{CO_2} in chronic metabolic acidosis. Kidney Int 22:311–314.

DuBose TD, Jr. (2008) Acidosis and alkalosis. In: Fauci AS, Braunwald E, Kasper DL, et al. (eds.), Harrison's Principles of Internal Medicine, 17th ed., McGraw Hill Medical, New York, pp. 287–296.

Fernandez PC, Cohen RM, Feldman GM. (1989) The concept of bicarbonate distribution space: the crucial role of body buffers. *Kidney Int* 36:747–752.

Kraut JA, Kurtz I. (2001) Use of base in the treatment of severe academic states. *Am J Kidney Dis* 38:703–727.

Moe OW, Rector FC Jr, Alpern RJ. (1994) Renal regulation of acid-base metabolism. In: Narins RG (ed.), *Maxwell & Kleeman's Clinical Disorders of Fluid and Electrolyte Metabolism*, 5th ed., McGraw-Hill, , New York, pp. 203–242.

Nahas GG. (1966) Current concepts of acid-base measurement. *Ann NY Acad Sci* 133:1–274.

Rastegar A. (2007) Use of the delta AG/delta HCO_3 ratio in the diagnosis of mixed acid-base disorders. *J Am Soc Nephrol* 18:2429–2431.

Seifter JL. (2004) Acid-base disorders. In: Goldman L, Ausiello D (eds.), *Cecil Textbook of Medicine*, 22nd ed., Saunders, Philadelphia, pp. 688–699.

3

Potassium Disturbances

James C. M. Chan

3.1 Introduction

Acute and significant elevation of serum potassium concentration (hyperkalemia of ≥ 6 mEq/L) is encountered in up to 2% of inpatients; a majority of these are due to drug-induced hyperkalemia. Significantly reduced serum potassium concentration (hypokalemia of <3 mEq/L) is often diuretic-induced or the result of chronic tubular dysfunction due to gene mutations. If severe, both hyperkalemia and hypokalemia can be life-threatening, and must be diagnosed and corrected promptly.

3.2 Hyperkalemia

Spurious hyperkalemia due to improperly collected and hemolyzed blood needs to be excluded (Table 3.1). True hyperkalemia is due to three major mechanisms:

- decreased renal excretion from the kidneys, whether caused by adrenal disorder or drug-induced
- increased release from cells
- increased intake of potassium.

3.2.1 *Significant Consequences*

3.2.1.1 *Myocardial*

- At serum potassium of 6 mEq/L, the electrocardiogram (ECG) shows T wave tenting.
- At 7 mEq/L, the ECG shows widening of the PR interval and QRS complex plus flattening of the P wave and appearance of the sine wave.

Table 3.1   Causes of hyperkalemia.

Spurious hyperkalemia	Ischemic venipuncture, hemolysis, thrombocytosis, leukocytosis, familial pesudohyperkalemia, infectious mononucleosis
True hyperkalemia	
Decreased renal function Prerenal azotemia	
Renal disorders	Acute and chronic kidney failure, hyporeninemia, hypoaldosteronism, interstitial nephritis, systemic lupus erythematosus, sickle cell disease, obstructive uropathy, pseudohypoaldosteronism, post-kidney transplantation, amyloidosis, lead nephropathy
Adrenal disorders	Addison's disease, 21-hydroxylase deficiency, corticosteroid methyloxidase deficiency
Medications	Converting enzyme inhibitors, angiotensin receptor blockers, nonsteroidal anti-inflammatory agents, spironolactone, triamterene, amiloride, heparin, cyclosporine or tacrolimus
Increased release from cells	Cell lysis: crush injury, tumor lysis, hemolysis, rhabdomyolysis Medications: beta-adrenergic blockers, digitalis, arginine, succinylcholine Insulin deficiency and hyperglycemia Familial hyperkalemic periodic paralysis Acidosis: metabolic and respiratory Hyperosmolality Exercise
Increased intake of potassium	Potassium salts, aged blood, potassium penicillin, geophagia

- At 8 mEq/L, the ECG shows the T wave merging with the markedly widened QRS complex, giving the mistaken impression of a ventricular arrhythmia.

3.2.1.2 *Neuromuscular*

- Cardiac arrhythmia
- Paresthesia

- Flaccid paralysis of skeletal muscles, ascending from the peripheral muscles to trunk and respiratory muscles.

3.2.2 Diagnostic Workup

After spurious hyperkalemia is excluded, determine if true hyperkalemia is due to kidney failure. A glomerular filtration rate (GFR) of ≤25% of normal is invariably associated with hyperkalemia. If GFR is normal, low renin and low aldosterone may be due to type 4 renal tubular acidosis. Normal renin but low aldosterone may be due to Addison's disease. Elevation of both renin and aldosterone point to end-organ resistance, for example in the case of pseudohypoaldosteronism or obstructive uropathy.

3.2.3 Treatment

The treatment chosen is dependent on the underlying cause and the ECG findings. For rapid stabilization of cell membrane, the following treatment options are recommended in preferred order of administration.

3.2.3.1 Rapid Removal

- Intravenous 10% calcium gluconate at a dose of 5 mL/kg body weight given over 5 min under ECG monitoring.
- Force potassium from the extracellular space into the intracellular space at a rapid rate.
- Glucose 10% at a dose of 5 mL/kg body weight and insulin 0.1 unit/kg intravenous drip over 60 min.
- Sodium bicarbonate at a dose of 2 mEq/kg body weight intravenous drip over 30 min.
- Salbutamol at a dose of 2 µg/kg/min intravenous drip over 20 min or nebulized at 20 mg over 20 min.

3.2.3.2 Removal of Potassium from the Body over Several Hours

- Sodium polystyrene sulfonate resin (Kayexalate) 20 g in 100 mL of 20% sorbitol given orally. This dose can be repeated in 6 h as needed.
- Alternatively, it can be given as a retention enema, at a dose of 50 g kayexalate in 50 mL of 70% sorbitol solution, and may be repeated

in 1 h. With the enema, the potassium begins to be lowered in 1 h, but the oral dose requires 2 h. The side effect is sodium retention and pulmonary edema in patients with pre-existing congestive heart failure and oliguria.

- Peritoneal dialysis or hemodialysis: 50% reduction of serum potassium concentration with every 12 h of peritoneal dialysis or every 2 h of hemodialysis.

3.3 Hypokalemia

A serum potassium concentration of <3.5 mEq/L is considered hypokalemia. Hypokalemia can be caused by one of, or a combination of, the following four mechanisms (Table 3.2):

- increased renal excretion from the kidneys or adrenal disorder
- increased gastrointestinal loss
- increased shift of potassium into the cells
- decreased intake of potassium.

In view of the fact that most cases of hypokalemia develop slowly, the body has time to adjust and symptoms are mild, affecting the neuromuscular junction (muscle weakness, parasthesia, constipation), kidneys (polydipsia, polyuria, nocturia), and cardiovascular system (ectopic beats). Severe hypokalemia increases the risks of atrial fibrillation, atrioventricular block, and ventricular fibrillation.

Chronic hypokalemia may give rise to irreversible interstitial nephritis and growth retardation. ECG shows the following anomalies: flattening of the T wave and the ST segment, increase of the PR intervals, and decrease of the QRS complex.

The diagnostic approach with a careful history, physical examination, and laboratory chemistry (including blood gas and pH determinations) is usually sufficient in most patients. If the dietary intake is adequate, a urinary potassium excretion of <20 mEq/L indicates proper renal conservation in response to hypokalemia; but if it is >20 mEq/L renal wasting is likely.

3.3.1 *Treatment*

The daily potassium requirement is 2 mEq/kg body weight per day. Hypokalemia is treated by first providing this normal daily requirement and simultaneously replacing the measured or estimated

Table 3.2   Causes of hypokalemia.

Increased excretion of potassium by the kidneys

Renal tubular disorders
  Renal tubular acidosis
  Bartter syndrome
  Liddle syndrome
  Calcium-losing tubulopathy
  Magnesium-losing tubulopathy
  11β-hydroxysteroid dehydrogenase deficiency

Adrenal disorders
  Idiopathic hyperaldosteronism
  Aldosterone-producing adenoma
  Hyperaldosteronism, adrenocortical carcinoma
  11-hydroxylase deficiency
  17-hydroxylase deficiency
  Dexomethasone-suppressible hyperaldosteronism

Increased gastrointestinal loss of potassium

  Vomiting
  Diarrhea
  Laxative abuse

Increased cellular uptake of potassium

  Acute myelogenous leukemia, treated megaloblastic anemia
  Hypothermia
  Familial periodic paralysis
  Medications: insulin, β-adregenic agonists, barium, toluene

Reduced intake of potassium

  Chronic alcoholism
  Anorexia nervosa
  Geophagia

---

amounts of potassium wasting; then, the underlying disorder of hypokalemia (Table 3.2) is treated.

3.4 Potassium Homeostasis

To further refine the estimation of potassium excretion, the transtubular potassium gradient (TTKG) is developed. It is calculated by the ratio of urine/plasma potassium divided by the urine/plasma osmolarity. To control variables in water reabsorption at the collecting duct and in sodium delivery at the distal tubule, the urine osmolarity must exceed the plasma osmolarity and the urinary sodium concentration must exceed 25 mmol/L.

3.4.1 *In Hyperkalemia*

- A TTKG of >11 suggests adequate aldosterone activity.
- A TTKG of <11 suggests hypoaldosteronism or receptor blockade.

3.4.2 *In Hypokalemia*

- A TTKG of <2 points to non-renal loss.
- A TTKG of >4 is suggestive of renal wasting of potassium.

Acknowledgment

This work was supported by National Institutes of Health grants DK50419 and DK07761.

Suggested Reading

Batlle D, Moorthi KM, Schueter W, Kurtzman N. (2006) Distal renal tubular acidosis and the potassium enigma. *Semin Nephrol* 26:471–478.
Evans KJ, Greenberg A. (2005) Hyperkalemia: a review. *J Intensive Care Med* 20:272–290.
Gill JR Jr, Santos F, Chan JCM. (1990) Disorders of potassium metabolism. In: Chan JCM, Gill JR Jr (eds.), *Kidney Electrolyte Disorders*, Churchill Livingstone, New York, pp. 137–170.

4

Sodium and Water Disturbances

Ramin Sam and Todd S. Ing

4.1 Urinary Dilution and Concentration

Kuhn and Ryffel first originated the concept of a countercurrent multiplier system for urinary concentration in 1942.

4.1.1 *The Countercurrent Exchange Mechanism*

4.1.1.1 *Proximal Convoluted Tubule*

- Its content is iso-osmolal to plasma.
- Seventy percent of the filtered load of sodium and water is reabsorbed here.
- Fluid (water and solutes) delivery to the ascending limb and beyond depends on how much sodium and water are reabsorbed by the proximal tubule.

4.1.1.2 *Descending Limb of Loop of Henle*

- Being permeable to water, it will allow water to leave the lumen and enter the hyperosmolal medulla, allowing its luminal content to have the same osmolality as the surrounding medulla.
- Its permeability to NaCl and urea is low.

4.1.1.3 *Thin Ascending Limb of Loop of Henle*

- It is impermeable to water.
- The fluid entering the ascending limb has a NaCl concentration of 600 mM and a urea concentration of 300 mM, as opposed to the surrounding medulla, which has a NaCl concentration of 300 mM and a urea concentration of 600 mM.

- NaCl leaves the lumen to enter the medulla, while urea leaves the medulla to enter the lumen.
- Whether movement of solutes in this segment is active or passive is still not clear.
- It is not vasopressin-responsive.

4.1.1.4 Thick Ascending Limb of Loop of Henle

- It is impermeable to water.
- Active transport of sodium, potassium, and chloride by the action of the $Na^+/K^+/2Cl^-$ pump is present.
- The NaCl reabsorption is regulated by vasopressin.
- It is poorly permeable to urea.

4.1.1.5 Distal Convoluted Tubule

- It is relatively impermeable to water.
- Active sodium reabsorption takes place here.
- The tubular fluid entering this segment has an osmolality of ~100 mmol/kg, while the fluid exiting this segment has an osmolality of ~50 mmol/kg.
- It is not vasopressin-responsive.

4.1.1.6 Collecting Ducts

- Water permeability depends largely on the presence of vasopressin, which increases water permeability 10-fold. In the absence of vasopressin, this segment becomes impermeable to water so that any hypo-osmolal tubular fluid can course through it and exit as dilute urine.
- Outer medullary collecting ducts are urea-impermeable, while inner medullary collecting ducts are moderately urea-permeable (regulated by vasopressin). Inner medullary collecting ducts are responsible for adding urea to the medulla (50% of inner medullary osmolality is due to urea).
- Aldosterone promotes the absorption of sodium variably coupled to potassium and hydrogen secretion at the cortical portion of this segment.
- Sodium reabsorption also takes place in the distal portion of the collecting ducts. This reabsorption is blocked by vasopressin.

4.1.1.7 Vasculature and Juxtamedullary Nephrons

- The vascular countercurrent flow is also important in maintaining the osmolality gradient in the renal medulla, and ultimately in influencing urinary concentration and dilution capacities.
- Juxtamedullary nephrons have long loops of Henle, which penetrate deeply into the medulla. The cortical nephrons have short loops. In humans, 85% of the nephrons have short loops while 15% have long ones. Nephrons with long loops have classically been thought to be important in the generation and maintenance of a hyperosmolal medulla. One recent study, however, found that papillectomized rat kidneys were able to excrete a maximally dilute urine, and thus the long-loop nephrons were thought not to be essential for the maximal generation and reabsorption of solute-free water.

4.1.1.8 The Role of Urea

Urea, highly concentrated at the inner medullary collecting ducts, diffuses into the medulla to contribute to its hyperosmolality. The latter promotes the absorption of water from (a) the water-permeable and solute-impermeable descending limb and (b) the vasopressin-sensitive collecting ducts when vasopressin is present.

4.1.1.9 The Role of the Vasa Recta

The vasa recta functions as a countercurrent exchanger that allows the preservation of interstitial hyperosmolality. Blood coming down the descending vasa recta becomes increasingly concentrated as water diffuses out of and solutes diffuse into this segment of the nephron. In the ascending vasa recta, the reverse process takes place so that solutes are trapped in the medulla to maintain its osmolality. An increase in medullary blood flow may "wash out" the medullary hyperosmolality, resulting in an impairment of concentrating capacity.

4.1.2 Arginine Vasopressin

- It is a peptide with a molecular weight of 1099 Da.
- Vasopressin is produced in the supraoptic and paraventricular magnocellular nuclei in the hypothalamus.

- A 1% change in plasma osmolality causes vasopressin release. Non-osmotic stimuli for vasopressin release include pain, emotional stress, hypotension, and hypovolemia (including reduced effective circulatory volume).
- Infusion of NaCl, sucrose, and mannitol into the internal carotid artery at an osmolality of 310 mmol/kg increases vasopressin release threefold. However, infusions of urea or glucose do not, as these solutes are ineffective osmoles by virtue of their ability to enter brain cells.
- V_2 (vasopressin) receptors are present on the basolateral membrane of collecting duct cells.

4.1.3 *Water Channels or Aquaporins*

- Embedded in cell membranes, aquaporins are proteins that regulate the flow of water. In the kidneys aquaporin 1 (AQP1) is present on both the apical and basolateral membranes of the proximal tubule and the descending limb of Henle. Without AQP1, there is diminished maximal urinary osmolality.
- Aquaporin 2 (AQP2), present only on the apical membrane of collecting ducts, is regulated by vasopressin. AQP2 is phosphorylated and moves to the luminal membrane upon binding of vasopressin to its receptor V_2.
- Aquaporin 3 and aquaporin 4 (AQP3 and AQP4) are present on the basolateral membrane of the principal cells of collecting ducts, but only AQP3 is regulated by vasopressin. AQP3 is predominantly expressed in the cortical medulla, while AQP4 is mainly expressed in the inner medulla.
- AQP2 levels can be measured in the urine to assess the activity of vasopressin.

4.1.4 *Free (or Solute-Free) Water and Osmolal Clearances*

If a person has a glomerular filtration rate (GFR) of 125 mL/min, then the daily GFR will be 180 L. Out of this amount, 178.5–179 L is reabsorbed by tubules and the collecting ducts, leaving 1–1.5 L to be excreted from the body as urine daily. Under ideal circumstances, 20 L of the 180 L of the glomerular filtrate can be excreted as free water in the urine. Free water is defined as water without any contained solutes. Free water clearance is defined as the amount of water to be subtracted from, or added to, a given urine in order to make the resultant solution (i.e. the "new urine") iso-osmolal with plasma.

Note that the "clearance" in free water clearance has a different meaning from the conventional clearance term in general use for solutes. For example, conventional renal solute clearance is defined as the volume of plasma from which a particular solute has been removed completely per unit time, or as the volume of plasma completely "cleared" of a particular solute per unit time. Thus, conventional renal clearance is calculated as: $C_{solute} = U_{solute} \times V/P_{solute}$, where C_{solute} represents the renal solute clearance; V, the urine flow rate; and U_{solute} and P_{solute}, the urinary and plasma levels of the solute, respectively. The "solute" in question in the instance of osmolal clearance is "osmoles".

4.1.4.1 *In the Case of a Dilute Urine*

In the case of a dilute urine (say, 10 mL in volume passed per min), all of the solute particles can virtually be confined to a smaller volume that is iso-osmolal with plasma (it happens to be 2 mL in volume/min in this instance), leaving behind 8 mL/min of pure urine water that is free of solutes. Since 8 mL/min of pure water (without solutes) needs to be subtracted from the 10 mL/min of the present dilute urine in order to make the remaining 2 mL/min solution (the "new urine") iso-osmolal with plasma, the 8 mL/min of pure water is known as a free water clearance while the 2 mL/min is known as an osmolal clearance. The above description can be expressed by the formula:

Urine volume (mL/min) = osmolal clearance (mL/min)
+ free water clearance (mL/min).

Free water clearance (mL/min) = urine volume (mL/min)
− osmolal clearance (mL/min)
= 10 mL/min − 2 mL/min
= 8 mL/min.

Note that the same osmolal clearance value can be obtained by using the conventional renal solute clearance formula mentioned above. Indeed, application of the conventional formula is the usual way to derive osmolal clearance.

With a dilute urine, free water clearance has a positive value. Positive free water clearance is denoted as C_{H_2O}.

4.1.4.2 *In the Case of a Concentrated Urine*

If an individual passes only 1 mL/min of concentrated urine which still contains the same amount of osmoles that the 10 mL/min of dilute urine in the previous example possesses, then the osmolal clearance is still the same as before, i.e. 2 mL/min. The following formulas still apply:

Urine volume (mL/min) = osmolal clearance (mL/min)
+ free water clearance (mL/min).

Free water clearance (mL/min) = urine volume (mL/min)
− osmolal clearance (mL/min).

Free water clearance = 1 mL/min − 2 mL/min
= −1 mL/min.

With the passage of a concentrated urine, free water clearance will have a negative value. This is because one needs to add free water to the original concentrated urine in order to make the "new urine" iso-osmolal with plasma. Negative free water clearance is denoted as $T^C_{H_2O}$.

4.1.4.3 *Electrolyte Free Water Clearance versus Free Water Clearance*

Recently, the concept of an "electrolyte free water clearance" has been developed. Urea is excluded from the formula for calculating this clearance because urea, when not introduced into the body abruptly, does not bring about water movement among body fluid compartments.

The formula for deriving electrolyte free water clearance is:

Urine volume (mL/min)
= electrolyte clearance (mL/min)
+ electrolyte free water clearance (mL/min).

Electrolyte free water clearance (mL/min)
= urine volume (mL/min) − electrolyte clearance (mL/min).

In this instance, electrolyte clearance (mL/min) is: $(U_{Na} + U_K)V/P_{Na}$, where U_{Na} represents urine sodium level; U_K, urine potassium level; P_{Na}, plasma sodium level; and V, urine flow rate.

If electrolyte free water clearance is positive, plasma sodium level will increase. On the other hand, if electrolyte free water clearance is negative, plasma sodium level will fall.

To summarize: Both free water clearance and electrolyte free water clearance are measures geared for the precise quantitation of water balance. When these clearances have a positive value in the face of a dilute urine, solute-free or electrolyte-free water is lost from the body and the remaining body fluids are concentrated. On the other hand, when the values are negative in the presence of a concentrated urine, there is a net effect of returning solute-free or electrolyte-free water to the body, thereby diluting body fluids.

4.1.4.4 *The Role of GFR and Proximal Tubular Reabsorption in the Formation of a Dilute or a Concentrated Urine*

Both glomerular filtration and proximal tubular reabsorption will determine how much sodium and water are delivered to the more distal parts of the nephron for the diluting or the concentrating mechanism to take place. For example, levels of cardiac output, renal blood flow, blood pressure, afferent and efferent arteriole tones, effective circulatory blood volume, renin/angiotensin/aldosterone, epinephrine/norepinephrine, atrial natriuretic and other hormones, as well as peritubular events can all influence GFR and proximal tubular reabsorption.

A diminished GFR and/or a rise in proximal tubular reabsorption may reduce the quantity of fluid delivered to the thick ascending limb and the distal tubule for solute-free water to be made by the absorption of sodium and chloride. Thus, the kidney's diluting capacity is impaired. In addition, similar reductions in fluid delivery to the water-impermeable ascending limb can limit the total amount of NaCl that can be transported to the medulla to increase the latter's osmolality. The resultant reduction in medullary hyperosmolality will impair the kidney's ability to produce a highly concentrated urine. This is because, in the face of a reduction in medullary hyperosmolality, less water will enter the medulla from the collecting ducts and leave a concentrated urine behind.

4.1.4.5 *How Does the Body Make a Dilute Urine?*

When an adequate quantity of fluid containing sodium, potassium, chloride, and water is delivered from the proximal tubule and the descending limb to the thick ascending limb, these electrolytes will be transported to the medulla through the action of the Na/K/2Cl pump. At the distal convoluted tubule, an active sodium transport delivering sodium and chloride to the interstitium also takes place. Since the thick ascending limb and the greater part of the distal tubule are impermeable to water, the fluid leaving the distal tubule will be hypo-osmolal as the result of the loss of solutes upstream. In the absence of vasopressin, water in the hypo-osmolal fluid that emerges from the distal tubule will not be absorbed. Thus, a dilute urine will be formed.

4.1.4.6 How Does the Body Make a Concentrated Urine?

Both the thick ascending limb and the collecting ducts are mainly responsible for urine concentration. By transporting sodium, potassium, and chloride (but not water) into the interstitium, the thick ascending limb is responsible for generating a hyperosmolal medulla. By making the collecting ducts very permeable to water, vasopressin fosters the absorption of water from the collecting ducts on account of the osmotic influence brought about by the hyperosmolality in the medulla. The loss of water, but not solutes, from the collecting duct fluid creates a concentrated urine. The latter can have a specific gravity as high as 1.035 and an osmolality as high as 1200 mmol/kg.

4.2 Diseases of Urinary Concentration and Dilution

4.2.1 Inability to Concentrate Urine (i.e. Passage of a Dilute Urine)

(i) Failure to produce vasopressin due to diseases of the posterior pituitary (central diabetes insipidus). These diseases include trauma, infections, granulomas, neoplasms, and vascular problems. Rarely, the disease is hereditary (autosomal dominant or autosomal recessive) in nature.

(ii) Suppression of vasopressin production by hypo-osmolality — psychogenic polydipsia (compulsive water drinking). Plasma hypo-osmolality suppresses vasopressin formation. Patients cannot pass concentrated urine because of lack of vasopressin.

(iii) Failure of collecting ducts to respond to vasopressin

- Congenital nephrogenic diabetes insipidus: The renal tubule is insensitive to vasopressin. Ninety percent of these patients have gene mutations in the vasopressin V_2 receptor; this inheritance is X-linked. The other 10% of patients have AQP2 gene mutations that exhibit autosomal recessive inheritance characteristics.

- Nephrogenic diabetes insipidus: Collecting ducts are damaged by various diseases in such a way that they do not respond to vasopressin. Examples of such diseases include amyloidosis, sickle cell disease, chronic hypokalemia, hypercalcemia, lithium toxicity, and ureteral obstruction. Chronic hypokalemia, hypercalcemia, lithium toxicity, and ureteral obstruction are associated with a defect in producing maximally concentrating urine because of a downregulation of AQP2 expression.

(iv) Decreased contact time between collecting duct fluid and medullary interstitium (osmotic diuresis). This is partially due to the rapid passage of collecting duct fluid down the duct lumen, thus preventing water from entering the hyperosmolal medullary interstitium even if vasopressin is present. The urine passed under such circumstances is often not much higher than iso-osmolality.

(v) Failure to provide osmoles for urine formation. Beer potomania is associated with passage of a dilute urine.

(vi) Note that, as in situations in which large amounts of dilute urine are excreted, the countercurrent multiplication mechanism is disrupted with consequent "washout"of the medullary hyperosmolality, adding one more reason to account for the failure to produce a concentrated urine.

4.2.2 *Inability to Dilute Urine*

(i) In the syndrome of inappropriate antidiuretic hormone (SIADH), there is failure to maximally dilute urine because of high levels of AQP2.

(ii) Patients with hypothyroidism and glucocorticoid deficiency also have increased AQP2 levels and an inability to maximally dilute their urines.

(iii) Congestive heart failure and cirrhosis of liver: A reduced effective circulatory volume causes increased sodium and water reabsorption from the proximal tubule, so that there is a reduction of fluid delivery to the distal nephron. In addition, vasopressin levels are high because of a reduced effective circulatory volume.

4.3 Hyponatremia

4.3.1 Definition (Table 4.1)

- Normal plasma sodium concentration ranges from 136 mmol/L to 145 mmol/L.
- Hyponatremia is often defined as a plasma sodium concentration of <135 mmol/L.
- Severe hyponatremia is defined as a plasma sodium concentration of <115 mmol/L.
- Acute hyponatremia is development of hyponatremia in <36–48 hours.

4.3.2 Incidence and Associated Findings

- Hyponatremia is the most common electrolyte abnormality in hospitalized patients, and has been reported to have a wide prevalence range of 3%–30%.
- In a report involving patients with a plasma sodium level of <120 mmol/L, the mortality rate was found to be 19%.
- Forty-six percent of hyponatremic patients have associated electrolyte abnormalities (hypophosphatemia, 17%; hypokalemia, 16%; hypomagnesemia, 15%; hyperkalemia, 6%).

4.3.3 Mechanism of Development

- In normal humans, plasma sodium concentration is quite stable and varies by only about 1% in an individual over long periods of time. This is due to the fact that a 1% change in plasma osmolality brings about changes in plasma vasopressin level and thirst.
- Hyponatremia can be due to a gain of water, a loss of sodium, or both, by the blood (almost always by the body too). This disorder is most often caused by a high water intake in the setting of an underlying defect in solute-free water excretion, which in turn is

Table 4.1 Definition of the dysnatremias.

	Hyponatremia (mmol/L)	Hypernatremia (mmol/L)
Cut-off value	<135	>145
Severe	<115	>160

most frequently caused by an appropriate or inappropriate secretion of the antidiuretic hormone (ADH).

- The osmotic threshold for arginine vasopressin (AVP, the ADH in humans) release is 280–290 mmol/kg; the threshold decreases with age and pregnancy.
- Each 1% rise in plasma osmolality causes a twofold-to-fourfold increase in ADH release. An 8% fall in plasma volume leads to an exponential increase in ADH release. Hypotension also serves as a potent stimulus for the release of the hormone.
- Older people are more prone to the development of hyponatremia, as they have 20% less total body water (the addition of a given amount of water can bring about a greater degree of hyponatremia when compared to a younger individual).
- Very low protein/osmole diets can cause hyponatremia because water intake can exceed the maximum volume of urine that can be excreted based on the amount of solutes available for urine formation. For example, in an individual, if the total amount of solutes available for excretion is 100 mmol per day and the osmolality of the maximally dilute urine is 50 mmol/kg, the body can only excrete a maximum of 2 L of water (i.e. urine) per day. If that individual consumes 3 L of water a day, 1 L will be retained.

4.3.4 Pseudohyponatremia (a.k.a. Spurious Hyponatremia)

- Plasma osmolality is normal despite the apparent hyponatremia (sodium is expressed in mmol/L of plasma).
- Pseudohyponatremia was originally described in the 1950s, when flame photometry was first used to determine plasma sodium concentration. Normally, 1 L of plasma contains 80 mL of space-occupying solids (mostly in the form of lipids and proteins) and $1000 - 80 = 920$ mL of water. Sodium is present in plasma water only, and not in plasma solids. The normal plasma sodium level is 140 mmol/L; however, this amount of sodium is present only in the 920 mL of plasma water and not in the 80 mL of plasma solids. The presence of 140 mmol of sodium in 920 mL of plasma water equates to that of $140 \times (1000/920) = 152$ mmol of sodium in 1000 mL (1 L) of plasma water. If a patient's plasma now contains more solids, e.g. 160 mL of lipids, there will be only $1000 - 160 = 840$ mL of water left per L of this new plasma. Since sodium is present only in the water of plasma, the total amount of sodium

present in 1 L of this new lipid-laden plasma (having only 840 mL of water) will be reduced to $140 \times (840/920) = 128$ mmol. However, the concentration of sodium per L (1000 mL) of plasma water will still be $128 \times (1000/840) = 152$ mmol, a value identical to the original level (see above).

Flame photometry measures only the sodium in a volume of plasma irrespective of the plasma's solid or water contents, and hence the apparents hyponatremia when sodium concentration is expressed in the normal fashion of mmol/L of plasma (e.g. 128 mmol/L of plasma in the above illustration). Since plasma osmolality (whose unit being mmol/kg water) measures the number of particles (such as urea, glucose, sodium, and other electrolytes) per kg of plasma water, this measure will also be normal in the present example.

- Pseudohyponatremia does not happen with direct potentiometry, which uses a sodium electrode to measure the sodium concentration of plasma water. However, the problem of pseudohyponatremia will persist when indirect potentiometry (currently used in >2/3 of laboratories in the US), which also employs a sodium electrode but a diluted sample of plasma for sodium measurement, is carried out. Since the plasma sample used for dilution has a lower sodium concentration (per unit volume, e.g. per L) to begin with, the sodium measurement problem underlying the pseudohyponatremia phenomenon is not addressed, but is perpetuated instead.
- Pseudohyponatremia happens in cases of severe hypercholesterolemia, hypertriglyceridemia, and hyperproteinemia. Hypertriglyceridemia is the one which is most often implicated. Severe hypercholesterolemia is an uncommon cause of pseudohyponatremia. Note that a rise in plasma lipids of 4.6 g/L leads to a decrease in plasma sodium level of approximately 1 mmol/L. Whether certain hyperproteinemias can cause pseudohyponatremia has recently been questioned. It is now thought that the M proteins of multiple myeloma do cause true hyponatremia, as these proteins are positively charged and thus less sodium particles are needed to bind to the negatively charged ions in the plasma. Similarly, whether infusion of immunoglobulin preparations can cause pseudohyponatremia has also been debated. Nevertheless, pseudohyponatremia is important because, if the entity is not recognized, mistaken treatment of this spurious hyponatremia with sodium-rich solutions might be carried out, with the resultant development of an iatrogenic hypernatremia. Normal plasma

osmolality in the face of hyponatremia should alert the physician to the probability of a diagnosis of pseudohyponatremia.

4.3.5 *True Hyponatremias*

4.3.5.1 *Translocational Hyponatremia*

Translocational hyponatremia is due to the movement of water from the intracellular space into the extracellular space. Total body sodium and total body water are normal. The plasma sodium level is low, while the plasma osmolality level is high.

Glucose, maltose, mannitol, and glycine can all raise plasma osmolality, but cannot enter cells (exception: glucose can enter brain cells even in the absence of insulin). As a result, water will be drawn from the cells into the plasma, diluting the sodium in plasma and causing hyponatremia. Note that the hyponatremia (defined as low plasma sodium concentration) in this setting is real and not spurious. Translocational hyponatremia is the only true hyponatremia associated with the exit of water from cells, whereas the other true hyponatremias are characterized by the entry of water into cells. A plasma glucose increment of 5.6 mmol/L (100 mg/dL) has been suggested to lower the plasma sodium level by 1.6 mmol/L. The entry of glucose into cells through insulin administration is followed by the return of the abstracted water to the cells, with a resultant restoration of normonatremia. Maltose, mannitol, and glycine can all be excreted in the urine or disposed of by renal replacement therapies.

4.3.5.2 *Euvolemic[a] Hyponatremia*

This type of hyponatremia, which has only mild volume excess, is due to water retention alone. Total body sodium is normal with a mild increase in total body water. Blood volume is only slightly on the high side because the small gain in water is distributed throughout the body's intracellular and extracellular compartments. Edema is commonly not evident clinically.

SIADH-related hyponatremia

This category of hyponatremia is the most common cause of hyponatremia in hospitalized patients, and SIADH is the most common

---

[a] "-volemic" refers to blood volume.

cause of this modest-volume-excess hyponatremia. Water retention (an increase of slightly less than 10% of total body water content and without prominent edema) rather than sodium loss is the main contributor to the development of hyponatremia in SIADH. The modest hypervolemia secondary to the water retention triggers the body's adaptive mechanisms, such as secretion of the atrial natriuretic peptide, suppression of aldosterone secretion, and reduction in the expression of AQP2 (the ADH-sensitive water channel in the collecting ducts), in an attempt to ameliorate the hypervolemia. Atrial natriuretic peptide enhances urinary sodium excretion by increasing glomerular filtration and by suppressing sodium absorption from the collecting ducts. In addition, volume expansion due to water retention per se can impair proximal sodium absorption.

There are four different patterns of ADH abnormalities in SIADH:

- Erratic ADH release pattern: ADH release is entirely independent of osmotic control.
- Reset osmostat pattern: There is an abnormally low osmotic threshold for ADH release, but an ability to excrete a maximally dilute urine if sufficiently water-loaded.
- ADH leak pattern: There is a sustained ADH release at an abnormally low osmotic threshold and normal increases in serum ADH levels with osmotic challenge.
- No detectable abnormality in serum ADH levels.

In SIADH, the plasma levels of sodium, osmolality, chloride, urea, creatinine, and uric acid are low. The urine osmolality may be either inappropriately high for the degree of hypo-osmolality or maximally dilute (e.g. urine osmolality as low as 50 mmol/kg in the case of reset osmostat). The urine sodium level usually reflects sodium intake, i.e. >20 mmol/L; however, should the patient become sodium- or volume-depleted, urine sodium concentration can reach very low levels. SIADH occurs when there is an inappropriate secretion of ADH or an ADH-like substance despite a low plasma osmolality and normovolemia (or mild hypervolemia).

SIADH is associated with various malignancies such as bronchogenic carcinoma, lymphoma, prostatic carcinoma, and pancreatic carcinoma. It is also seen with pulmonary disorders such as pneumonia, lung abscess, bronchiectasis, tuberculosis, cystic fibrosis, and positive-pressure breathing. Central nervous system (CNS) causes include cerebrovascular accidents, infections, head trauma, subdural hematoma, delirium tremens, multiple sclerosis, and porphyria. SIADH can also occur in the elderly without an apparent cause (suggesting abnormal vasopressin secretion) and in patients with AIDS. Some medications also induce SIADH (see below).

The diagnosis of SIADH should be suspected in a hyponatremic patient who does not have hypovolemia, edematous disorders, hypoadrenalism, hypothyroidism, or renal failure while also not receiving certain hyponatremia-inducing drugs. In patients with a resetting of the osmostat (regarded by some as one subtype of SIADH; please see above), the plasma osmolality threshold for ADH secretion is lowered, thus bringing about a hyponatremia that is asymptomatic and does not require treatment.

Beer potomania

Beer potomania ("poto" = drinking, "mania" = craze) falls somewhere between hypovolemic and mildly hypervolemic hyponatremia. It was first described in the 1970s and is unique to beer drinkers. The cause of the hyponatremia is a very low osmolal intake, since beer does not have much in the way of sodium, protein, or other solutes. Patients are at an extreme risk if their hyponatremia is rapidly corrected. It is suggested that the patient does not feed (or feeds minimally) in the first 24 hours after presentation, as a large osmolal intake can lead to a more rapid correction of the hyponatremia. Apart from patients with beer potomania, 70% of chronic alcoholic patients have hyponatremia. Severe hyponatremia is often associated with other electrolyte abnormalities such as hypokalemia, hypomagnesemia, and hypophosphatemia.

Exercise-associated hyponatremia

Many patients with this disorder have gained weight from their baseline due to excessive drinking of hypo-osmolal fluids. Urine sodium concentration is usually less than 30 mmol/L. A delayed presentation of hyponatremia can be seen after a marathon and is thought to be due to the delayed absorption of hypo-osmolal fluid from the gastrointestinal tract. Hyponatremia is directly related to water ingestion (main cause of hyponatremia), duration of the marathon, and low body mass index, although loss of sodium in sweat also plays a part in the development of the hyponatremia. Since tissue hypoxia may complicate strenuous exercise, it is possible that hypoxia may worsen neurologic outcomes. The exercise-induced non-osmotic release of vasopressin may further impair renal water excretion.

Conventional sports drinks are not protective of the development of hyponatremia, as these fluids are hyponatric. Ingestion of a large volume of fluids during marathons is not recommended anymore; rather, thirst should be used as a guide to fluid consumption. The clinical manifestations include non-cardiogenic pulmonary edema as a result of raised intracranial pressure secondary to cerebral edema. Nausea, vomiting, seizure, respiratory arrest, and death may occur.

Hypothyroidism

Severe hypothyroidism is thought to be a rare cause of hyponatremia. Intrarenal mechanisms and a persistant vasopressin release may be the causes for the hyponatremia. The combination of primary hypoaldosteronism and hypothyroidism can lead to severe hyponatremia.

Psychiatric disorder

About 20% of psychiatric patients have polydipsia. If water intake exceeds a patient's ability to excrete free water, hyponatremia can result. In these patients, the secretion of ADH is suppressed. Patients with psychogenic polydipsia usually have diurnal variation in plasma sodium concentrations, with higher levels in the morning than at night. Before psychogenic polydipsia is diagnosed, infiltrative diseases of the CNS such as sarcoidosis should be excluded first as these diseases can lead to abnormal thirst. In certain patients, hyponatremia as a result of the consumption of pharmacologic agents such as thiazide and carbamazepine rather than as a result of psychogenic polydipsia per se remains a possibility. Clozapine has been used successfully to treat psychogenic polydipsia.

Hospital-acquired hyponatremia

Hospital-acquired hyponatremia — especially of the postoperative variety — is common, but most episodes are mild and asymptomatic. Postoperative hyponatremia can occur with transurethral resection of the prostate. Use of sodium-poor irrigation fluids has been incriminated in most instances; thus, normal saline should be the preferred solution for irrigation. Severe hyponatremia in healthy women after elective surgery under general anesthesia has been reported. Urine findings have suggested the diagnosis of SIADH. There are multiple stimuli for vasopressin secretion in the postoperative state in the form of recent anesthesia, nausea, vomiting, pain, and analgesic administration. These patients developed cerebral edema along with manifestations of seizures, hypoxia, and neurologic damage. Twenty-seven percent of the patients died and 60% ended up in a persistent vegetative state. The patients gained an average of 7.5 L of fluids after surgery. Use of hyponatric and/or sodium-free solutions will worsen the situation.

Pregnancy

The occurrence of hyponatremia during labor has been reported and is related to hypo-osmolal fluid intake.

Mutation of vasopressin receptor

The nephrogenic syndrome of inappropriate antidiuresis is a newly described syndrome that is thought to be caused by a mutation of V_2 receptor that constitutively activates the latter receptor in the absence of ADH. It has been described in children with hyponatremia. ADH levels are undetectable.

Medication-induced hyponatremia

- Non-steroidal anti-inflammatory drugs (NSAIDs) can also potentiate the antidiuretic effect of ADH and cause hyponatremia.
- Hyponatremia is well described with selective serotonin inhibitor therapy. In one study of 15 patients, 40% developed hyponatremia after a 2-week course. Hyponatremia is three times more common with selective serotonin receptor inhibitor (SSRI) therapy than with other antidepressants. The risk of hyponatremia is greatest in the first week of therapy and in elderly women. Hyponatremia has also been reported with selective norepinephrine receptor inhibitors such as duloxetine, atomoxetine, and venlafaxine. In one study of 58 patients, the use of these drugs caused hyponatremia in 17% of the patients.
- Carbamazepine, oxcarbazepine, and valproic acid have also been reported to cause hyponatremia.
- Ecstasy seems to cause a unique syndrome of severe hyponatremia associated with increased intracranial pressure, noncardiogenic pulmonary edema, and high mortality rates. Most reported cases have been in postmenopausal women.

- Severe hyponatremia with seizures has been reported after polyethylene glycol-based bowel cleansing for colonoscopy.
- True hyponatremia with intravenous immunoglobulin (IVIG) treatment is now thought to occur because of the accumulation of a sucrose carrier in commercial IVIG preparations. Also, it comes in 2.33 L of sterile water if 2 g/kg (6%) IVIG is given to a 70-kg man.
- Hyponatremia has been reported with the use of ciprofloxacin, desmopressin, amiodarone, tacrolimus, theophylline, and camphor intoxication. Other commonly used drugs that can cause hyponatremia include acetaminophen, narcotics, chlorpropamide, cyclophosphamide, vincristine, clofibrate, nicotine, oxytocin, haloperidol and amitriptyline. The suggested causes for these medication-related hyponatremias include the production of ADH or ADH-like substances as well as intrarenal mechanisms.

4.3.5.3 Hypovolemic Hyponatremia

- Hypovolemic hyponatremia is due to both sodium and water deficits: total body sodium ↓↓, total body water ↓.
- Non-blood body fluids, such as urine, vomitus, diarrheal fluid, and sweat, do not ordinarily contain sodium in a concentration higher than that of plasma. Consequently, the loss of these hyponatric fluids from the body can bring about hypernatremia because the loss of water exceeds that of sodium (from the viewpoint of plasma). However, if these sodium and water losses are accompanied by a level of water intake adequate enough to convert the loss of water to be less than that of sodium but not adequate enough to correct the hypovolemia, hypovolemic hyponatremia can result.
- In the face of extrarenal losses, sodium and water are conserved by the kidneys, resulting in a reduction in urine sodium concentration to <10 mmol/L. In contrast, with renal losses, the capacity of the kidneys to conserve sodium is impaired; hence, the urine sodium level will often be >20 mmol/L.
- Diuretic therapy: With hypovolemic hyponatremia due to diuretic therapy, the urine sodium level can be elevated when the diuretic is in effect; yet when the effect of the diuretic wears off, the urine sodium value can become low if there is volume depletion. The majority of diuretic-induced hyponatremia cases are related to the use of thiazides. Underweight elderly women appear to be especially susceptible to this electrolyte disorder, especially if they increase their fluid intake after the initiation of therapy. Eleven percent to

33% of inpatient geriatric patients developed hyponatremia after the initiation of thiazide therapy in one study. The concomitant presence of diuretic-induced hypokalemia and metabolic alkalosis is common. Acting on the distal convoluted tubule, thiazides cause hyponatremia because they suppress the reabsorption of sodium and chloride, thus allowing these electrolytes to remain in the tubular fluid and impairing the formation of a solute-poor, dilute urine (i.e. reducing solute-free water clearance). Other reasons for the development of hyponatremia include reduced delivery of fluid to the diluting segments and increased secretion of vasopressin, both mechanisms being related to the diuretic-induced volume depletion and leading to the reduction of solute-free water clearance. It is likely that any accompanying hypokalemia, might help to promote the development of hyponatremia although the underlying mechanism for such an association is unknown.

Hyponatremia often occurs shortly after starting the diuretic (usually within 2 weeks), and recurrence of hyponatremia often takes place if drug therapy is resumed after prior stoppage. Hypovolemia is often not clinically apparent and the most frequent symptoms include malaise, dizziness, and vomiting. If their hyponatremia is corrected rapidly, these patients are at a high risk of developing neurological manifestations. Loop diuretics causes hyponatremia much less often because they affect not only the diluting, but also the concentrating, ability of the ascending limb.

- Salt-losing renal diseases: Certain renal diseases can be associated with loss of sodium in the urine. These renal ailments include chronic advanced renal failure (with GFR <20 mL/min; being the most common cause), proximal renal tubular acidosis, medullary cystic disease, polycystic kidney disease, chronic pyelonephritis, analgesic nephropathy, and obstructive nephropathy. The degree of sodium wasting varies widely.

- Osmotic diuresis: Examples of osmotic diuresis comprise mannitol diuresis, glucose diuresis due to diabetic hyperglycemia, and urea diuresis due to relief of urinary obstruction or recovery from acute kidney injury. Urine resulting from osmotic diuresis usually possesses an osmolality not too distant from that of plasma. Since osmotic diuresis urine contains a substantial amount of the solute responsible for the diuresis, the level of sodium in the urine will necessarily be less than that in the plasma. Since water loss is in excess of sodium loss, hypernatremia should be the rule rather than the exception. However, if a patient consumes a large amount of water to combat the accompanying hypovolemia, hypovolemic hyponatremia can occur.

- Cerebral salt wasting causes hyponatremia, extracellular fluid (ECF) contraction, and renal sodium wasting in the setting of intracranial disease. Although the urine sodium level is usually >20 mmol/L, cerebral salt wasting can be associated with a low urine sodium concentration if sodium intake is low.

- With hypovolemic hyponatremia, clinical manifestations of volume depletion are often seen along with elevations in serum levels of urea and creatinine.

4.3.5.4 Hypervolemic Hyponatremia

Hypervolemic hyponatremia is due to both sodium and water retention: total body sodium ↑; total body water ↑↑. The following conditions are associated with the retention of both sodium and water. However, the retention of water is greater than that of sodium — hence, hyponatremia.

- Five percent to 20% of patients with congestive heart failure have hyponatremia, which is an independent predictor of mortality. Hyponatremia is often mediated by both a reduced delivery of tubular fluid to the distal diluting segments as a result of increased proximal tubular reabsorption, and an increased production of vasopressin. Both of these steps lower free water excretion. A low cardiac output reduces arterial filling and the effective circulatory blood volume. A fall in this latter volume is sensed by the aortic and carotid sinus baroreceptors; the latter's impulses then stimulate vasopressin release.

- Thirty percent to 35% of cirrhotics also have hyponatremia, which is also a strong poor prognostic factor. It is suggested that, in patients with advanced cirrhosis, splanchnic arterial vasodilatation brings about arterial underfilling (i.e. reduced effective circulatory volume), with a resultant activation of the neurohumoral axis of norepinephrine, renin/angiotensin/aldosterone, and non-osmotic stimulation of vasopressin. It is likely that an augmented formation of vasopressin plays a large part in causing the impairment of free water excretion, while intrarenal mechanisms causing a decreased fluid delivery to the distal nephron play a smaller role.

- Hyponatremia in patients with the nephrotic syndrome also occurs, but is not as common. Some hypoalbuminemic patients have low blood volume, but high total body water content. A high vasopressin plasma level has been found in these patients. Other nephrotic patients with poor renal function have a high blood volume. The pathogenesis of their hyponatremia is unknown, but may be related to decreased renal mass (please see below).

- Patients with severe renal failure are unable to excrete sodium and free water in the normal manner because of the reduction in renal mass. Hyponatremia will occur if there is an excess of water over sodium in the body.

4.4 Complications of Hyponatremia

- The main concerns with hyponatremia are CNS-related. The abrupt lowering of plasma osmolality in acute hyponatremia leads to the entry of water into the brain, bringing about brain edema and a syndrome known as hyponatremic encephalopathy. This syndrome has been reported with plasma sodium levels as high as 128 mmol/L.
- Rhabdomyolysis has also been reported with hyponatremia.
- When hyponatremia is due to the acute lowering of extracellular osmolality, e.g. with the infusion of massive amounts of hypo-osmolal solutions, hemolysis can occur.

4.5 Risk Factors for Hyponatremic Encephalopathy

Children, hypoxic patients, and premenopausal women in the post-operative state are at a heightened risk for the development of hyponatremic encephalopathy, have a higher chance of encountering a poor outcome, and require prompt medical attention. To begin with, a child has a higher ratio of brain size to cranial vault size than an adult; in addition, a child has less brain atrophy. As a result of these factors, symptoms from hyponatremia can develop more rapidly and tolerance to cerebral edema can be reduced. Hypoxia impairs the body's adaptive response to hyponatremia, and can worsen the effects of hyponatremia and cause cerebral edema. With respect to the susceptibility of premenopausal women, female hormones may inhibit the adaptive decrease in brain volume as a response to acute hyponatremia. Other patients who are highly susceptible to hyponatremic encephalopathy include elderly persons on diuretic therapy and patients with psychogenic polydipsia.

4.6 Treatment of Hyponatremias (Other than Translocational Hyponatremia)

In the management of hyponatremia, plasma potassium levels should be assessed often; and potassium preparations should be administered in the face of hypokalemia. This is because hypokalemia can promote the exit of intracellular potassium into the ECF along with the entry of ECF sodium into the cells, thus worsening hyponatremia.

4.6.1 Euvolemic Hyponatremia

4.6.1.1 Symptomatic Euvolemic Hyponatremia

Acute

If hyponatremia develops within 48 hours (i.e. the hyponatremia is acute) and the patient is symptomatic with a plasma sodium level of <120 mmol/L, then the general consensus is that these patients' hyponatremias should be corrected relatively quickly. Children, young women, and postoperative patients appear to be more susceptible to rapidly progressive hyponatremic encephalopathy; consequently, prompt treatment of their hyponatremia is particularly indicated. Severe acute symptomatic hyponatremia should be treated rapidly at a rate of 1–3 mmol/L/h increase in plasma sodium level; correction by <3–4 mmol/L/day has been associated with a worse outcome. Use of 3% saline solution, preferably in combination with a potent loop diuretic to prevent extracellular volume overload, is often favored. Intravenously administered osmotic diuretics such as urea and mannitol could also be used, but experience in using these agents is limited.

Chronic

Chronic hyponatremia is often defined as hyponatremia that has lasted for >48 hours. Over this period, the original brain cell swelling secondary to the initial acute hyponatremia has subsided. This dissipation of swelling to return to the original size is due to the extrusion of electrolytes and organic solutes, an adaptive effort of the brain cells to lower their osmolality in order to adjust to the new hypo-osmolal extracellular environment. Animal studies have suggested that a rapid correction of hyponatremia in such a setting can bring about a greater loss of water from brain cells than from their counterparts in a normonatremic individual. The pathogenetic mechanism underlying this phenomenon is believed to be as follows: there are less electrolyte and organic solutes in chronic hyponatremic brain cells to resist cell shrinkage in the event of a rapid increase in plasma sodium level; such a marked brain cell shrinkage can lead to the development of the osmotic demyelination syndrome.

Chronic hyponatremic patients who are more susceptible to this syndrome include patients receiving diuretic therapy and those suffering from malnutrition, chronic alcoholism, beer potomania, advanced liver disease, severe hypokalemia, or profound hyponatremia (plasma sodium level <105 mmol/L). Most demyelinating lesions are present in the central pons, the medulla oblongata, and the mesencephalon. Clinical features include upper motor neuron manifestations, pseudobulbar palsy, spastic quadriparesis, and mental disorders ranging from mild confusion to coma. Some patients with osmotic demyelination do survive. Demyelination is diagnosed by a magnetic resonance imaging (MRI) finding of hyperintense lesions on T2-weighted images; however, positive MRI findings are generally seen only 3–4 weeks after the correction of hyponatremia and after the onset of neurologic manifestations. This demyelination syndrome usually has a biphasic clinical presentation, with an initial improvement in the neurological status (as hyponatremia improves) followed by a worsening of mental function. Uremia and infusion of myoinositol or glucocorticoids may protect against demyelination.

The possibility of encountering the osmotic demyelination syndrome has complicated the treatment of chronic symptomatic hyponatremia. It is believed that in order to minimize the development of this syndrome, both the rate of correction and the absolute change in plasma sodium concentration should receive careful attention. There is controversy as to how fast chronic symptomatic hyponatremia should be treated. Some authors have recommended that the plasma sodium value should be rectified by a correction rate of not more than 0.5 mmol/L per hour, and by an absolute change in plasma sodium concentration of not more than 12 mmol/L in the first 24 hours, and not more than 18 mmol/L in the first 48 hours. Other authors have suggested that the maximal rate of correction can be 1–2 mmol/L per hour, as long as the absolute change does not exceed 25 mmol/L over the first 48 hours. A reasonable approach would seem to be:

- In patients who are only minimally symptomatic, one should proceed with a slower rate of 0.5 mmol/L or less per hour.

- In patients who exhibit more severe neurological manifestations, a correction rate of 1–2 mmol/L per hour would appear to be appropriate.
- In patients who are comatose or seizing and in imminent danger of tentorial herniation or respiratory arrest, a correction rate of even 3–5 mmol/L per hour would be justified.

It should be noted that acute treatment should be discontinued once any of the following three endpoints has been reached:

- The patient's symptoms are abolished.
- A safe plasma sodium level (usually >120 mmol/L) is at hand.
- A total increase in sodium level of 20 mmol/L has been achieved.

Subsequent treatment should consist of slower-acting therapies such as fluid restriction, oral repletion, and diuretic therapy, depending on the etiology of the hyponatremia.

There are a number of formulas to determine the quantity of NaCl required for administration or the amount of free water required for removal in order to raise the plasma sodium value to a desired level. One simple formula to gauge the approximate amount of NaCl needed is (note that 1 mmol NaCl has 1 mmol Na):

$$\text{mmol Na required} = \text{TBW} \times \Delta[\text{Na}]$$
$$\text{mmol Na required} = 0.6 \times \text{weight in kg} \times \Delta[\text{Na}]$$
$$\Delta[\text{Na}] = \text{desired [Na]} - \text{current [Na]},$$

where TBW is the total body water. The saline solution conventionally used is of the 3% variety (513 mmol NaCl/L).

Although infused sodium is largely restricted to the ECF, total body water is used for the above calculation because any change in ECF sodium concentration causes a prompt water shift from the intracellular fluid (ICF). The above, very-approximate formula does not take into consideration ongoing urinary, alimentary, or insensible free water, sodium, and potassium loss as well as various intakes; thus, frequent monitoring of plasma electrolyte levels, urinary electrolyte values, and urine output is mandatory. Administration of the 3% saline solution should be adjusted in accordance with current laboratory findings, should inadvertent overshooting of the plasma sodium level occur, relowering of the level by the use of desmopressin has been shown to prevent the occurrence of brain lesions in humans. Finally, the management of symptomatic hyponatremic patients should prefer-ably be carried out in an intensive care unit.

4.6.1.2 Asymptomatic Euvolemic Hyponatremia

Hyponatremia in patients with asymptomatic hyponatremia is usu-ally chronic in nature. Asymptomatic patients with euvolemic hyponatremia should be managed with water restriction only, even if the plasma sodium value is very low. Should water restriction be unsuccessful, other means can be tried. Demeclocycline can inhibit the renal effect of vasopressin and increase solute-free water excre-tion. The drug can be used as a second-line agent to treat hyponatremia. However, demeclocycline can cause azotemia and photosensitivity, and is contraindicated in patients with renal or liver disease because of its accumulation in the body and its nephrotoxic-ity potential. Orally administered urea at a dose of 30–60 g daily has been used successfully to treat SIADH; this is because, with urea-induced osmotic diuresis, water is lost in excess of sodium. Other osmotic agents such as mannitol can also be used. A combination of furosemide therapy (40 mg by mouth daily) and high NaCl intake (200 mmol daily) has also been found to be effective in the manage-ment of asymptomatic SIADH.

Vasopressin receptor antagonists (vaptans) are newer drugs that inhibit the action of vasopressin. There are four vasopressin receptors (V_{1a}, V_{1b}, V_2, and V_3), of which only V_2 is present in the kidneys. Being nonpeptides, V_2 vaptans can be given orally and have longer half-lives. However, nonpeptide antagonists can penetrate the blood-brain barrier and thus may cause CNS side effects. Vaptans are metabolized by the cytochrome CYP3A4 pathway, and thus drug–drug interaction is a concern. Conivaptan, another vaptan, is given intravenously and is the only vaptan approved by the US Food and Drug Administration. SIADH is the ideal indication for treat-ment with vaptans. Vaptans should be avoided in hypovolemic patients. Patients on vaptan therapy should be monitored closely for the rate of correction of plasma sodium levels. To date, no cases of demyelination have been reported. Two other new vaptans, lixivaptan and tolvaptan, have been shown to increase plasma sodium levels in patients with euvolemic hyponatremia and hypervolemic hypona-tremia. Further studies are required to determine the precise role that these novel drugs play in the overall management of non-hypovolemic hyponatremic patients.

4.6.2 Hypovolemic Hyponatremia

Treatment often consists of replacement of lost sodium and water with isotonic saline. If clinically feasible, oral sodium chloride and water can be given instead for mild cases. The recommended rate and magnitude of sodium correction (see above) should still be observed.

The rate of correction must be adjusted to prevent the occurrence of demyelination (see above). Hyponatremia due to the cerebral salt-wasting syndrome can be treated with fludrocortisone.

4.6.3 Hypervolemic Hyponatremia

- Water restriction: Apart from treatment of the underlying condition (e.g. improving cardiac function in heart failure), water restriction is indicated.
- Diuretics: Potent loop diuretics can often increase solute-free water and sodium excretion in edematous states.
- Hypertonic saline: In severely hyponatremic (e.g. plasma sodium <110 mmol/L) patients with CNS symptoms, judicious administration of small quantities of 3% saline (50–100 mmol of NaCl) along with the use of a potent loop diuretic may be required.
- Renal replacement therapies: Hemodialysis, peritoneal dialysis, hemofiltration, and hemodiafiltration using dialysate/replacement fluid sodium levels higher than that in the plasma can all be used effectively in severely hyponatremic patients. In addition, the ultrafiltration capacity of these procedures can often be utilized to remove excess fluid from these patients.
- V_2 receptor antagonists: The use of these antagonists to treat hyponatremia due to, for example, congestive cardiac failure and cirrhosis of liver, is under investigation.
- The recommended rate and magnitude of sodium correction (see above) should still be observed.

4.7 Hypernatremia

4.7.1 Definition (Table 4.1)

- Hypernatremia is defined as a plasma sodium concentration of >145 mmol/L.
- Severe hypernatremia is defined as a plasma sodium value of >160 mmol/L.

4.7.2 Incidence

- Patients presenting with hypernatremia account for only 0.2% of total hospital admissions.
- One percent of hospitalized patients are hypernatremic, and these hypernatremic patients are usually intubated and in the intensive care unit.
- One study found that 32% of patients with hypernatremia were hypernatremic on admission, while 60% developed it during their hospital stay.

4.7.3 Prognosis

- The mortality rate in general is about 40%.
- Serious hypernatremia has a 60%–70% mortality rate.
- Patients who are hypernatremic on admission have a better prognosis than those with hospital-acquired hypernatremia.

4.7.4 Mechanism of Development

- Hypernatremia can be due to loss of water, gain of sodium, or both. Loss of water is the more common denominator.
- Many patients with hypernatremia have either a decreased sense of thirst or an inability to access water, as hyperosmolality — ordinarily such a strong stimulus for thirst — is mediated via the hypothalamic thirst center.
- Fifty percent of patients with hypernatremia on admission and 89% of those who develop hypernatremia after admission have a urinary concentrating defect. The most common causes of a concentrating defect are renal insufficiency, diuretic therapy, and solute diuresis [such as diuresis due to glucose (e.g. in hyperglycemic states), mannitol, glycerol, or urea (urea diuresis being secondary to protein loading, urea administration, hypercatabolism, relief of urinary obstruction, recovery from acute kidney injury, or absorption of digested blood proteins in the face of gastrointestinal bleeding)]. With solute diuresis, water loss is in excess of sodium loss in the nonconcentrated urine because a large fraction of the osmoles in the urine is now made up by the solute responsible for the diuresis, leaving little room for sodium to be excreted.
- Classically, hypernatremia has been assumed to be hypovolemic in the majority of patients. More recently, however, it is realized that

the occurrence of severe hypernatremia without volume depletion is not uncommon. In fact, in a recent study, only 41% of patients with hypernatremia were hypovolemic, whereas 51% were euvolemic.

4.7.5 Spurious Hypernatremia

Spurious hypernatremia has been described when blood is drawn from venous dialysis catheters housing a citrate lock, which consists of a high concentration of trisodium citrate.

4.7.6 True Hypernatremia

4.7.6.1 Euvolemic Hypernatremia

- Total body water ↓, total body sodium normal.
- Common causes include hypodipsia, diabetes insipidus (central and nephrogenic), and some of the extrarenal disorders of a milder nature that are listed in Sec. 4.4.6.2. With these causes, mainly water rather than sodium is lost. Since total body sodium tends to be normal, blood volume is better maintained. However, if water deficit is severe, euvolemia may progress to hypovolemia. The urine sodium level is variable.

4.7.6.2 Hypovolemic Hypernatremia

- Total body water ↓↓, total body sodium ↓.
- Renal causes include osmotic diuresis, loop diuretic therapy, postobstructive diuresis, and intrinsic renal disease. The urine sodium level is >20 mmol/L.
- Extrarenal causes include (a) skin losses via sweating (hot weather, exercise, cystic fibrosis) and burns; and (b) alimentary losses via vomiting, diarrhea, and fistula output. The urine sodium level is <10 mmol/L.
- With both renal and extrarenal causes, water loss is in excess of sodium loss.

4.7.6.3 Hypervolemic Hypernatremia

- Total body water ↑ or normal, total body sodium ↑↑.
- Common causes include mineralocorticoid excess, Conn's syndrome, Cushing's syndrome, Liddle's syndrome, licorice gluttony, and excessive sodium chloride and/or sodium bicarbonate administration

(the total body water will be normal if no water is taken along with these sodium salts). The urine sodium level is >20 mmol/L.

4.7.7 Common Causes (Table 4.2)

- The typical patient presenting with hypernatremia is a nursing home patient who is afflicted by dementia or is somehow unable to access water. This person truly has volume depletion and has usually developed hypernatremia over a long period of time. Eighty-three percent of these patients have an underlying infectious process.
- Hypernatremia is common in the intensive care unit. Most of these patients have underlying renal insufficiency with an inability to concentrate their urine. Commonly, these patients are hypervolemic, as large volumes of intravenous fluids have been given at the beginning of their illness. In a 1943 study, the authors stated that large amounts of isotonic saline given to oliguric or anuric patients suffering from acute kidney injury had little effect on the subsequent rise of plasma sodium concentration; however, with improvement in renal function, excretion of a large volume of urine — characterized by excessive loss of water over that of sodium — did lead to hypernatremia if the water was not replaced. It was suggested that as urine output increases, water intake should also be raised and sodium intake should be avoided.
- Hypodipsic hypernatremia is seen in children and adults with various congenital and acquired diseases of the brain.
- Central diabetes insipidus is a well-described cause of hypernatremia. In one study, only 6 (6%) out of 103 patients with hypernatremia had central diabetes insipidus. The water deprivation test is not required in a patient with hypernatremia, but is indicated in a patient with polyuria and normal plasma sodium level. Nephrogenic diabetes insipidus is most often seen with lithium therapy; however, demeclocycline therapy, foscarnet therapy, hypercalcemia, hypokalemia, sickle cell ailments, amyloidosis, and other tubulointerstitial diseases are other common causes.
- Cases of inadvertent infusion of 5% saline instead of 5% dextrose solution, leading to severe hypernatremia (plasma sodium value as high as 216 mmol/L), have been reported. For this reason, use of the 5% saline solutions has been abandoned in favor of the 3% variety. Nevertheless, excessive administration of the latter can still cause hypernatremia.
- Hypertonic sodium bicarbonate infusions using solutions contained in ampoules (44.6 mmol or 50 mmol in 50 mL) can lead to

Table 4.2   Causes of hypernatremia.*

Inadequate water consumption

Hypothalamic disorders
Impaired thirst

Failure to ingest water
Impairment of consciousness
Mental illness

Physical weakness and/or dearth of care
Infants and other very young persons
Cachexia
Debilitating illness
Paralysis
Postanesthesia

Extrarenal water loss

Insensible loss
Sweat/perspiration
Heat
Fever
Severe exercise
Cystic fibrosis
Burns
Mechanical respiration
Hyperventilation

Alimentary loss
Vomiting
Nasogastric aspiration
Diarrhea
Sodium phosphate laxatives or enemas
Lactulose or sorbitol therapy

Peritoneal cavity loss
Loss of water in excess of sodium with the use of hyperosmolal
glucose-enriched peritoneal dialysis solutions

Renal water loss

Osmotic diuresis
Glucose
Urea
Mannitol
Glycerol

(*Continued*)

Table 4.2 *(Continued)*

Vasopressin problems
Lack of vasopressin
  Central diabetes insipidus
Nonresponsiveness to vasopressin
  Nephrogenic diabetes insipidus
    Congenital
    Lithium
    Demeclocycline
    Amyloidosis
    Hypokalemia
    Hypercalcemia
    Relief of urinary obstruction
    Tubulointerstitial diseases

Sodium gain
Excessive sodium intake
  NaCl
  NaHCO$_3$
  Bleach or sodium phosphate ingestion
  Mistaken use of NaCl instead of sugar for infant feeding
  Drinking sea water during shipwreck or drowning
  Parenteral hypertonic sodium chloride or bicarbonate solutions
  Addition of hypertonic sodium bicarbonate solutions to normal saline
    to treat metabolic acidosis
  Use of high-sodium dialysate/replacement fluid in renal replacement
    therapies

Excessive renal sodium absorption
  Conn's syndrome
  Cushing's syndrome
  Liddle's syndrome
  Corticosteroid therapy (especially fludrocortisone)
  Licorice ingestion

---

*Adapted from Table 14: Causes of Hypernatremia, page 46 of the Nephrology Section of MKSAP 12, 2001.

hypernatremia, and thus iso-osmolal solution of sodium bicarbonate should be used preferentially (except in emergency resuscitation situations). Moreover, the inadvertent addition of such sodium bicarbonate preparations to normal saline (the sodium level of which is already 154 mmol/L) in an attempt to treat metabolic acidosis has brought about hypernatremia.

- Cases of severe hypernatremia associated with massive ingestion of salt intake (e.g. mistaken use of salt instead of sugar in infant food, since some salt and sugar preparations look alike) or drowning in seawater have been reported.
- Peritoneal dialysis patients using dialysates containing large amounts of glucose are prone to hypernatremia. The high-glucose dialysates extract more water than sodium from the blood, resulting in hypernatremia. Other renal replacement therapies using high-sodium dialysate/replacement fluids can also cause hypernatremia.

4.7.8 *Adaptation of Brain to Chronic Hypernatremia*

- Brain cells accumulate solutes to increase intracellular osmolality in an attempt to counteract the osmotic effects of the hypernatremia (and the hyperosmolality) and to restore the intracellular fluid volume towards normal.
- In the first 24 hours, brain cells accumulate sodium, potassium, and chloride. However, during this time, restoration of the brain cell volume is incomplete.
- It takes up to 2 days for brain cells to accumulate enough organic solutes (known as idiogenic osmoles) to raise intracellular osmolality in order to counterbalance the effects of the hypernatremia. These idiogenic osmoles include taurine, glutamine, glutamate, methylamines, and myoinositol. Because of their accumulation, brain cell volume can eventually become normal.

4.7.9 *Complications*

- Plasma sodium concentration determines intracellular fluid volume. Thus, an increase in plasma sodium levels leads to shrinkage of brain cell volume and secondary neurological symptoms. The latter include lethargy, weakness, irritability, seizures, stupor, coma, and death. Myelinosis of the brain has also been described in a diabetic patient suffering from both marked hypernatremia and severe hyperglycemia.
- Severe hypernatremia (plasma sodium concentration > 170 mmol/L) has also been reported to cause high plasma creatine phosphokinase values as a result of muscle damage and rhabdomyolysis.
- Rapid correction of chronic hypernatremia causes a sudden lowering of plasma osmolality and consequent brain edema due to the entry of water into the normal-sized but still hyperosmolal brain cells.

4.7.10 Treatment

4.7.10.1 Euvolemic Hypernatremia

Water replacement is recommended. If a large amount of electrolyte-free water in the form of 5% dextrose solution is given to treat marked hypernatremia due to severe central diabetes insipidus with massive output of dilute urine, one should bear in mind the possibility of causing a dextrose-induced hyperglycemia. The latter can bring about an osmotic diuresis. As more 5% dextrose solution is given to replace urine output, a vicious cycle of "diuresis → dextrose infusion → hyperglycemia → glucose diuresis → hypernatremia → dextrose infusion → hyperglycemia …" is established.

Vasopressin preparations are not able to overcome the osmotic diuretic effects of hyperglycemia. Insulin therapy is required to control this iatrogenic hyperglycemia. Under such circumstances, the intravenous administration of ¼ saline solution or even pure water to combat the water deficit has been suggested. Note that central diabetes insipidus will respond to vasopressin preparations, whereas nephrogenic diabetes insipidus will not.

4.7.10.2 Hypovolemic Hypernatremia

Hypotonic saline is the agent of choice under most circumstances. Oral repletion of water and sodium is suggested if the condition is mild and not urgent.

4.7.10.3 Hypervolemic Hypernatremia

Treat the primary disease where appropriate. For hypernatremia due to excessive sodium administration, the combination of water replacement and diuretic therapy is often advised.

4.7.10.4 General Therapeutic Recommendations

- Whenever possible, water deficit should be treated with water administered via the oral or gastric route.
- In acute hypernatremia (hypernatremia developing within hours), reducing the plasma sodium value by 1 mmol/L/h has been suggested. This more rapid correction is feasible because the adaptive response of the shrunken brain cells has not been accomplished, and these shrunken cells can now resume their normal

size resulting from water entry consequent to the correction of hypernatremia. However, the above approach is controversial because some authors believe that the correction rate should still be at a slower rate of 0.5 mmol/L/h over 48–72 hours.

- It has been suggested that in the treatment of chronic hypernatremia, the plasma sodium level should be reduced by 0.5 mmol/L/h. The goal of treatment should be a plasma sodium concentration in the neighborhood of 145 mmol/L. This slower correction approach is recommended because faster corrections can bring about cerebral edema due to the entry of water into brain cells that have already resumed their normal volume as a result of the accumulation of electrolytes and the generation of idiogenic osmoles.

- Patients with intravascular volume depletion manifesting as hypotension or orthostasis may require normal saline infusion to replenish the volume deficit first. The water deficit can be addressed after the ECF volume has been restored.

- The most common mistake in the treatment of hypernatremia is that the treatment is not adequate enough to correct the high plasma sodium concentration.

- Solute-free water deficit can be used to determine how much water is required to correct the hypernatremia. A very approximate measure of solute-free water deficit can be calculated as follows. Since it is assumed that there is no loss of sodium, the following formula holds:

Current TBW × current plasma [Na] = new TBW × new plasma [Na]

Water deficit
= new TBW − current TBW
= (current TBW × current plasma [Na]/new plasma [Na]) − current TBW
= current TBW {(current plasma [Na]/new plasma [Na]) − 1}
= 0.5 (weight in kg){(current [Na]/145) − 1} if the patient is quite dehydrated and the desired new plasma [Na] is 145 mmol/L,

where TBW is the total body water. TBW correlates with muscle mass, and therefore decreases with advancing age and wasting. TBW also correlates with the degree of dehydration. In addition, the value is lower in women than in men. By evaluating the above variables, a value between 40% and 60% of current body weight can be used as a rough estimate of total body water.

Suggested Reading

Alquire PC, Epstein PE (eds.). (2006) Nephrology section. In: *MKSAP14 — Medical Knowledge Self-Assessment Program*, American College of Physicians, Philadelphia, PA, pp. 6–11.

Berl T, Schrier RW. (2003) Disorders of water metabolism. In: Schrier RW (ed.), *Renal and Electrolyte Disorders*, 6th ed., Lippincott Williams & Wilkins, Philadelphia, PA, pp. 1–63.

Fukagawa M, Kurokawa K, Papadakis MA. (2008) Fluid and electrolyte disorders. In: McPhee SJ, Papadakis MA, Tierney LM Jr (eds.), *Current Medical Diagnosis and Treatment 2008*, 47th ed., McGraw Hill, New York, NY, pp. 757–784.

Hatem CJ, Kettyle WM (eds.). (2001) Nephrology section. In: *MKSAP12 — Medical Knowledge Self-Assessment Program*, American College of Physicians, Philadelphia, PA, pp. 32–38.

Narin RG (ed.). (1994) *Maxwell and Kleeman's Clinical Disorders of Fluid and Electrolyte Metabolism*, 5th ed., McGraw-Hill, New York, NY, pp. 45–127.

Turchin A, Seifter JL, Seely EW. (2003) Mind the gap. *N Engl J Med* **349**: 1465–1469.

Verbalis JG. (2007) The syndrome of inappropriate antidiuretic hormone secretion and other hypoosmolar disorders. In: Schrier RW (ed.), *Diseases of the Kidney and Urinary Tract*, 8th ed., Wolters Kluwer Health/Lippincott Williams & Wilkins, Philadelphia, PA, pp. 2214–2248.

5

Hypercalcemia, Hypocalcemia, and Hypomagnesemia

Peter G. Kerr

5.1 Introduction

Abnormalities of calcium and magnesium are often linked, particularly as hypomagnesemia may compound hypocalcemia. Each will be dealt with individually, with comments added about their interactions.

Most calcium exists in bone, with a small proportion in the extracellular fluid (ECF). This turns over daily with an absorption of about 4 mmol per day from the gut and an excretion of a similar amount in the urine. Calcium homeostasis is summarized in Fig. 5.1.

In terms of assessing the serum calcium level, two options are available: total calcium and ionized calcium. The extracellular distribution of calcium is shown in Fig. 5.2. Total calcium includes protein-bound calcium; as this predominantly involves albumin binding, it is traditional to correct the serum calcium for the albumin level. The calculation then provides a serum level, as if the serum albumin was 40 g/L. A typical calculation would be:

$$\text{serum Ca (mmol/L)} + (40 - \text{serum albumin [g/L]} \times 0.02)$$
$$= \text{corrected serum calcium (mmol/L)}$$

or

$$\text{serum Ca (mg/dL)} + (4.0 - \text{serum albumin [g/dL]} \times 0.8)$$
$$= \text{corrected serum calcium (mg/dL)}.$$

The alternative — ionized calcium — represents the non-protein-bound component and does not require correction for albumin levels.

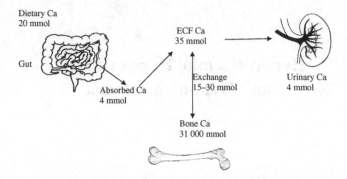

Fig. 5.1   Calcium homeostasis in human subject.

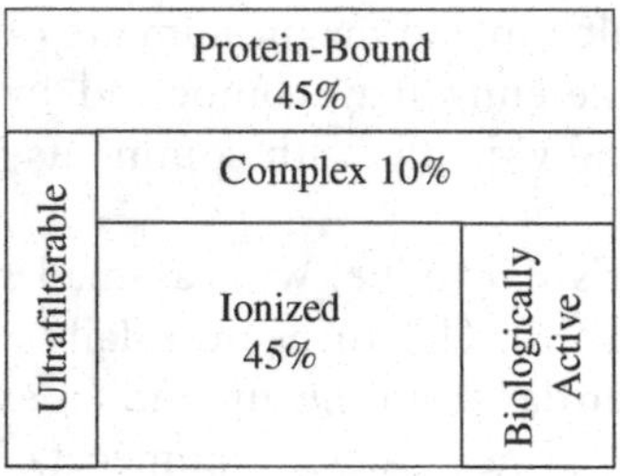

	Protein-Bound 45%	
Ultrafilterable	Complex 10%	Biologically Active
	Ionized 45%	

Fig. 5.2   Extracellular distribution of calcium.

5.2 Hypercalcemia

Elevated serum calcium may be due to a number of disease states or, commonly, iatrogenic causes. The common etiologies are outlined in Table 5.1.

5.2.1 *Clinical Manifestations*

- The level of serum calcium at which symptoms develop varies markedly. Generally, symptoms are evident at serum calcium > 3.0 mmol/L (12 mg/dL).
- "Stones, bones, moans, and groans" is a common memory aid for hypercalcemia (see below).
- Patients are often seemingly depressed and may have nonspecific aches and pains, especially abdominal pain. Bone pain may be a feature.

Table 5.1   Causes of hypercalcemia.

Disease states
   Primary hyperparathyroidism
   Malignancy (especially metastatic bone disease)
   Granulomatous disease (especially sarcoidosis)
   Immobilization
   Other (endocrinopathies, familial hypercalcemia)

Iatrogenic causes
   Excess administration of vitamin D, calcium, or parathyroid hormone
   Other drugs (lithium, thiazides, aminophylline)
   Milk-alkali syndrome

- Mental functioning is slowed, and fatigue and muscle weakness are common.
- Constipation is very common.
- Nausea, vomiting, and development of peptic ulceration may occur.
- Polyuria and polydipsia are also common, and volume depletion with acute renal impairment may occur.
- Renal calculi and nephrocalcinosis are common with prolonged hypercalcemia.

5.2.2 *Management — General Principles*

- Asymptomatic, mild hypercalcemia may not require specific therapy.
- Generally, when the calcium level exceeds 3.0 mmol/L, treatment is indicated.
- Treat the underlying condition where and when possible.

5.2.3 *Management of Acute, Symptomatic Hypercalcemia*

- Intravenous normal saline to establish a diuresis (except in patients with established acute or chronic renal failure) — aim upwards of 5 L of urine per day.
- Frusemide (but not thiazides) may be used in patients with renal or cardiac dysfunction.
- Bisphosphonates assist by inhibiting osteoclast function, and their effect is maintained for at least some weeks. Most commonly, pamidronate intravenously at a single dose of 30–90 mg is used.

- Calcitonin only has a brief action and is not often used alone.
- Glucocorticoids are often effective, especially in hematological malignancies and granulomatous disease. The doses vary according to local protocols and disease states (e.g. prednisolone, 20–50 mg/day; dexamethasone, 4–16 mg/day).
- Hemodialysis or peritoneal dialysis with low calcium dialysate is particularly useful in patients with renal failure.
- Cinacalcet, a calcimimetic agent (typical starting dose, 30–60 mg/day) which rapidly drops the serum parathyroid hormone level, may be useful in patients with primary hyperparathyroidism.

5.3 Hypocalcemia

The effects of hypocalcaemia vary greatly, depending in part on the chronicity of the situation. The serum pH also influences the protein binding of calcium, with alkalosis (e.g. during hyperventilation) increasing the protein binding and diminishing the level of available calcium — hence, symptoms of hypocalcemia in this situation. The common etiologies are outlined in Table 5.2.

Table 5.2   Causes of Hypocalcemia.

Acute causes
  Neck surgery (e.g. radical neck dissection, thyroid surgery, parathyroid surgery), often, but not necessarily, with inadvertent parathyroid tissue removal or destruction
  Inadequate replacement of calcium (e.g. in post-parathyroid surgery)
  Drugs (bisphosphonates, calcimimetics, mithramycin, calcitonin, foscarnet, phenytoin)
  Citrate infusion (usually very-short-duration hypocalcemia)
  Excessive phosphate (tumor lysis, laxatives)
  Acute pancreatitis

Chronic causes
  Hypoparathyroidism (surgical, irradiation, gene defects, autoimmune, etc.)
  Parathormone resistance (pseudohypoparathyroidism and pseudopseudohypoparathyroidism)
  Hypomagnesemia
  Vitamin D deficiency
  Secondary hyperparathyroidism/Bone and mineral metabolic disorder of chronic kidney disease

Causes with no net change in calcium
  Hypoalbuminemic states (e.g. nephrotic syndrome)
  Hyperventilation

5.3.1 *Clinical Manifestations*

Acute changes in calcium are likely to produce the following symptoms:

- Neuromuscular irritability
- Tetany
- Seizures
- Paresthesia
- Respiratory distress
- Prolonged QT interval on electrocardiogram (ECG).

Severe hypocalcemia may precipitate acute respiratory arrest via tetany and laryngospasm.

Neuromuscular irritability may be demonstrated by:

- Chvostek's sign (a twitch of the facial muscles induced by tapping over the facial nerve at the angle of the jaw); or
- Trousseau's sign (carpal spasm induced by inflating a BP cuff above systolic for 3 min).

Neither sign is particularly reliable.

5.3.2 *Management*

- Acute, symptomatic hypocalcemia requires rapid treatment.
- A calcium salt should be infused intravenously, typically 100–200 mg elemental calcium over 5–10 min.
- Options include 10% calcium gluconate (90 mg elemental calcium per 10 mL) or 10% calcium chloride (360 mg elemental calcium per 10 mL); 10 mL of 10% calcium gluconate as a slow bolus is safe in most situations. An infusion of 10–20 mg/kg over the next 4–6 h may then be added, as required.
- The former is more commonly used, as it is less irritating to peripheral veins. However, calcium chloride is useful for administration post-parathyroidectomy via a central line when large quantities may be needed.
- If the clinical response is poor, administer 5–10 mmol intravenous magnesium chloride (usually available as 1 mmol/mL) or magnesium sulfate (usually available as 2 mmol/mL) over 5–10 min (see also Sec. 5.4.2).

Chronic hypocalcemia is usually managed with oral calcium supplementation, often with oral vitamin D. The form of the latter will depend on whether there is coexistent chronic renal failure, wherein 1,25 dihydroxyvitamin D (calcitriol) is usually used.

5.4 Hypomagnesemia

Hypomagnesemia represents the total body deficiency of magnesium, but, like potassium, only represents the severe end of the spectrum of magnesium deficiency. Magnesium is a predominantly intracellular ion, with only about 1% existing in the extracellular compartment. The common etiologies are outlined in Table 5.3.

5.4.1 *Clinical Manifestations*

- Frequently asymptomatic
- Cardiac arrhythmias (including ventricular ectopy, tachycardia, and fibrillation; prolonged QT interval and torsades de pointes on ECG).
- Neuromuscular irritability (mimicking hypocalcemia)
- Hypokalemia
- Hypocalcemia

The neuromuscular irritability is often due to combined hypomagnesemia and hypocalcemia. Attempts to treat the hypocalcemia may prove difficult until the magnesium is also replaced. Hypokalemia

Table 5.3   Causes of hypomagnesemia.

Extrarenal
    Nutritional (chronic alcoholism, parenteral nutrition, refeeding
      syndrome)
    Intestinal malabsorption (inflammatory bowel disease, coeliac disease, etc.)
    Chronic diarrhea
    Cutaneous (severe burns)
    Redistribution (especially post-parathyroidectomy)

Renal
    Polyuria
    Diuretics (especially loop diuretics)
    Hypercalcemia
    Tubular nephrotoxins (cisplatin, amphotericin B, aminoglycosides,
      calcineurin inhibitors such as cyclosporin and tacrolimus)
    Familial
    Bartter/Gitelman syndromes

---

and hypomagnesemia may coexist, especially in patients receiving diuretics. As with hypocalcemia, hypokalemia in the presence of hypomagnesemia may be resistant to treatment unless the magnesium is concomitantly treated.

5.4.2 *Management*

- Management in acute situations (e.g. seizure activity, tetany, arrhythmias) is required.
- Intravenous magnesium may be replaced using (a) 2.465 g/5 mL $MgSO_4 \cdot 7H_2O$, which provides 2 mmol (4 mEq) of ionic magnesium per mL; or (b) 480 mg/5 mL $MgCl_2 \cdot 6H_2O$, which provides 1 mmol (2 mEq) of ionic magnesium per mL.
- Administering 2–4 mmol of elemental magnesium in 5% dextrose is recommended over 10–30 min, and may be repeated every 6 h.
- Alternatively, an infusion of 20 mmol (40 mEq) may be administered over 3–4 hours diluted in 5% dextrose.

Oral replacement salts of magnesium are readily available for less acute situations, and are dosed according to the response.

Suggested Reading

Brenner BM. (2008) Chapter 16: Disorders of calcium, magnesium and phosphate balance. In: *Brenner & Rector's The Kidney*, 8th ed., Saunders Elsevier, Philadelphia, pp. 588–611.

Schrier RW. (2002) Chapter 6: Disorders of calcium, phosphorus, vitamin D, and parathyroid activity. Chapter 7: Normal and abnormal magnesium metabolism. In: *Renal and Electrolyte Disorders*, 6th ed., Lippinicott, Williams & Wilkins, Philadelphia, pp. 241–348.

6

Acute Renal Failure

Kar Neng Lai

6.1 Definition

Acute renal failure (ARF) is characterized by an abrupt and sustained decline in the glomerular filtration rate (GFR) leading to uremia. Biochemically, most studies define ARF as a serum creatinine of 180–270 µmol per L, or a twofold increase of baseline creatinine. Oliguria (urine output <15 mL/h) is a feature in many patients. Nonoliguric renal failure is seen in those with:

- nephrotoxic damage
- severe burns
- oliguric renal failure treated by aggressive management with fluids and diuretics.

A recent international, interdisciplinary consensus panel, the Acute Dialysis Quality Initiative (ADQI) group (www.adqi.net), has classified ARF or acute kidney injury (AKI) according to the change from baseline serum creatinine or urine output. The ADQI workgroup considered the definition of AKI to require the following features:

- ease of use and clinical applicability
- high sensitivity and specificity for different populations and research questions
- consideration of creatinine change from baseline
- implementation of classification for acute-on-chronic renal disease.

This group then formulated a multi-level classification system (RIFLE) defining three grades of increasing severity of AKI as risk (R), injury (I), and failure (F) as well as the two outcome variables of loss (L) and end-stage kidney disease (E) (Fig. 6.1).

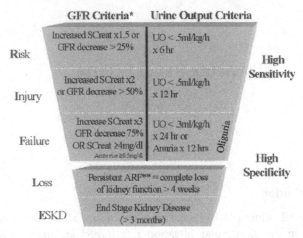

Fig. 6.1 Proposed classification scheme for acute renal failure (ARF). The classification system includes separate criteria for creatinine and urine output (UO). A patient can fulfill the criteria through changes in serum creatinine (SCreat) or changes in UO, or both. The criteria that lead to the worst possible classification should be used. Note that the F component of RIFLE (Risk of renal dysfunction, Injury to the kidney, Failure of kidney function, Loss of kidney function, and End-stage kidney disease) is present even if the increase in SCreat is under threefold, as long as the new SCreat is greater than 4.0 mg/dL (350 µmol/L) in the setting of an acute increase of at least 0.5 mg/dL (44 µmol/L); the designation RIFLE-F$_C$ should be used in this case to denote acute-on-chronic disease. Similarly, when the RIFLE-F classification is achieved by UO criteria, a designation of RIFLE-F$_O$ should be used to denote oliguria. The shape of the figure denotes the fact that most patients (high sensitivity) belong to the mild category, including some without actually having renal failure (less specificity). In contrast, at the bottom of the figure, the criteria are strict and therefore specific, but some patients will be missed. GFR: glomerular filtration rate. [From Bellomo R *et al. Crit Care* 2004; 8: R204–R212, used with permission.]

The two clinical outcomes in RIFLE criteria are separated to acknowledge the important adaptations which occur in end-stage renal disease that are not seen in patients with ARF. A unique feature of the RIFLE classification is that it provides for three grades of severity of renal dysfunction on the basis of a change in serum creatinine, reflecting changes in the GFR or in the duration and severity of decline in urine output from the baseline. The RIFLE criteria have the advantage of providing diagnostic definitions for the stage at which kidney injury can still be prevented (risk stratum), the stage when the kidney has already been damaged (injury), and the stage when renal failure is established (failure). One limitation of the RIFLE criteria is that it provides no insight into the pathophysiology of increased serum creatinine or oliguria, or both, despite the fact that different pathophysiologic mechanisms could have different outcomes. The RIFLE criteria have been tested in clinical practice and seem to be at least coherent with regard to the outcome of the patient in different settings of ARF, including sepsis and cardiac surgery.

Although the RIFLE criteria allow diversification in the definition of AKI, making it possible to identify more exactly than before the degree of renal injury, it is clear that other important variables describing the type of patient are not included. Suggested modifications include (a) the origin of the patient, (b) the most important causal factors that are responsible for AKI, and (c) the pre-existing kidney function.

6.2 Incidence and Prevalence

- Community-acquired ARF is present in 1% of all hospitalized patients; and hospital-acquired ARF, in nearly 5% of hospitalized patients.
- Around 15% of critically ill patients have ARF.
- The incidence has not decreased in the last two decades.

6.3 Classification and Causes

The classification of ARF into prerenal, intrinsic renal, and postrenal forms (Table 6.1) is convenient for most purposes. Although this classification is helpful in formulating a diagnostic approach, it does not take into account the fact that ARF is often multifactorial. For example, in postsurgical ARF fluid depletion, systemic infection and nephrotoxic drugs may play a role and require specific treatment in addition to measures such as dialysis and nutrition. ARF may also complicate chronic renal failure.

Prerenal failure is predominantly due to acute circulatory failure or low systemic perfusion, and is characterized in the early stages by:

- a lack of structural damage
- retention of the ability to concentrate the urine
- rapid reversibility, provided the circulatory failure is corrected promptly and completely
- occasionally, maintenance of blood pressure within the normal range

Table 6.1   Common causes of acute renal failure (ARF).

Prerenal (ischemic)	
Extracellular volume depletion	Gastrointestinal loss, urinary loss, burns, third-space fluid loss
Intravascular volume loss	Sepsis, hemorrhage, hypoalbuminemia
Effective volume depletion from arterial underfilling	Heart failure, cardiac tamponade, massive pulmonary embolism, cardiac surgery, peripheral vasodilation
Renal (intrinsic)	
Ischemic acute tubular necrosis	Shock, trauma, sepsis, hypoxia
Nephrotoxic acute tubular necrosis	Antibiotics, analgesics, contrast media, heavy metal, solvents, paraproteins, paraquat, organophosphate
Glomerulonephritis	Acute diffuse proliferative or crescentic nephritis
Acute pyelonephritis	
Acute interstitial nephritis	Antibiotics, analgesics, leptospirosis, legionella, viral infections
Vasculitis	Polyarteritis and its variants
Intratubular obstruction	Myeloma (Bence Jones protein), urate, tumor lysis syndrome, rhabdomyolysis
Coagulopathies	Acute cortical necrosis, hemolytic-uremic syndrome, thrombotic thrombocytopenic purpura, postpartum renal failure, snake bite
Intrarenal hemodynamic changes	Afferent arteriolar vasoconstriction: nonsteroidal anti-inflammatory drugs, cyclooxygenase-2 inhibitors, cyclosporine, tacrolimus
	Efferent arteriolar vasodilatation: angiotensin-converting enzyme inhibitors (ACEIs), angiotensin receptor blockers (ARBs)
Postrenal	
Renal tract obstruction	Stones, tumor (prostatic or pelvic), prostatic hypertrophy, periureteric fibrosis, bladder dysfunction, urethral stricture, papillary necrosis, retroperitoneal lymphoma, post-irradiation
Miscellaneous	
Metabolic disorder	Hypercalcemia, hepatorenal syndrome, tumor lysis syndrome
Major vessel occlusion	Renal artery thrombosis, renal vein thrombosis

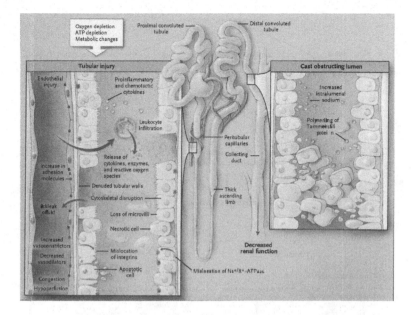

Fig. 6.2 Mechanism of ischemic acute tubular necrosis. Tubular injury is a direct consequence of metabolic pathways activated by ischemia, but is potentiated by inflammation and microvascular compromise. The inset shows shedding of epithelial cells and denudation of the basement membrane in the proximal tubule, with backleak of filtrate (inset, left) and obstruction by sloughed cells in the distal tubule (inset, right). [From Abuelo JG. *N Engl J Med* 2007; 357: 797–805, used with permission.]

Failure to restore adequate renal blood flow leads to structural changes referred to as acute tubular necrosis (ATN). ATN can also be caused by a wide variety of drugs and other nephrotoxins. Tubular damage appears to be central to both forms. The mechanism of ATN is summarized in Fig. 6.2, and the pathophysiological events are depicted in Fig. 6.3.

6.4 Diagnosis

In hospital practice, ARF is often diagnosed during the treatment of other medical illnesses, either on the basis of rising plasma creatinine or falling urine output. When the diagnostic clue is a rise in plasma creatinine, a careful examination of the clinical and therapeutic situation over the preceding few days will usually uncover the causes of renal failure

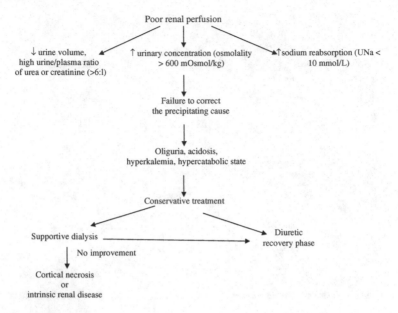

Fig. 6.3 A simplified flow diagram of the pathophysiologic events in prerenal ARF.

(e.g. infection, fluid depletion, or the use of nephrotoxic drugs), all of which can usually be treated appropriately. Such patients may not be oliguric and may often be managed without dialysis. Patients presenting with a sudden onset of oliguria or recognition of oliguria in hospital, however, usually have a serious prerenal cause of renal failure — most commonly septicemia, acute cardiac failure, serious volume depletion, or a combination of these. Obstructive etiology should be excluded in elder male patients. Although the causes are often clearly apparent, renal failure may ensue if they cannot be promptly controlled.

In patients presenting with renal failure outside hospital practice, the first task is to distinguish between the large majority of patients with ATN and those with less common conditions (e.g. acute nephritis, vasculitis, multiple myeloma, drug-induced renal failure, or urinary tract obstruction) for whom active intervention may be successful in halting the progress of the disease. The most important distinguishing features are revealed by:

- history (including predisposing factors (Table 6.2), recent drug intake (Table 6.3), and drug abuse (Table 6.4))

Table 6.2   Predisposing factors of ARF.

Metabolic
    Old age
    Diabetes mellitus
    Hypercalcemia
    Chronic renal failure

Vascular
    Atherosclerosis
    Malignant or accelerated hypertension
    Renal artery stensois
    Hepatorenal syndrome

Medication
    Nonsteroidal anti-inflammatory drugs
    Cyclosporine or tacrolimus
    ACEIs and ARBs
    Cyclooxygenase-2 inhibitors
    Contrast agents

Circulatory
    Sepsis
    Major trauma or burns
    Dehydration

Table 6.3   Drugs causing ARF.

Acute interstitial nephritis (often with tubular damage)
    Allopurinol
    Antivirals (indinavir, atazanavir, adefovir, tenofovir, abacavir)
    Cephalosporins
    Cimetidine
    Phenytoin
    Diuretics
    Non-steroidal anti-inflammatory drugs
    Penicillins
    Proton pump inhibitor
    Rifampicin
    Sulphinpyrazone
    Sulphonamides

Tubular necrosis
    Aminoglycosides
    Amphotericin B

(Continued)

Table 6.3 (*Continued*)

Cephalosporins
Cisplatin
Co-trimoxazole
Cyclosporine
Lithium
Methyldopa
Radiographic contrast media

Obstructive uropathy
Papillary necrosis
   Analgesics
   Antivirals (indinavir)

Urate obstruction
   Cytotoxic drugs

Intratubular crystal obstruction
   Sulphonamides (sulphadiazine)
   Antivirals (acyclovir, indinavir)

Periureteric fibrosis
   Methysergide

Renal vasculitis
   Amphetamines
   Penicillins
   Sulphonamides

Intrarenal hemodynamic changes
Afferent arteriolar vasoconstriction
   Non-steroidal anti-inflammatory drugs, cyclooxygenase-2
    inhibitors, cyclosporine, tacrolimus

Efferent arteriolar vasoconstriction
   ACEIs and ARBs

Hypercatabolism
   Tetracyclines

- physical examination
- urine examination for red blood cells, white blood cells, cast, crystals, and myoglobin
- urine biochemistry and osmolality (Table 6.5)
- plain radiograph of the kidneys and renal ultrasound to detect kidney sizes and exclude obstructive uropathy.

Table 6.4   Renal failure due to drug abuse.

Cocaine
  Rhabdomolysis, malignant arteriosclerosis

Heroin
  IgM mesangioproliferative glomerulonephritis, focal glomerulosclerosis,
  diffuse sclerosis

Glue sniffing
  Acute tubular necrosis

Hydrocarbon
  Acute tubular toxicity

Methylenedioxymethamphetamine (Ecstasy)
  Rhabdomyolysis, accelerated hypertension

6.4.1 *Biomarkers for Early ARF*

Clinically available markers now employed in defining ARF include plasma blood urea nitrogen and creatinine, urine output, and urinary clearance of other markers of tubular injury. Most of these markers, although easily available and clinically relevant, may not be a true reflection of renal function in critically ill patients. As the GFR falls, tubular secretion of creatinine increases, leading to a relatively smaller rise in plasma creatinine. Plasma creatinine levels can thus underestimate the degree of renal impairment or overestimate the GFR during the evolution of ARF. Unlike in the steady renal state, GFR estimates based on plasma creatinine values are not accurate and lead to falsely high GFR estimations in ARF.

Patients with oliguric ARF have a poorer prognosis compared to patients with nonoliguric ARF. Severe renal impairment can occur despite adequate or even excess urine output. In a critically ill but volume-repleted and hemodynamically stable patient, low urine output can serve as a sensitive clinical marker for the development of ARF and has a good positive predictive value. Due to interventions in the intensive care unit (ICU), the negative predictive value of urine output is rather poor.

Hence, a quest for new ARF biomarkers for detecting early tubular injury is an important area of clinical research. Serum and urine biomarkers such as cystatin C, neutrophil gelatinase-associated lipocalin (NGAL), interleukin-18, and kidney injury molecule-1 (KIM-1) may be of potential clinical significance, and are summarized in Table 6.6.

Table 6.5 Urine diagnostic indices in ARF.

	Urine (Na) (mmol/L)	Urine osmolality (mOsm/kg)	Urine/Plasma creatinine	Fractional excretion Na (%)	Urine sediment
Prerenal oliguria	<20	>450	>40	<1	Hyaline cast
ATN	>40	<350	<20	>3	Heme granular casts
Obstruction	>40	<350	<20	>3	Inactive
Acute glomerulonephritis	<20	>400	>40	<1	RBCs, RBC casts, active
Acute interstitial nephritis	>40	<350	<20	>3	RBCs, WBCs, eosinophils (Hansel's secretion stain)

Note: ATN: acute tubular necrosis; RBCs: red blood cells; WBCs: white blood cells.

Table 6.6 Promising biomarkers for ARF in different clinical settings.

Biomarker	Sample source	Kidney transplant	Contrast nephropathy	Sepsis	Cardiac surgery	Commercial assay
Cystatin C	Plasma	Intermediate	Intermediate	Intermediate	Intermediate	Dade Behring
NGAL	Plasma	Early	Early	Early	Early	AntibodyShop
NGAL	Urine	Early	Early	Early	Early	AntibodyShop
IL-18	Urine	Intermediate	Absent	Intermediate	Intermediate	Medical and Biological Laboratories
KIM-1	Urine	Not studied	Not studied	Not studied	Intermediate	None

Theoretically, serial measurement of a biomarker could help clinicians detect early disease and follow the response to treatment once the disease is advanced. Further research studying these biomarkers of prognosticating value in patients with ARF will be of importance.

6.5 Management

Treatment of ARF depends on a rapid and accurate diagnosis. If an underlying cause is found, the treatment is usually obvious, such as stopping the hemorrhage, correcting the sepsis, removing the drugs responsible for acute interstitial nephritis, or relieving the obstruction in postrenal ARF. If renal impairment is advanced, however, it may be necessary to treat the metabolic, fluid, and electrolyte disturbances before diagnostic procedures can be arranged. The discussion below is confined to the general treatment of prerenal, postrenal, and intrinsic ARF, and the management of the sequelae which are common to all forms of renal failure. Management of specific forms of ARF, including contrast-related nephropathy, hepatorenal syndrome, rhabdomyolysis, and ARF in bone marrow transplant, is discussed in Chapter 9.

6.5.1 *Prerenal ARF*

6.5.1.1 *True Volume Depletion or Hypovolemia*

Immediate treatment is directed toward replenishing volume deficits.

- For volume deficits due to hemorrhage, administer packed red blood cells and beware of hyperkalemia associated with stored blood.
- For volume deficits not predominantly due to hemorrhage, administer 0.9% normal saline (NS) intravenously.
- The amount of intravenous fluid and the rapidity of fluid administration depend on the clinical situation.
- Bolus (500–1000 mL over 60 min) can be given to a stable young patient; a smaller amount (250–500 mL) should be given to elderly patients or those with cardiopulmonary diseases.
- No continuous infusion should be ordered.
- Fluid replacement should be continued until euvolemia is achieved, as judged by blood pressure, pulse, skin turgor, jugular venous pressure, and urine output.

- For patients who require vigorous resuscitation, aggressive fluid replacement should be given preferably under the monitoring system of either a central venous catheter (reading not >5 cm of water for central venous pressure) or a Swan–Ganz catheter (reading not >15 cm of water for pulmonary artery wedge pressure).
- A Swan–Ganz catheter is indicated in the presence of pulmonary disease, valvular heart disease, or an unstable cardiovascular system.
- Electrolyte deficits (potassium in the first week, phosphate and magnesium thereafter) must be monitored and replaced if necessary.

6.5.1.2 *Effective Volume Depletion from Arterial Underfilling*

ARF in this setting is a secondary problem related to primary cardiac or liver diseases. The therapeutic approach is directed at treating the underlying cause. Supportive treatment is recommended if the primary disease fails to respond immediately.

Heart failure

- Diuretics in combination with digitalis to improve cardiac output
- Reduced cardiac loading with nitrates, hydralazine, ACEIs, or ARBs
- Hemofiltration or ultrafiltration if heart failure is drug-resistant

Liver disease (see also Chapter 9)

- Sodium restriction
- Aldosterone antagonist (monitor the serum potassium)
- Cautious loop diuretic
- Large-volume paracentesis with albumin infusion in severe ascites
- Transjugular intrahepatic portosystemic stent shunt
- Liver transplantation

6.5.2 *Postrenal ARF*

- Following a diagnosis of obstructive uropathy — delineation of the outflow tract by antegrade urography, retrograde urography, ureterogram, cystoscopy, or computed tomography (CT) scanning to demonstrate the site of obstruction.

- Foley catheter drainage for acute obstruction secondary to prostatic hypertrophy and bladder outlet obstruction.
- Urological consultation for ureteral drainage or stent as indicated.
- Radiological consultation for antegrade drainage if ureteral drainage or stent fails.

6.5.3 Intrinsic Renal ARF

6.5.3.1 *Primary Renal Diseases: Glomerulonephritis and Vasculitis*

- Immunological markers, including complements, may be helpful in making the diagnosis.
- Renal biopsy is frequently required for establishing a definitive diagnosis before the initiation of specific treatment such as immunosuppression or plasma exchange.

6.5.3.2 *Acute Interstitial Nephritis*

- Remove the agent that has been identified as the cause of acute interstitial nephritis.
- To speed up the recovery, one may consider a high-dose, short-term prednisolone treatment (1 mg/kg/day for 1–2 weeks with diminishing doses for a further 2–3 weeks) in patients with moderate to severe renal impairment or in whom renal impairment has been present for weeks (though not evidence-based). A confirmatory renal biopsy should be performed prior to steroid treatment. The typical features are interstitial eosinophilic infiltrate and tubular necrosis with normal glomeruli.

6.5.4 Supportive Therapy for All Forms of Established ARF

6.5.4.1 *Fluid Balance*

- Daily (or more frequent) clinical assessment of extracellular fluid volume status, fluid balance measurements, and body weight is recorded.
- If clinically euvolemic, daily fluid replacement is determined by measured losses and 500 mL for insensible losses.
- Dietary sodium restriction is prescribed.
- Hyponatremia may signify excessive free water administration.

6.5.4.2 *Hyperkalemia*

- Hyperkalemia is life-threatening and is a treatment priority if the serum potassium exceeds 7 mmol/L, particularly when electrocardiogram (ECG) changes are present.
- Typical ECG findings reveal widening of the QRS complex, reduction of atrial activity, and high T wave peaks. A further rise in serum potassium may cause ventricular tachycardia or fibrillation. Continuous cardiac monitoring is needed and cardiac resuscitation equipment should be available.
- Care should be taken, however, not to correct hyperkalemia too quickly if the patient is receiving digitalis preparation.
- Treatment for hyperkalemia is discussed in Chapter 3. Dialysis should be started as soon as possible if conservative management fails to correct the hyperkalemia and the patient remains oliguric.

6.5.4.3 *Fever*

- Febrile patients should have regular chest radiographs and cultures of urine, sputum, and other sites (e.g. wound drainage); frequent inspection of indwelling catheters; and frequent blood cultures.
- Not infrequently, fever is due to opportunistic infections from the respiratory or gastrointestinal tract.
- Broad-spectrum antibiotics may be needed if the patient develops symptoms of bacteremia/septicemia while pending for culture report.
- Unexplained fever, particularly when accompanied by toxic manifestations (e.g. hypotensive episodes, disorientation), strongly suggests an undetected abscess which requires drainage.
- Abdominal ultrasound and CT scanning are invaluable in localizing such collections before needle aspiration or surgical drainage, which should not be delayed as persistent sepsis prevents resolution of ATN.

6.5.4.4 *Drug Dosage*

- Drug dosages must be adjusted based on the measured or best estimate of creatinine clearance.
- Certain medications need dosage adjusted if the patient is receiving dialysis: no drug should be prescribed without knowing the effect of renal failure on its dose requirements.

- Commonly used drugs, such as narcotic analgesics and sedatives, will accumulate in patients with ARF and should therefore not be added to the drug list simply for convenience.
- Adequate drug levels (especially antibiotics) must be achieved to produce the required therapeutic effect, and the appropriate dose interval must be allowed to ensure that persistently high levels do not cause drug toxicity (guidelines given in Chapters 31 and 32).

6.5.4.5 Nutrition

- ARF is a hypercatabolic state, often with negative protein balance.
- Other contributory factors to hypercatabolism include sepsis, surgery, multi-organ failure, uremia, and acidosis: these need to be effectively treated before the catabolic process is controlled.
- In the hypercatabolic state, nutritional support is needed to prevent a negative protein balance.
- Provision of adequate calories (25–30 kcal/kg/day and 1 g/kg/day of protein) will reduce protein breakdown, reduce mortality, and improve the rate of recovery.
- Enteral feeding is the preferred method of nutritional support.
- Parenteral nutrition may be required if the patient has severe gastrointestinal upset or abdominal operation. Catheter-induced sepsis, hyperglycemia, hepatic derangement, and hyperkalemia are recognized risks of parenteral nutrition.
- Dialysis support is needed if the patient remains oliguric despite a large volume of hyperalimentation supplement (>2 L/day).

6.5.4.6 Dialysis

- The indications for acute dialysis are discussed in Chapter 12, and the hemofiltration treatment is discussed in Chapter 16.
- Peritoneal dialysis is less frequently used in ARF; patients with a low catabolic rate and high urine output can be managed by peritoneal dialysis.
- In patients who are hemodynamically stable, continuous renal replacement therapy offers no advantage over intermittent renal replacement therapy with respect to patient outcome.
- The advantages and limitations of continuous renal replacement therapy (hemofiltration or hemodiafiltration) are outlined in Table 6.7.

Table 6.7 Continuous renal replacement therapy versus intermittent renal replacement therapy.

Advantages
  Better hemodynamic stability
  Controlled fluid removal and electrolyte adjustment
  Facilitates parenteral hyperalimentation
  Better acid-base balance

Limitations
  Continuous anticoagulation
  Immobilization and risk of hydrostatic pneumonia
  Large lactate load — bad for patients with hepatic impairment

---

6.6 Prevention and What to Avoid

6.6.1 *Protection of Renal Perfusion*

The most important steps in preventing prerenal ARF and ATN are the avoidance of hypotension and renal ischemia as well as the rapid correction of hypovolemia. It is often possible to interrupt the chain of events, leading to tubular damage.

Patients undergoing major surgery or suffering from severe trauma are at risk of ARF. This can often be avoided by careful planning to preserve renal perfusion and urine output. A good example of the benefits of planning and an aggressive approach to resuscitation in patients with posttraumatic renal failure is the treatment of crush syndrome following natural disasters. Rapid evacuation of such patients, restoration of fluid volume with central pressure measurements, careful monitoring of blood and urine biochemistry as well as blood gases, and administration of bicarbonate and mannitol according to a set protocol can prevent ARF in many patients. The predisposing factors outlined in Table 6.2 (especially nephrotoxic drugs) should be avoided.

Another commonly avoidable cause of reduced renal perfusion and renal failure is dehydration due to the administration of potent diuretics to patients with unrecognized volume depletion and oliguria. In patients with septicemia, early treatment of the infection and volume expansion will often prevent ATN.

6.6.2 *Therapy with No Proven Benefit in ATN or Established Renal Failure*

- High-dose diuretics is not associated with improved patient outcome in ARF, despite the conversion from oliguric to nonoliguric renal failure in a proportion of patients.

- No evidence suggests that renal-dose dopamine (1–3 μg/kg/min) alters the patient outcome, despite temporary natriuresis and increased urine output.
- Intravenous fluid challenge.

6.7 Recovery from Acute Tubular Necrosis

Failure to recover from ATN within 2–3 weeks is usually evidence of an underlying problem, with persistent or recurrent infection being the most common one. If no further improvement occurs after 4–6 weeks, cortical necrosis with a permanent loss of glomerular function should be considered.

Improvement in serum biochemistry is often delayed for up to 1 week after an increase in urine output is noted. This may be followed by marked diuresis, which may be due to fluid retention during the oliguric phase of renal failure, or failure of the damaged tubules to conserve sodium and water. Intravenous fluid and electrolyte therapy may be required to prevent volume depletion, hypokalemia, and hypomagnesemia. Hypercalcemia is common in the recovery phase of severe, traumatic renal failure and renal failure associated with myoglobinuria. Dialysis should be continued until there is a spontaneous drop in creatinine and urea levels, and careful fluid management continued until urine volumes have returned to normal values and the risk of fluid and electrolyte depletion is no longer present.

6.8 Prognosis

The mortality in patients with ATN requiring dialysis depends on the cause of renal failure and the incidence of complications. Patients with nonoliguric ARF have a lower mortality (10%–40%), in part because they have a less severe underlying disease or have been treated more promptly or more aggressively. A particularly high mortality (80%–90%) is found in older patients and those with:

- multiple trauma
- severe burns
- severe pancreatitis
- hepatorenal syndrome
- intra-abdominal sepsis
- pre-existing cardiovascular disease
- toxins such as paraquat

6.9 Future Novel Treatments

It is unlikely that targeting events which occur late in ARF or even a single pathway will be effective. Novel compounds have been tested in selected clinical settings complicated by ARF; these include antiapoptotic caspase inhibitors, antiseptic activated protein C, and anti-inflammatory adenosine receptor agonists. New strategies targeting multiple pathways or combination therapy are attractive options that require stringent scrutiny by well-designed clinical trials.

Suggested Reading

Abuelo JG. (2007) Normotensive ischemic acute renal failure. *N Engl J Med* 357:797–805.

Devarajan P. (2007) Emerging markers of acute kidney injury. *Contrib Nephrol* 156:203–212.

Jo SK, Rosner MH, Okusa MD. (2007) Pharmacologic treatment of acute renal injury: why drugs haven't worked and what is on the horizon? *Clin J Am Soc Nephrol* 2:356–365.

Kellum J, Leblanc M, Venkataraman R. (2007) Acute renal failure. *Am Fam Physician* 76:418–422.

Kellum J, Venkataraman R. (2007) Defining acute renal failure: the RIFLE criteria. *J Intensive Care Med* 22:187–193.

Rabindranath K, Adams J, Macleod AM, Muirhead N. (2007) Intermittent versus continuous renal replacement therapy for acute renal failure in adults. *Cochrane Database Syst Rev* 3:CD003773.

Van Biesen W, Vanholder R, Lameire N. (2006) Defining acute renal failure: RIFLE and beyond. *Clin J Am Soc Nephrol* 1:1314–1319.

7

Selected Glomerular Disorders

Kar Neng Lai

This chapter discusses principally seven important primary or secondary glomerulopathic entities. The pathophysiological events are different for each one, and treatment regimes are targeted to prevent the development of chronic renal failure.

7.1 Minimal Change Nephropathy (MCN)

- Otherwise known as lipoid nephrosis, MCN is most often seen in children, but is also responsible for 15% of adult cases of idiopathic nephrotic syndrome.
- It presents as nephrotic syndrome; hematuria or acute renal impairment is rare.
- T-cell-related mechanisms are suggested with a lymphokine called glomerular permeability factor.
- Raised CD8 lymphocytes and reduced CD4 lymphocytes are observed.
- Glomerular permselectivity is predominantly charge-selective.
- Beware of secondary MCN (Table 7.1).

7.1.1 Consequences of Proteinuria Complicating Nephrotic Syndrome

- Sodium retention due to activation of the renin-angiotensin-aldosterone system by hypovolemia and decreased sensitivity to atrial natriuretic peptide.
- Hypercoagulable state due to (a) hemoconcentration and hyperviscosity, (b) increased platelet aggregation secondary to thrombocytosis and release of β-thromboglobulin, (c) increased factor V and VII production with urinary loss of protein S, (d) reduction of antithrombin III, and (e) hypertriglyceridemia.

109

Table 7.1 Secondary MCN with identifiable extraglomerular disease process.

Neoplasia
Hodgkin's lymphoma
Non-Hodgkin's lymphoma
Drugs
Daunomycin
Interferons
Lithium
Non-steroidal anti-inflammatory agents
Infections
Atopy

- Hyperlipidemia.
- Increased susceptibility to infection.
- Urinary loss of thyroid-binding globulin, T3, and T4, with normal free T4 and thyroid-stimulating hormone (TSH).
- Reduced serum iron and copper due to loss of binding proteins.
- Increased serum level and toxicity of protein-bound drug.

7.1.2 Treatment

7.1.2.1 First Attack

- The first line of therapy for MCN is steroids.
- Since MCN is exquisitely responsive to steroid treatment, the disappearance of proteinuria in children is frequently considered diagnostic of MCN.
- Treatment recommendation for the first attack of MCN in children is 2 mg/kg/day of prednisone/prednisolone (not exceeding 60 mg/day) for 6–8 weeks.
- Due to the lower incidence of complete remission and slower response to therapy, the duration of treatment in adults can be extended up to 16 weeks and a dose of 1 mg/kg/day is commonly used in adults.
- Complete remission occurs within 8 weeks in 93% of children with MCN; whereas in adults, complete remission is achieved only in 51%–76% of patients within 8 weeks and 76%–96% within 16 weeks.

7.1.2.2 Steroid-Resistant and Frequently Relapsing MCN

Frequent relapse

- Treatment by alkylating agents such as cyclophosphamide (2 mg/kg/day) or chlorambucil (0.15 mg/kg/day) with tapering alternate-day prednisone for 8 weeks achieves a remission rate of 63% at 10 years.
- Side-effects of cyclophosphamide include bone marrow suppression, increased infection, hemorrhagic cystitis, bladder cancer, infertility, and secondary malignancy.
- Chlorambucil may have a higher risk of malignancy.

Steroid-dependent MCN

- The treatment of choice is cyclophosphamide for 8 weeks or cyclosporine (6 mg/kg/day for children and 5 mg/kg/day for adults) for 6–12 months.

Steroid-resistant MCN

- Cyclosporine for 6 months with gradual tapering by 25% every 2 months until complete discontinuation is recommended.
- A 60% response rate has been reported.
- Cyclosporine A is safer than repeated courses of cyclophosphamide.

Other therapies

- The use of mycophenolate mofetil (MMF) (1–2 g/day) is limited in experience, but is well tolerated in patients.
- Levamisole (2.5 mg/kg/alternate day) is used in children with a high relapse rate when discontinued.

7.2 Idiopathic Membranous Nephropathy

- This is one of the most common causes of nephrotic syndrome, with peak incidence in the fourth-to-sixth decade of one's life.
- It has a variable natural history, with up to 30% of patients having spontaneous complete remission of proteinuria usually within the first 2 years of presentation, while the remaining 70% will either have persistent proteinuria or slow progression to end-stage renal disease.

- Once the diagnosis is made, the management of symptoms related to proteinuria and hypertension is mandated in almost all patients.
- Symptomatic treatment consisting of angiotensin receptor blockers (ARBs) or angiotensin-converting enzyme inhibitors (ACEIs) is preferred for controlling proteinuria and hypertension, and statins for hyperlipidemia.
- Identification of clinical parameters that bear poor prognostic outcome is important for selecting patients to receive appropriate immunosuppressive therapy and for avoiding overtreatment that may lead to undesirable side-effects.
- Poor prognostic parameters include male gender, increasing age, nephrotic-range proteinuria, the ratio of IgG to α-1-microglobulin excretion in urine, focal segmental glomerulosclerosis, and impaired renal function at presentation.
- It is logical to adopt a more aggressive approach in immunosuppressive therapy for those patients with medium to high risk, while a symptomatic approach is appropriate for those with low risk of renal progression.
- Beware of secondary membranous nephropathy (Table 7.2).

Table 7.2   Secondary membranous nephropathy.

Neoplasia
   Solid tumors (lung, colon, breast, kidney, stomach)
   Hodgkin's lymphoma
   Non-Hodgkin's lymphoma

Infections
   Hepatitis B and C
   Malaria
   Syphilis or leprosy
   Schistosomiasis

Multi-system disease
   Systemic lupus enythematosus
   Rheumatoid arthritis
   Autoimmune thyroiditis
   Dermatitis herpetiformis
   Sarcoidosis

Drugs and toxins
   Captopril
   Gold
   D-penicillamine
   Non-steroidal anti-inflammatory agents

7.2.1 Treatment

The treatment algorithm is outlined in Fig. 7.1. Most reported treatment regimes improve proteinuria, but only cytotoxic agents improve renal survival in limited randomized controlled trials.

7.2.1.1 Cytotoxic Agents

- Alternating monthly steroids and alkylating agents for 6 months. Steroid: 1 mg/kg/day (up to 60 mg/day) for the month; alkylating agents: either chlorambucil (0.15 mg/kg/day) or cyclophosphamide (2 mg/kg/day). With declining renal function, treatment may be continued up to 1 year.

7.2.1.2 Calcineurin Inhibitor

- Cyclosporine (5 mg/kg/day) or tacrolimus (0.05/mg/day) for adults for up to 12 months. There is a high relapse rate with discontinuation of therapy.

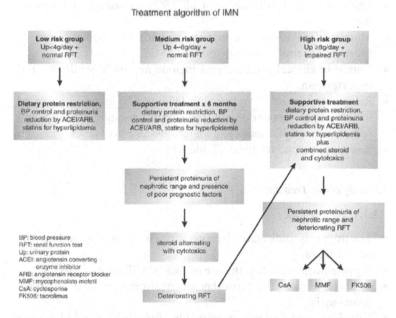

Fig. 7.1 Treatment algorithm for idiopathic membranous nephropathy (IMN). ACEI, angiotensin-converting enzyme inhibitor; ARB, angiotensin receptor blocker; BP, blood pressure; CsA, cyclosporine; FK506, tacrolimus; MMF, mycophenolate mofetil; RFT, renal function test; Up, urinary protein. [From Lai KN. *Kidney Int* 2007; 71: 841–843, used with permission.]

7.2.1.3 Mycophenolate Mofetil

- Dosage of 0.5–2 g/day — limited experience, but well tolerated.

7.2.1.4 Rituximab

- A monoclonal anti-CD20 antibody, with success in isolated case reports.

7.3 Focal Segmental Glomerulosclerosis (FSGS)

- This is not a disease, but rather a lesion with no definite prognostic value.
- It has five histological variants: FSGS "not otherwise specified" (classic FSGS), perihilar variant, cellular variant, tip variant, and collapsing variant.
- The only predictive prognostic element is the response of proteinuria to treatment, irrespective of histology.
- The common denominator of all FSGS variants is a podocyte disease.
- Mutations of various structural proteins in podocyte lead to sporadic or familial steroid-resistant FSGS.
- Common clinical presentations include nephrotic syndrome and hypertension.
- Relapse of nephrotic syndrome and glomerular lesions is observed in 30% of patients undergoing renal transplantation for FSGS, and recurrence of FSGS leads to allograft loss in 5% of cases.
- Beware of secondary FSGS (Table 7.3).

7.3.1 Specific Treatment

7.3.1.1 First Attack

- Treatment is indicated if proteinuria is persistent and in the nephrotic range.
- If proteinuria < 2 g/day, the use of ACEIs/ARBs is preferred.
- Steroids remain the mainstay of treatment in case of heavy proteinuria.
- Full-dose prednisolone (1 mg/kg/day for adult) should be given for 8–12 weeks to achieve the highest remission rate (~30%).
- In case of even partial remission, a slow tapering dose over months is preferred to avoid a rebound effect.

Table 7.3   Secondary FSGS.

Reduced nephron number
  Morbid obesity
  Reflux nephropathy
  Renal dysplasia
  Renovascular disease
  Single kidney (congenital or acquired)

Glomerular disease and obsolescence
  Alport's syndrome
  Diabetic nephropathy
  Heroin-associated nephropathy
  HIV-associated nephropathy
  Sickle cell disease

Alkylating agents

- Either cyclophosphamide or chlorambucil can be used.
- It is to be considered in patients who are steroid-dependent or have experienced multiple relapses.
- It may yield a long-lasting remission.
- Steroid resistance is highly predictive of resistance to alkylating agents in FSGS.

Cyclosporin A

- It is good as a steroid-sparing agent in steroid-dependent FSGS.
- Low-dose cyclosporin (5 mg/kg/day) with steroid has been tried in steroid-resistant FSGS with variable results.
- In case of cyclosporin dependency, the dose should be tapered to avoid calcineurin inhibitor-related nephrotoxicity.

Tacrolimus and MMF

- Experience is limited to case reports or non-randomized clinical trials with extremely small patient samples.

7.4 IgA Nephropathy (IgAN)

- IgAN is a disease caused by abnormal glycosylation of the IgA molecule.
- The importance of genetic factors in the regulation of serum IgA responses in IgAN has been highlighted in studies of familial

IgAN. Unaffected family members of patients with IgAN have been shown to have high levels of total serum IgA, IgA immune complexes, and exaggerated production of IgA by cultured peripheral blood B lymphocytes. So far, a candidate gene for the pathogenesis remains undefined.

- Recurrence of IgAN in the renal allograft due to the immuno-chemical abnormality of the IgA molecule has an incidence of 5–15%, given the different criteria for allograft renal biopsy.
- Its renal pathology is similar to that of Henoch–Schönlein purpura nephritis.
- It runs a relentless progressive clinical course, with end-stage renal failure in 30% of patients over 30 years.
- Acute renal failure is uncommon, except in the crescentic form of IgAN.
- Poor predictive prognostic factors include male gender, hypertension, impaired renal function at presentation, glomerulosclerosis, tubulointerstitial fibrosis, and nephrotic-range proteinuria (except for the overlapping syndrome of IgAN and lipoid nephrosis).
- Mesangial binding of polymeric IgA in IgAN leads to a variable degree of glomerular injury. The pathologic changes in the tubulointerstitium are mediated through humoral factors including tumor necrosis factor-α and angiotensin II.
- Differential expression of angiotensin II receptors in glomerular mesangial cells, podocytes, and tubular epithelial cells supports the therapeutic potential of renin-angiotensin blockade.
- Beware of secondary IgAN (Table 7.4).

7.4.1 *Treatment*

There is still no treatment known to modify mesangial deposition of IgA, i.e. the essential pathogenetic process of IgAN. Available treatment options are mostly directed at the downstream immune and inflammatory cascades in the glomerulus and the tubulointerstitium, which often results in renal scarring. The clinical course differs between different ethnic groups and is apparently affected by the criteria of renal biopsy. Table 7.5 outlines the treatment recommendation according to clinical features.

Patients with slowly progressive IgAN are characterized by hypertension, proteinuria > 1g/day, or reduced glomerular filtration rate (GFR) at the time of diagnosis. Specific treatment strategies in this group of patients remain contentious. Clinical trials are difficult to conduct, as the natural clinical course is slowly progressive and a fall in serum

Table 7.4   Secondary IgAN.

Multi-system disease
  Henoch–Schönlein purpura
  Celiac disease
  Dermatitis herpetiformis
  Crohn disease
  Seronegative arthropathy (ankylosing spondylitis,
    Reiter syndrome, psoriasis)
  Behcet's disease
  Sicca syndrome

Neoplasia
  IgA monoclonal gammopathy
  Mucin-secreting carcinoma
  Carcinoma of the lung, larynx, pharynx, pancreas
  Mycosis fungoides
  Sezary syndrome

Infections
  Hepatitis B
  Leprosy
  Toxoplasmosis
  HIV infection

Others
  Chronic liver disease (including alcoholic liver disease)
  Portosystemic shunt
  Familial immunothrombocytopenia
  Pulmonary hemosiderosis

---

creatinine is not infrequently observed only 10 years after first presentation. The paucity of good clinical trials highlights the uncertainty in determining the best treatment and for how long. The scale of benefit of immunosuppressive drugs in suppressing clinical nephritis or improving outcome is unmatched by the use of renin-angiotensin inhibitors alone. A treatment algorithm according to the clinical status is outlined in Fig. 7.2. The following treatments modulating immune and inflammatory injury were previously studied in limited randomized controlled trials or open studies.

7.4.1.1 *Corticosteroids*

- These should only be considered when there is continued proteinuria (> 2g/day) despite tight blood pressure control and maximal

Table 7.5 Treatment options for IgAN according to clinical features.

Clinical presentation	Treatment options
Recurrent macrohematuria with preserved kidney function	No specific treatment
Proteinuria <1 g/day ± microhematuria	No specific treatment
Proteinuria >1 g/day ± microhematuria	Renin-angiotensin blockade with ACEIs and ARBs
Nephrotic syndrome/Nephrotic-range proteinuria	
With minimal change histology (overlapping syndrome)	0.5–1 mg/kg/day prednisolone for up to 8 weeks (treating as MCN)
With structural glomerular changes (proliferation, sclerosis)	No specific treatment
Acute renal failure	
Crescentic IgAN (active lesion with no chronic fibrosis)	
Induction (~8 weeks)	0.5–1 mg/kg/day prednisolone and 2 mg/kg/day cyclophosphamide
Maintenance	Prednisolone in reducing dose and 2.5 mg/kg/day azathioprine
Hypertension	Target BP of 120/75 mmHg if proteinuria >1 g/day Prefer ACEIs and/or ARBs

renin-angiotensin blockade. Pulse steroid is not recommended, and low-dose oral prednisolone (20 mg/day at induction; 5–10 mg/day for maintenance) for 6 months can be tried.

7.4.1.2 *Cytotoxic Drugs (Cyclophosphamide)*

• No consistent benefit.

7.4.1.3 *Fish Oil*

• No consistent benefit.

7.4.1.4 *Mycophenolate Mofetil*

• Dosage of 0.5–2 g/day — limited experience, but well tolerated. Conflicting results are demonstrated, with benefits in Asian

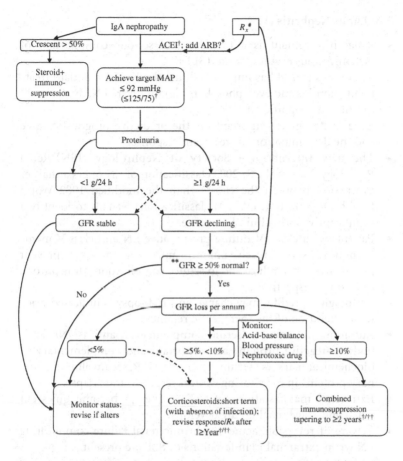

Fig. 7.2 An algorithm of recommended treatment options for IgAN. [†]Therapy with efficacy of evidence base grade 1 data; [*]therapy with high *a priori* evidence to use, but not tested independently in randomized controlled trials; [††]remission in microhematuria and proteinuria 6 months after starting immunosuppressive drugs; [**]no evidence that immunosuppressive drugs can benefit declining function in patients starting therapy with a > 50% loss in GFR. Broken lines denote less frequently encountered scenarios. MAP: mean arterial pressure.

patients. Reduced binding of IgA to cultured mesangial cells was observed in one recent clinical trial.

7.4.1.5 *Coagulation-Modifying Agents*

- No consistent benefit, despite promising data in earlier trials.

7.5 Lupus Nephritis (LN)

- Renal involvement is a frequent and serious complication of systemic lupus erythematosus (SLE).
- Although survival has improved dramatically with standard treatment (steroids and cyclophosphamide) for severe LN, drug-related toxicities are significant.
- Renal histology is important for the predictive prognostic value and the determination of treatment response.
- The new International Society of Nephrology (ISN)/Renal Pathology Society (RPS) 2003 classification of LN offers a sharper distinction between the classes than the modified 1982 World Health Organization (WHO) classification, yet fails to identify a significantly worse clinical outcome.
- Patients with class IV diffuse proliferative LN and class V membranous LN should receive immunosuppressive therapy to prevent progressive renal failure and to reduce complications of nephrotic syndrome, respectively.
- Histological grading may change and re-biopsy is indicated prior to an alteration of the therapeutic regime.
- Autoimmune markers (serum complement 3, anti-dsDNA antibody, C-reactive protein) are important and complementary to biochemical markers (serum creatinine, GFR, serum albumin, urinary protein) in monitoring clinical response and relapse.
- Extrarenal manifestations of SLE frequently become quiescent when end-stage renal failure develops.
- Beware of reversible acute-on-chronic renal failure complicating LN when extrarenal manifestations of SLE are present.

7.5.1 *Treatment*

7.5.1.1 *Class IV Diffuse Proliferative LN*

Treatment of class IV LN comprises two phases: induction with aggressive suppression of autoimmune injury, and maintenance to prevent relapse with less toxicity. A treatment algorithm of the induction and maintenance therapy is outlined in Fig. 7.3.

Prospective induction trials reveal:

- Oral cyclophosphamide is as effective as intravenous cyclophosphamide.
- Low-dose intravenous cyclophosphamide (500 mg every 2 weeks for a total of 6 doses) is as effective as high-dose intravenous

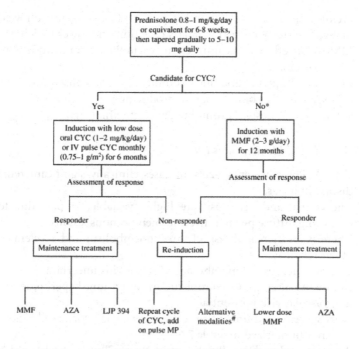

Fig. 7.3 Treatment algorithm for diffuse proliferative LN. *Previous serious toxicities to CYC, severe cytopenia, patient's reluctance, etc. #Alternative treatments including MMF, cyclosporine A, immunoadsorption, intravenous immunoglobulin. AZA, azathioprine; MP, methylprednisolone; CYC, cyclophosphamide; MMF, mycophenolate mofetil. [From Lai KN *et al. Nephrology* 2005; 10: 180–188, used with permission.]

cyclophosphamide (six monthly pulses of 0.5–1 g/m² followed by two quarterly pulses) with less infection and lower toxicities.
- MMF is as effective as intravenous cyclophosphamide, but with lower toxicities.
- Rituximab has been reported to achieve some success in isolated case reports or small-scale open studies.

Prospective maintenance trials reveal:

- Oral cyclophosphamide is as effective as intravenous cyclophosphamide.
- Low-dose intravenous cyclophosphamide (500 mg every 2 weeks for a total of 6 doses) is as effective as high-dose intravenous

cyclophosphamide (six monthly pulses of 0.5–1 g/m² followed by two quarterly pulses) with less infection and lower toxicities.
- MMF is as effective as intravenous cyclophosphamide, but with lower toxicities.
- LJP 394 (Riquent, abetimus sodium), which consists of four dsDNA helices to bind antibody-producing B cells, shows no consistent benefit despite promising data in the first trial.

7.5.1.2 Class V Membranous LN

- Class V LN represents ~20% of cases clinically significant renal disease in lupus.
- The course and prognosis are highly variable, in part due to coexisting diffuse proliferative and membranous lesions.
- There is an increased risk of thromboembolism and accelerated atherosclerosis.
- Optimal therapy for membranous LN remains uncertain.
- Adjunctive therapy to control the hypertension, hyperlipidemia, and vascular risk is essential.
- Retrospective and uncontrolled treatment trials for membranous LN are summarized in Table 7.6.
- A recent trial with small patient sample of Class IV + Class V LN receiving multi-target therapy (Prednisone 0.6–0.8 mg/kg/day, MMF 1 g/day and tacrolimus 4 mg/day) showed a higher complete remission rate (65%) at 9 months as compared with intravenous cyclophosphamide (Bao H, *et al.* JASN, 2008).

7.6 Diabetic Nephropathy (DN)

- Type 1 diabetes mellitus (DM) is due to autoimmune-mediated islet B cell destruction, often in young patients, and accounts for 5%–10% of all diabetics.
- Type 2 DM is a heterogeneous condition characterized by insulin resistance and islet failure, often in patients >40 years, and accounts for 90% of all diabetics.
- Both types of DM, if poorly controlled, will reach stage 3 renal disease (microalbuminuria and hypertension) in 10 years and progress to stage 5 (end-stage renal failure) in 20–25 years.
- Both types of DM with nephrotic-range proteinuria, if not receiving renin-angiotensin blockade, have a 50% chance of progressing to end-stage renal failure in 2 years.

Table 7.6 Retrospective and uncontrolled treatment trials for membranous LN.

Treatment regime	Patient number	Mean follow-up (months)	Results
Chlorambucil + methylprednisolone alternating every month for 6 months vs. methylprednisolone (retrospective)	19	83	Steroid + chlorambucil: CR, 63%; PR, 36%; relapse, 9% Steroid alone: CR, 37%; PR, 12%; relapse, 87%
Azathioprine + prednisone for 12 months; indefinite maintenance with low-dose prednisone and azathioprine (open label)	38	90	CR, 67%; PR, 22%; relapse, 19% after mean 90 months; decline of GFR, 13%
Sequential therapy — induction: oral cyclophosphamide for 6 months + prednisolone; maintenance: azathioprine (uncontrolled)	20	74	CR, 55%; PR, 35%; relapse, 40% after mean 47 months; renal function, stable
Cyclosporin + prednisolone (retrospective)	24	16	CR, 52%; PR, 43%; relapse, 33% after withdrawal of cyclosporin
Mycophenolate mofetil (6 months) + prednisone + aggressive blood pressure and lipid control with ACEI and/or ARB + statin (uncontrolled)	13	15	CR, 69%; PR, 15%
Steroid + tacrolimus (0.1–0.2 mg/kg/day) for 6 months (uncontrolled)	18	12	CR, 28%; PR 50% at 3 months

CR: complete response; PR: partial response.

- Over 90% of DN cases have retinopathy and/or neuropathy; the absence of retinopathy may suggest a coexisting glomerular disease, and renal biopsy may be indicated.

7.6.1 *Treatment*

- Prevention is important and annual screening for proteinuria/microalbuminuria (expressed as albumin/creatinine ratio) should be performed.
- Blood pressure control targeted at 120/80 mmHg or lower.
- Glycemic control with HbA1c < 7%
- Correction of hyperlipidemia with LDL cholesterol < 2.6 mmol/L
- Maximal blockade of the renin-angiotensin system by ACEI and/or ARB for (a) blood pressure control, (b) reduction of proteinuria, (c) correction of intrarenal hypertension, (d) anti-inflammatory action, and (e) stopping of fibrogenic activities.

7.7 Anti-Neutrophil Cytoplasmic Antibody (ANCA)-Associated Systemic Vasculitis (AASV)

- Glomerulonephritis occurs in Wegener's granulomatosis (85%), microscopic polyangiitis (90%), and Churg–Strauss syndrome (<10%).
- Common presentations are acute renal failure and pulmonary hemorrhage.
- ANCA positivity with antigen specificity is important in diagnosis and monitoring of clinical course (response and relapse).
- ANCAs are necessary, but not sufficient, for the development of the clinical syndromes in AASV; and preparatory signals (e.g. inflammation following infection) must reach adequate threshold levels to allow high-titer ANCAs to induce full clinical expression.

7.7.1 *Treatment*

As in LN, treatment of AASV comprises two phases: induction with aggressive suppression of autoimmune injury, and maintenance to prevent relapse with less toxicity. A treatment algorithm of the induction and maintenance therapy recommended by the British Society of Rheumatology is outlined in Fig. 7.4.

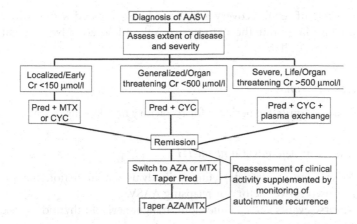

Fig. 7.4 Treatment algorithm for ANCA-associated systemic vasculitis (AASV) adopted from recommendation by the British Society of Rheumatology and British Health Professionals in Rheumatology. Pred, prednisolone/prednisone; MTX, methotrexate; CYC, cyclophosphamide; AZA, azathioprine; Cr, serum creatinine. [Adopted with modification from Lapraik C *et al. Rheumatology* 2007; 46: 1615–1616, used with permission.]

7.7.1.1 *Corticosteroids*

- These are usually given as daily oral prednisolone/prednisone.
- Initially, a higher dose (1 mg/kg/day up to 60 mg) is given.
- Sometimes, intravenous methylprednisolone (250–500 mg) is given as the loading dose.

7.7.1.2 *Intolerance of Cyclophosphamide*

- Alternative treatment such as methotrexate, azathioprine, or mycophenolate mofetil may be used.

7.7.1.3 *Mycophenolate Mofetil*

- This is used for maintenance therapy, with a variable relapse rate of 9%–43% obtained from trials with small sample size.

7.7.1.4 *Plasma Exchange*

- This is used in patients whose serum creatinine >500 μmol/L.

- The rate of renal recovery is higher when compared with methyl-prednisolone, but the patient survival and severe adverse event rates are similar.

7.7.1.5 *Rituximab*

- This has limited experience for refractory or relapsing AASV.

7.7.1.6 *Alemtuzumab (Campath-1H)*

- This is a lymphocyte-depleting antibody used in induction therapy.
- It is used for refractory or relapsing AASV.
- Adverse events such as infection, malignancy, and thyroid disease are common.
- Relapses are common.

7.7.1.7 *Co-trimoxazole*

- This reduces the incidence of relapse in Wegener's granulomatosis with 800 mg sulfamethoxazole and 160 mg trimethoprim twice daily.

Suggested Reading

Ballardie FW. (2007) Quantitative appraisal of treatment options for IgA nephropathy. *J Am Soc Nephrol* 11:2806–2809.

Lai KN. (2007) Membranous nephropathy: when and how to treat. *Kidney Int* 71:841–843.

Lai KN, Tang SC, Mok CC. (2005) Treatment of lupus nephritis: a revisit. *Nephrology* 10:180–188.

Lapraik C, Watts R, Bacon P, *et al.* (2007) BSR and BHPR guidelines for the management of adults with ANCA associated vasculitis. *Rheumatology* 46:1–11.

Meyrier A. (2004) Nephrotic focal segmental glomerulosclerosis in 2004: an update. *Nephrol Dial Transplant* 19:2437–2444.

Saha TC, Singh H. (2006) Minimal change disease: a review. *South Med J* 99:1264–1269.

Waldman M, Appel GB. (2006) Update on the treatment of lupus nephritis. *Kidney Int* 70:1403–1412.

8

Hypertension and Renal Disease in Pregnancy

Susan Hou

This chapter covers two separate but related areas of renal disease. Hypertension is a common pregnancy complication in healthy women and in women with essential hypertension. Management of most hypertensive pregnant women should result in a healthy mother and baby.

Pregnancy in women with pre-existing renal disease can be harrowing for both the mother and the doctors, but increasingly results in healthy infants. Pregnancy is typically complicated by hypertension, worsening proteinuria, and prematurity with or without worsening renal function (Table 8.1).

8.1 Hypertension in Pregnancy

There is a decrease in systolic blood pressure of about 9 mmHg and in diastolic blood pressure of 17 mmHg during pregnancy. The lowest blood pressure is seen between 16 and 20 weeks of gestation, and the blood pressure gradually increases toward term. Hypertension is the most common medical problem occurring during pregnancy.

8.1.1 Classification

8.1.1.1 Preeclampsia

- Preeclampsia is defined by a triad of hypertension, proteinuria, and edema after the 20th week of pregnancy.
- It occurs in 2% to 7% of nulliparous women. Seizures (eclampsia) may occur at blood pressures lower than would be worrisome in the general population. The general principles of treatment are outlined in Table 8.2.

Table 8.1   Risk factors for preeclampsia.

Primigravida
Extremes of (childbearing) age
Pre-existing hypertension
Pre-existing renal disease
Diabetes
Different father
Twin gestation
Hydatidiform mole
Fetal hydrops

Table 8.2   Treatment of preeclampsia.

Admission to hospital
Anticonvulsants: magnesium sulfate
Antihypertensive agents: hydrazine and labetalol
Indications for delivery
   >36 weeks of gestation
   HELLP syndrome
   BP > 160/110 after 24 h of hospitalization
   Proteinuria > 3 g/24 h
   Rising serum creatinine
   Headache, blurred vision, scotomata, right upper quadrant pain, clonus

BP: blood pressure.

- A 30-mm increase in systolic blood pressure and a 15 mmHg rise in diastolic blood pressure are significant, and patients often start from a low baseline.
- The most common signs of severe preeclampsia are microangiopathic hemolytic anemia, elevated liver enzymes (sometimes over 1000 IU), and low platelets, collectively referred to as the HELLP syndrome. It is a multisystem disease affecting many organ systems (Table 8.3). The definitive treatment for preeclampsia is delivery.

8.1.1.2 *Chronic Hypertension*

- Chronic hypertension is estimated to occur in 1% to 5% of pregnancies and is associated with increased risk of superimposed preeclampsia, abruptio placentae, and increased neonatal morbidity and mortality.

Table 8.3   Manifestations of HELLP syndrome.

Disseminated intravascular coagulation	21%
Pulmonary edema	8%
Acute renal failure	16%
Ascites	8%
Laryngeal edema	1%
Subcapsular hematoma of the liver	1%
Blindness	1%
Adult respiratory distress syndrome	1%

- The diagnosis is easiest if a history of hypertension before pregnancy is available or if hypertension occurs before 20 weeks of gestation. Almost half of the women with preexisting hypertension will experience a pregnancy-related drop in blood pressure between 13 and 20 weeks of gestation, and the diagnosis of essential hypertension will not be apparent if the woman is first seen during that period.

8.1.1.3 *Chronic Hypertension with Superimposed Preeclampsia*

- The risk of severe hypertension in the third trimester is highest in women who do not have a mid-trimester drop in blood pressure or in those who have an increase in blood pressure. Blood pressures are often higher than seen in simple preeclampsia.

8.1.1.4 *Gestational Hypertension*

- Gestational hypertension is the development of hypertension without proteinuria during the third trimester in a previously normotensive woman. The hypertension generally resolves within 10 days postpartum. There is an 80% chance of recurrence in subsequent pregnancies and a risk of developing hypertension later in life.

8.1.1.5 *Secondary Hypertension*

All secondary forms of hypertension can occur during pregnancy.

- Pheochromocytoma is rare in pregnancy as it is in general, but carries a 50% mortality rate if undiagnosed. The diagnosis can be made by 24-h urine measurements of epinephrine and norepinephrine. These values are within normal limits in normal and preeclamptic pregnancy, but are increased twofold to fourfold for 24 h after a seizure.

- Cocaine intoxication usually presents with hypertension and signs of sympathetic hyperactivity similar to a pheochromocytoma. Cocaine use is more common than pheochromocytoma and can be detected on toxicology screening. Cocaine use may be associated with renal failure from rhabdomyolysis or with abruptio placentae.
- Other secondary causes of hypertension may occur in pregnancy, but specific diagnosis is rarely urgent unless the blood pressure cannot be controlled.
- If a potassium-sparing agent is needed, amiloride rather than spironolactone should be used.

8.1.2 *Management*

8.1.2.1 *Home Blood Pressure Monitoring*

Since blood pressure may rise abruptly, women at risk for preeclampsia should be continued for monitoring 6 weeks postpartum.

8.1.2.2 *Antihypertensive Drugs*

<u>Angiotensin-converting enzyme inhibitors and Angiotensin receptor blockers</u>

- It has been recognized for many years that these drugs cause renal dysplasia, oligohydramnios, pulmonary hypoplasia, poor ossification of the fetal skull, and contractures when used in the late second and third trimesters.
- There is now one study which indicates an increase in congenital anomalies when used in the first trimester. These drugs should be stopped when the patient decides to conceive.

<u>Diuretics</u>

- There is a general reluctance to use diuretics in pregnant women, although at one time they were widely used in the hope that they would prevent preeclampsia and they were safe in low doses.

- There are concerns about diuretics: the physiologic volume expansion of pregnancy is slightly decreased by diuretics. Preeclampsia is associated with volume contraction relative to normal pregnancy. Intravascular volume contraction and electrolyte abnormalities may occur in the fetus.
- In women with pre-existing renal disease, however, it may be impossible to control blood pressure without diuretics.

Methyldopa

- This drug has been used in pregnant women for over 40 years. Careful developmental testing of children at age 4 years shows no detrimental effect.

Calcium channel blockers

- Once reserved for refractory hypertension in pregnancy, calcium channel blockers are now widely used as a first-line drug for the treatment of hypertensive pregnant women. Nifedipine is the most widely used, but felodipine, isradipine, and nimodipine have also been used. No increase in congenital anomalies was seen in studies of women who received calcium channel blockers.
- This group of drugs interacts with magnesium, so care should be used in starting magnesium in a woman taking calcium channel blockers.
- Children at 18 months show no developmental problems.

Hydralazine

- This has been used for 40 years and is safe, but is not effective as a single agent when given orally.

Labetalol and beta blockers

- There have been several case reports of neonatal bradycardia, hypoglycemia, and respiratory depression associated with β-blockers, but these problems are generally easily managed by the neonatologist.
- There are mixed data concerning whether β-blockers are associated with intrauterine growth restriction.
- Labetalol combines α- and β-blockade, and has been widely used as first-line therapy for hypertension in pregnancy because it has been associated with less adrenergic blockade in the newborn.

8.1.3 Treatment of Severe Hypertension

8.1.3.1 Hydralazine

- Intravenous hydralazine in doses of 5–10 mg every 20–30 min is the drug of first choice for hypertensive crisis in pregnancy.

8.1.3.2 Labetalol

- Intravenous labetalol is the second most commonly used regimen for treating hypertensive emergencies in pregnant women. It is given either as a 20-mg loading dose followed by 20–30 mg every 30 min or at a 1–2-mg/min drip.

8.1.3.3 Nifedipine

- Short-acting nifedipine has fallen out of use in the general population. However, there are some centers where it is used for the treatment of severe hypertension in pregnant women.

8.2 Renal Disease in Pregnancy

8.2.1 Lupus Nephritis

Of all renal diseases in pregnancy, lupus nephritis is the most variable in its course.

- Remission for 6 months prior to conception is associated with a lower risk of lupus flares, but these still occur in one third of patients.
- Lupus flares occur in 23%–64% of patients with lupus nephritis and can be seen in different lupus renal histological gradings.
- Lupus nephritis that presents during pregnancy is commonly of class IV type, but a biopsy is needed to confirm the pathological grading.
- Steroids and azathioprine are usually used during pregnancy, but cyclophosphamide has sometimes been used after 20 weeks of gestation. There is no experience with rituximab (anti-CD20).
- Fetal problems associated with a lupus mother include:

    (i) recurrent spontaneous abortion with anticardiolipin and antiphospholipid antibody
    (ii) congenital heart block in women with anti-SSA antibody

(iii) rash and thrombocytopenia from maternal IgG (usually resolves within 6 months).

8.2.2 *Other Renal Diseases*

For renal diseases other than lupus nephritis, the most important predictor of pregnancy complications is renal function at the time of conception. All women with renal disease have an increased risk of hypertension, worsening proteinuria, and premature delivery. If the serum creatinine is greater than 1.4 mg/dL, renal disease progresses more rapidly than it would have without pregnancy, causing the woman to require dialysis or transplant earlier. Once the kidney function begins to deteriorate, unless from preeclampsia, it does not generally improve with termination of the pregnancy.

- Hypertension in women with renal disease: The same monitoring and medications are used in women with renal disease as in chronic hypertension, but diuretics may be necessary.
- Nephrotic syndrome: Increased proteinuria may lead to profound hypoalbuminemia and massive edema may occur. Salt restriction should be started at the beginning of pregnancy. Low doses of diuretics are probably safe, but the effects of the high doses needed to diurese a person with nephrotic syndrome are unknown. Heparin does not cross the placenta and it has been widely used in pregnancy, but its efficacy in preventing thrombosis in women with nephrotic syndrome has not been studied. Treatment of hyperlipidemia should be delayed until after delivery.
- Worsening renal function: Increasing proteinuria, or even a rise in serum creatinine, that is not associated with preeclampsia is not a reason to terminate a previable pregnancy. Dialysis should be initiated at a glomerular filtration rate (GFR) of around 20 mL/min.

8.2.3 *Renal Transplant*

- Fertility: Fertility is usually restored by kidney transplant. A transplant recipient should wait at least a year posttransplant before planning a pregnancy so that she is past the peak risk for acute rejection and cytomegalovirus (CMV) infection. Renal function should be stable preferably with a serum creatinine below 1.5 mg/dL, but certainly below 2 mg/dL.

- Medications: Prednisone, azathioprine, cyclosporine, and tacrolimus have all been used in pregnancy, and continuation of these drugs is preferable for the baby to prevent acute rejection. Continuation of drugs to prevent acute rejection is better for the baby than risking losing the kidney. Indirectly, it is still probably better for the baby to have a mother who is not on dialysis.
- Mycophenolate mofetil may cause birth defects and should be avoided. There is little experience with sirolimus.
- Angiotensin-converting enzyme inhibitors and cholesterol-lowering drugs should be stopped before conception.
- Graft function: Graft survival and acute rejection rates are similar to women who have not been pregnant, as long as guidelines are followed and there is close monitoring.
- Infection in transplant recipients: About 40% of women develop urinary tract infection. CMV, toxoplasmosis, herpes simplex, and listeria infections are of concern for the baby.

8.2.4 Dialysis

- Fertility and outcome: Estimates of the frequency of conception in dialysis patients range from 0.3% per year in Belgium to 1.8% per year in Saudi Arabia. The likelihood of having a surviving infant is about 50% in women who reach the second trimester. Intensive dialysis (20–24 h a week) can improve the survival rate to 75%. There is a recent report of 100% surviving infants born to women doing nocturnal dialysis averaging 48 h per week.
- Dialysis modality: Conception is half as common in peritoneal dialysis patients as in hemodialysis patients. The infant survival rate is the same as for women treated with standard hemodialysis, but lower than for those treated with intensive hemodialysis.
- Dialysate composition: Intensive dialysis requires adjustments of calcium, phosphorus, and bicarbonate in the hemodialysate bath. Vitamin supplementation, especially folate, should be increased fourfold.
- Anemia: Erythropoietin requirements may double, since plasma volume increases and red cell production does not. Anemia may develop in other women with renal insufficiency who become pregnant.
- Prematurity: About 80% of infants born to dialysis patients, are premature, and premature birth is the major reason for fetal loss. Obstetricians should treat a dialysis patient as a patient who has already had several second trimester losses using cervical cerclage

and/or progesterone, depending on the usual practice at their institution.

- Fetal monitoring: Monitoring of fetal well-being should start as soon as the results can be interpreted. After birth, infants will experience an osmotic diuresis and volume status should be monitored in a high-risk nursery.

8.2.5 *Indications for Biopsy*

- New onset lupus
- Unexplained acute renal failure
- Nephrotic syndrome where treatment is being planned
- Rarely, to distinguish between preeclampsia and another renal problem

8.2.6 *Acute Renal Failure (Table 8.4)*

Acute renal failure in pregnant women, which used to account for 20%–40% of all acute renal failure cases, has become exceedingly rare with good obstetric care and legalization of abortion. Third trimester acute renal failure is still occasionally seen.

- Uterine infection or severe pyelonephritis can result in acute renal failure.
- HELLP syndrome can be complicated by acute renal failure. The renal failure is generally reversible if the woman does not have an underlying renal disease.
- Hemolytic-uremic syndrome is less common and can be difficult to distinguish from HELLP syndrome. It is treated with plasmapheresis, with variable results.
- Acute fatty liver of pregnancy presents as liver failure with incidental renal failure. Care is directed at the liver failure, and may be supportive or may require liver transplant.

Table 8.4 Causes of acute renal failure in pregnancy.

Sepsis (septic abortion and pyelonephritis)
Preeclampsia/HELLP syndrome
Hemolytic-uremic syndrome
Acute fatty liver of pregnancy
Obstetric catastrophe: abruptio placentae, amniotic fluid embolus

- Obstetric catastrophes including hemorrhage, abruptio placentae, or amniotic fluid embolus may lead to renal failure. During pregnancy, the kidneys are at more risk for cortical necrosis than in other settings with acute renal failure.

Suggested Readings

Hou S. (1999) Lupus in pregnancy. In: Lewis EJ, Schwartz MM, Korbet SM. (eds.) *Lupus Nephritis*, Oxford University Press, Oxford, pp. 262–283.

Jones DC, Hayslett JP. (1996) Outcome of pregnancy in women with moderate or severe renal insufficiency. *N Engl J Med* **335**:226–232.

McKay DB, Josephson MA, Armenti VT, *et al.* (2005). Reproduction and transplantation: report on the AST Consensus Conference on Reproductive Issues and Transplantation. *Am J Transplant* **5**:1592–1599.

Sibai B, Dekker G, Kupferminc M. (2005) Pre-eclampsia. *Lancet* **365**:785–799.

Sibai BM. (1996) Drug therapy: treatment of hypertension in pregnant women. *N Engl J Med* **335**:257–265.

Sibai BM, Ramadan MK, Salama M, *et al.* (1993) Maternal morbidity and mortality in 442 pregnancies with hemolysis, elevated liver enzymes and low platelets (HELLP syndrome). *Am J Obstet Gynecol* **169**:1000–1006.

9

Selected Problems in General Nephrology

Kar Neng Lai

This chapter discusses principally four important clinical settings that may lead to acute renal failure (ARF). The pathophysiological events are different, and preventive measures must be observed to reduce the risk of development into established ARF.

9.1 Hepatorenal Syndrome (HRS)

Hepatorenal syndrome occurs in patients with severe liver failure. Two forms of HRS are recognized (Table 9.1). Not all concomitant renal and liver failures are due to HRS, a condition in the appropriate patho-physiological setting diagnosed by the exclusion of other causes of ARF. More common causes of combined renal and liver failure include:

- acute tubular necrosis secondary to hypovolemia (hemorrhage, burns, fluid loss from kidney or gut)
- acute tubular necrosis complicating sepsis or multi-organ failure
- glomerular disorder (hepatitis C-related cryoglobulinemic mesangiocapillary glomerulonephritis)
- infection (leptospirosis, herpes simplex type 2, fulminant hepatitis A)
- medication (flavonoid, cyclosporine, tacrolimus).

The diagnostic criteria for HRS are listed in Table 9.2.

9.1.1 *Pathophysiology*

ARF in HRS is essentially prerenal in nature with arterial underfilling due to effective volume depletion. Renal histology is normal, and biopsy is unnecessary and hazardous. Kidneys from HRS patients

Table 9.1   Classification of HRS.

Type 1
  ARF is the main presenting feature
  Rapid deterioration of renal function
  Profound oliguria or anuria
  Short median survival (2 weeks)

Type 2
  Refractory ascites is the main presenting feature
  Protracted clinical course
  Progressive renal impairment
  Longer median survival (6 months)

Table 9.2   Diagnostic criteria of HRS.[a]

Major criteria	Supplementary information
Severe liver failure (acute or chronic)	Usually with portal hypertension
Serum creatinine $\geq$133 μmol/L or creatinine clearance <40 mL/min	
Absence of other causes of renal failure	No evidence of obstruction or parenchymal disease on ultrasound; proteinuria <500 mg/L
Absence of ongoing infection or fluid loss	
Absence of a sustained improvement in renal function following diuretic withdrawal and administration of 1.5 L of isotonic saline	
Additional criteria	
Oliguria	
Urine Na$^+$ <10 mmol/L	
Urine osmolality > plasma osmolality	
Urine red blood cells <50 per high power field	
Serum Na$^+$ <130 mmol/L	

[a] Adopted from the International Ascites Group (www.icascites.org).

function satisfactorily when transplanted to other patients with end-stage renal failure.

Portal hypertension is the main factor responsible for the development of splanchnic arterial vasodilatation, which is caused mainly by increased production of extrahepatic nitric oxide. Bacterial infections, particularly spontaneous bacterial peritonitis, and large-volume paracentesis without plasma expansion are triggers that worsen splanchnic vasodilatation and decrease cardiac output. The vasodilatation caused by pooling blood in the splanchnic bed triggers compensatory responses by activating the renin-angiotensin-aldosterone system, the sympathetic nervous system, and arginine vasopression. These lead to retention of sodium and water. Vasoconstriction plays an important role in the decreased renal perfusion that leads to functional renal failure. In the early stages of the disease, renal perfusion is maintained by the increased production of local renal vasodilators; however, as the disease progresses, the circulating and local vasoconstrictors overcome the effect of renal vasodilators, leading to severe renal vasoconstriction and a reduction in the glomerular filtration rate (GFR) and ultimately causing HRS. The proposed pathophysiological mechanism is summarized in Fig. 9.1.

9.1.2 Management

9.1.2.1 Prevention

- Overdiuresis — stop all diuretics
- Large-volume (>5 L) paracentesis without concurrent plasma expansion
- Sodium ($Na^+ < 80$ mmol/day) and fluid (<1 L/day) restriction
- Treatment of any precipitating factors such as gastrointestinal bleeding and sepsis (especially spontaneous bacterial peritonitis).

9.1.2.2 Pharmacologic Treatment

Systemic vasoconstrictors are used to counteract the splanchnic vasodilatation and hence reduce the intense renal vasoconstriction. Terlipressin, a vasopressin analog, is the most commonly used one.

- Terlipressin (0.5–1 mg/4–6 h IVI) administered with albumin 20–40 g daily for a maximum of 15 days or until serum creatinine falls to <133 μmol/L
- Improvement of GFR, raised arterial pressure, increased urine output
- Reduced mortality by 34% (Cochrane Database 2006)

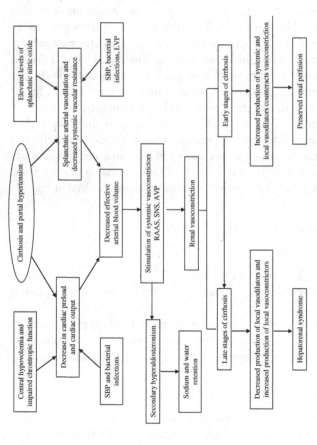

Fig. 9.1 The pathogenesis of HRS and its precipitating factors.

Abbreviations: AVP, arginine vasopressin; LVP, large-volume paracentesis; RAAS, renin-angiotensin-aldosterone system; SBP, spontaneous bacterial peritonitis; SNS, sympathetic nervous system. [Adopted with modification from Cardenas A, Gines P. *Nat Clin Pract Gastroenterol Hepatol* 2006; 3: 338–348, used with permission.]

- Response in type 2 HRS slightly better than in type 1 HRS
- Ischemic adverse effects averaging between 10% and 25%

In countries where terlipressin is unavailable, alternative include noradrenalin (1–10 µg/min); octreotide, an inhibitor of glucagon and another vasodilator peptide release (100–200 µg SC tds); and midodine, an α-agonist (7.5–12.5 mg PO tds) — all used in combination with albumin. Renal vasodilators such as dopamine, fenoldopam, and prostaglandins or endothelin-A antagonist are of no therapeutic benefit in HRS.

9.1.2.3 *Transjugular Intrahepatic Portosystemic Shunt (TIPS)*

- TIPS reduces portal pressure, suppresses a putative hepatorenal flux, and improves the circulating volume and cardiac output.
- It does not normalize the clinical, biochemical, and neurohumoral parameters.
- It prolongs survival enough either for liver transplantation or, if the patient is not a transplant candidate, to stay off dialysis.
- It may aggravate hepatic encephalopathy.
- It may worsen an existing hyperdynamic circulation or precipitate acute heart failure.
- It has been used in combination following initial pharmacologic treatment with systemic vasoconstrictor.

9.1.2.4 *Renal Replacement Therapy*

- Renal replacement therapy partially corrects the biochemical parameters, but does not improve patient outcome.

9.1.2.5 *Molecular Adsorbent Recirculating System (MARS)*

- MARS removes albumin-bound toxins (e.g. bile salts) and water-soluble cytokines.
- It serves as a bridge to transplantation in clinical trials.

9.1.2.6 *Liver Transplantation*

- Liver transplantation is the treatment of choice, but is limited by the supply of donor livers.
- Renal impairment may persist 1 month posttransplantation.

- Posttransplantation reversal of HRS may be only 60%, especially with marginal liver.
- Predictors of renal recovery include younger recipients, young donor, nonalcoholic liver disease, and low posttransplantation bilirubin.

9.2 Contrast-Induced Nephropathy (CIN)

CIN is defined as ARF with a 25% elevation of serum creatinine or an absolute increase in serum creatinine of 44 μmol/L 2 to 7 days following intravascular administration of radiocontrast in the absence of other identifiable causes of renal failure. The incidence is between 1.6% and 2.3%. Intra-arterial administration of radiocontrast might be more likely to lead to CIN than the intravenous route. The pathogenesis is believed to be (a) oxidant injury to proximal tubular cells and (b) contrast osmolarity, altering the afferent/efferent tone and thus perfusion. CIN is generally nonoliguric and reversible, and serum creatinine returns to normal within 14 days. Registry data report that the incidence of CIN requiring dialysis is 0.4%. The risk factors that bear important preventive measures are depicted in Table 9.3.

9.2.1 Preventive Measures

9.2.1.1 General

- Identify the risk factors listed in Table 9.3.

Table 9.3 Risk factors for CIN.

Patient-related	Non-patient-related
Anemia	Contrast viscosity
Chronic renal impairment	Contrast volume
Congestive heart failure or poor left ventricular function	High osmolar contrast
	Ionic contrast
Dehydration	Intra-arterial administration
Diabetes mellitus	Co-administration of
Elderly	non-steroidal anti-
Emergency procedures	inflammatory drugs
Hypotension	(NSAIDs)
Hypertension	
Intra-aortic balloon pump	

- Stop diuretics, NSAIDs, angiotensin-converting enzyme inhibitors, and angiotension receptor blockers if possible 2 days before the procedure.
- Avoid admitting high-risk patients as day cases.
- Vasodilators such as dopamine and calcium channel blockers have no therapeutic value.

9.2.1.2 *Hydration*

- The clinical state of hydration should be carefully examined before fluid is prescribed to prevent CIN.
- Intravenous hydration is superior to oral hydration.
- 0.9% NaCl normal saline (1 mL/kg/h) for 12 h pre-procedure and 12 h post-procedure (recommended).
- 0.45% NaCl half-normal saline and 2.5% half-dextrose (1 mL/kg/h) for 12 h pre-procedure and 12 h post-procedure.
- 1.26% $NaHCO_3$ (3 mL/kg/h = 0.45 mmol/kg/h) for 1 h pre-procedure and 6 h during and post-procedure.

9.2.1.3 *Antioxidants*

- Most data are based on the use of *N*-acetylcysteine, while information on ascorbic acid is limited.
- Meta-analyses reveal a borderline renoprotective effect of *N*-acetylcysteine. Increased serum creatinine due to interference with tubular handling independently of GFR has been reported.
- For prophylaxis: 600 mg PO bd on the day prior to and the day of the procedure.
- For co-intervention: infusion of 1 mg/kg/h in 0.9% NaCl saline 12 h pre-procedure and 12 h post-procedure.
- For prophylaxis: ascorbic acid 3 g PO 2 h before and 2 g PO bd the day after the procedure.

9.2.2 *Suggested Management Strategy*

Given the low incidence of CIN, a management strategy should be adopted for prescribing any prophylactic treatment (Fig. 9.2). The use of the smallest possible dose of low- or iso-osmolar contrast media, volume expansion, stopping of nephrotoxic drugs, and avoiding the use of repeat contrast injections within 48 h remain the most effective approach to reduce the risk of CIN.

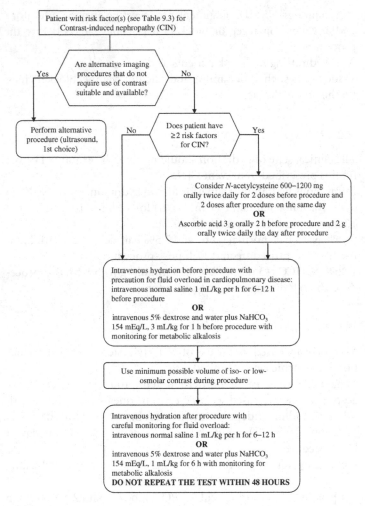

Fig. 9.2 Strategy for management of patients with risk factors for CIN.

9.3 Rhabdomyolysis

Rhabdomyolysis is caused by traumatic or nontraumatic muscle injury, resulting in release of muscle contents including myoglobin. Myoglobin, a heme pigment, is nephrotoxic, and its intratubular precipitation leads to obstruction and oxidative tubular dysfunction. Nontraumatic causes account for half of the patients with rhabdomyolysis, and

Table 9.4 Causes of rhabdomyolysis.

Physical trauma	Drugs and toxins
Compartment syndrome	Alcohol, amphetamine, cocaine,
Crush injury	ecstasy, heroin
Delirium tremens	Antimalarials
Electric shock	Statins and fibrates
Excess exertion	Snake and insect venoms
Malignant hyperthermia	Zidovudine
Neuroleptic malignant syndrome	
Prolonged immobilization	Electrolyte disturbance
NSAIDs	Hypernatremia
Sepsis and shock	Hyponatremia
Sickle cell disease	Hypokalemia
Status asthmaticus	Hypocalcemia
Status epilepticus	Hypophosphatemia
Infection	Endocrine disorders
Gas gangrene	Hyperglycemic emergencies
HIV and Coxsackie	Hypothyroidism
Malaria	
Tetanus, legionella, salmonella	
Myopathies	
Polymyositis/Dermatomyositis	
Inherited myopathies	

causes are summarized in Table 9.4. Characteristic laboratory findings include:

- a heme-positive urine in the absence of red blood cells
- pigmented granular cast
- urine positive for myoglobin
- rapid rise of serum creatinine, creatine phosphokinase, and lactate dehydrogenase; hyperuricemia; hyperphosphatemia; hyperkalemia; hypocalcemia; and increased anion gap
- mild disseminated intravascular coagulopathy (decreased platelets and raised D-dimers).

9.3.1 *Management*

Management for rhabdomyolysis is mainly preventive:

- Ensure adequate hydration to counteract hypovolemia, as a large quantity of fluid is retained in inflamed muscles.

- Maintain urine output > 150 mL/h in nontraumatic situations or even up to 300 mL/h in traumatic injuries. Continue this regime until urinary myoglobin is undetectable.
- Mannitol as an osmotic diuretic must be given with caution due to an increased osmolar gap that may worsen ARF. Mannitol may be given as an infusion (10 mL/h of 15% mannitol) or as a bolus (12.5 g in 250 mL of 5% dextrose solution infused over 2 h).
- Alkalinization with sodium bicarbonate may cause symptomatic hypocalcemia.
- With established ARF, follow the treatment outlined in Chapter 6.
- Hypocalcemia does not require correction unless symptomatic, and beware of rebound hypercalcemia in the recovery phase.

9.4 ARF in Hematopoetic Cell Transplant (HCT)

Approximately 90% of patients have a doubling of serum creatinine after allogeneic HCT due to (a) the nature of the underlying disease, (b) toxicity of anticancer therapy, (c) toxicity of immunosuppressive therapy, and (d) toxicity of antibiotics. The incidence is lower with autologous transplantation or nonmyeloablative HCT. Those patients requiring supportive dialysis have a high mortality. The renal settings unique to HCT according to the time of presentation are summarized in Table 9.5.

Table 9.5 Renal settings unique to HCT according to the time of presentation.

Immediate (days 1–7)
    Tumor lysis syndrome
    Stored marrow toxicity

Early (days 7–21)
    Acute tubular necrosis due to vomiting and diarrhea
    Cyclosporine or tacrolimus toxicity
    Hepatic veno-occlusive disease
    Nephrotoxic antimicrobials
    Sepsis

Late (4 weeks to 1 year)
    Bone marrow transplantation-associated hemolytic-uremic syndrome
    Calcineurin inhibitor nephrotoxicity

Suggested Reading

Gluud LL, Kjaer MS, Christensen E. (2006) Terlipressin for hepatorenal syndrome. *Cochrane Database Syst Rev* 4:CD005162.

Kellum J, Leblanc M, Venkataraman R. (2007) Acute renal failure. *Am Fam Physician* 76:418–422.

Noël C, Hazzan M, Noël-Walter MP, Jouet JP. (1998) Renal failure and bone marrow transplantation. *Nephrol Dial Transplant* 10:2464–2466.

Senzolo M, Cholongitas E, Tibballs J, Burroughs A, Patch D. (2006) Transjugular intrahepatic portosystemic shunt in the management of ascites and hepatorenal syndrome. *Eur J Gastroenterol Hepatol* 11:1143–1150.

Thomsen HS. (2007) Current evidence on prevention and management of contrast-induced nephropathy. *Eur Radiol* 17(Suppl 6):F33–F37.

Thomsen HS, Morcos SK, Barrett BJ. (2008) Contrast-induced nephropathy: the wheel has turned 360 degrees. *Acta Radiol* 49:646–657.

Van Praedt JT, De Vriese AS. (2007) Prevention of contrast-induced nephropathy: a critical review. *Curr Opin Nephrol Hypertens* 16:336–347.

Wadoi HM, Mai ML, Ahsan N, Gonwa TA. (2006) Hepatorenal syndrome: pathophysiology and management. *Clin J Am Soc Nephrol* 1:1066–1079.

10

Urinary Tract Infections

Evan J. C. Lee

Infection of the urinary tract is common in clinical practice. The usual cause is bacterial infection, and the most common organism is *E. coli*. Diagnosis is made easily and treatment with appropriate antibiotics is then instituted. There are different settings in which urinary tract infection (UTI) occurs (Table 10.1). Once diagnosis is confirmed, the decisions to be made are when to treat, which antibiotics to use, which route of administration to use, and for how long the treatment should be administered.

10.1 Asymptomatic Bacteriuria

Bacteriuria is often detected in the asymptomatic patient. The presence of bacteriuria does not require treatment, except in the pregnant patient.

10.1.1 *Screening for Bacteriuria*

In pregnancy, bacteriuria is associated with an increased risk of acute pyelonephritis if left untreated. It is considered not cost-effective to screen for asymptomatic bacteriuria, except in pregnancy.

10.2 Acute Cystitis

This occurs commonly in females in the reproductive age group. The symptoms are clinically distressing, but patients often respond quickly to appropriate antibiotic treatment.

Table 10.1 Clinical syndromes of UTI.

Asymptomatic bacteriuria
Acute cystitis
Recurrent cystitis
Acute pyelonephritis
Infection associated with obstructed urinary tract or stones
Infection associated with indwelling urinary catheters

10.2.1 *Clinical Symptoms*

Clinical symptoms are characterized by:

- frequency of micturition
- dysuria
- urgency of micturition

There may/may not be a febrile response.

10.2.2 *Diagnosis*

Diagnosis is made by:

- clinical symptoms
- presence of pyuria in the urine microscopic examination
- bacteriuria on culture of the urine.

10.2.3 *Treatment*

Treatment is with broad-spectrum antibiotics covering the spectrum of bacteria originating from the colon. Effective treatment protocols are summarized in Table 10.2.

If there has been no response within 48 h, antibiotics should be reviewed with reference to the urine bacteriological cultures.

10.3 Recurrent Cystitis

Recurrent episodes of cystitis are occasionally encountered.

Table 10.2 Antibiotic treatment of acute cystitis.

Single-dose therapy
  Oral amoxicillin 3 g
  Oral co-trimoxazole 4 tabs
  IM kanamycin 500 mg

10–14-day therapy (oral)
  Co-trimoxazole 2 tabs 12 hourly
  Amoxycillin 250 mg 6 hourly
  Ciprofloxacin 250 mg 6 hourly
  Cephalexin 250 mg 6 hourly

10.3.1 *Recurrent Cystitis in Women*

In women, the presence of vesicoureteric reflux should be considered. Often, however, it occurs commonly in women with normal urinary tracts. In these cases, treatment with prophylactic antibiotics may be useful. The common prophylactic regimes are:

* oral cephalexin (250 mg), or
* oral co-trimoxazole (one tab) after sexual intercourse or at bedtime.

Recurrent cystitis is common in women, especially those of reproductive age (two or three attacks per year). No radiological examination is required in contrast to male patients.

10.3.2 *Prevention of Recurrent Cystitis in Women*

In women, some simple measures have been found to be useful in reducing the frequency of episodes of cystitis. Cleaning the perineum after defecation in an anterior-posterior direction can often be useful. In women of the reproductive age group, cystitis is often related to sexual intercourse. In such cases, measures such as emptying the bladder after sexual activity or a dose of co-trimoxazole after sex can often prevent attacks.

10.3.3 *Recurrent Cystitis in Men*

In men who have developed acute cystitis (or recurrent cystitis), the possibility of prostatitis should be considered in men over the age of

50 years. If not treated with appropriately, there may be recurrent infection. In these instances, the organism is usually the same. Treatment should be with antibiotics that penetrate the prostate and are of adequate duration; these should be given for 6 weeks (see Table 10.3). In young males with repeated UTI, radiological examination is indicated to exclude any anatomical abnormalities.

10.4 Acute Pyelonephritis

Acute pyelonephritis is a serious medical illness that may lead to dehydration, sepsis, or even acute renal failure.

10.4.1 *Diagnosis*

Diagnosis is suspected in the presence of symptoms of fever, flank pain, and signs of costovertebral tenderness. Occasionally, there is a history of preceding symptoms of cystitis, i.e. frequency of micturition and dysuria. Urine should be examined for pyuria and bacteriuria as well as antibiotic susceptibility.

10.4.2 *Treatment*

Treatment can be with oral or parenteral antibiotics (Table 10.4). If the patient is systemically ill with a high fever and having chills and rigors, parenteral antibiotics should be used. Antibiotics should be given for a minimum of 7–14 days. With appropriate treatment, the symptoms usually subside in 3–4 days. Not infrequently, due to severe systemic symptoms and gastrointestinal upset, intravenous antibiotics and adequate intravenous fluid replacement should be administered in the initial phase of acute pyelonephritis.

10.5 Infection Associated with Obstruction or Stones

If urinary infection is associated with an obstructed urinary tract, surgical relief of the obstructed system should be considered.

The presence of urinary tract stones may be a cause for persistent pyuria. If there is recurrent or relapsing UTI as evidenced by clinical features of infection and bacteriuria, then treatment is necessary. In these cases, stones often need to be surgically treated before the infection can be resolved.

Table 10.3 Treatment of prostatitis and prostatic abscess.

Subset	Usual pathogens	Preferred IV therapy	Alternate IV therapy	PO therapy or IV-to-PO switch
Acute prostatitis/ Acute prostatic abscess	Entero-bacteriaceae	Quinolone[a] (IV) × 2 weeks or Ceftriaxone 1 g (IV) q24h × 2 weeks	TMP-SMX 2.5 mg/kg (IV) q6h × 2 weeks or Aztreonam 2 g (IV) q8h × 2 weeks	Quinolone[a] (PO) × 2 weeks or Doxycycline 200 mg (PO) q12h × 3 days, then 100 mg (PO) q24h × 11 days or TMP-SMX 1 SS tablet (PO) q12h × 2 weeks
Chronic prostatitis	Entero-bacteriaceae	IV therapy not applicable	Quinolone[a] (PO) × 1–3 months or Doxycycline 100 mg (PO) q24h × 1–3 months or TMP-SMX 1 DS tablet (PO) q12h × 1–3 months	Quinolone[a] (PO) × 1–3 months or Doxycycline 100 mg (PO) q24h × 1–3 months or TMP-SMX 1 DS tablet (PO) q12h × 1–3 months

Duration of therapy represents total time IV, PO, or IV + PO. Most patients on IV therapy who are able to take PO medications should be switched to PO therapy soon after clinical improvement (usually <72 h).

TMP-SMX: trimethoprim-sulfamethoxazole. SS: single strength. DS: double strength.

[a] Ciprofloxacin XR 1000 mg (PO) q24h or ciprofloxacin 400 mg (IV) q12h or levofloxacin 500 mg (IV or PO) q24h or gatifloxacin 400 mg (IV or PO) q24h.

Table 10.4 Treatment of acute pyelonephritis.

Oral antibiotics
  Co-trimoxazole 2 tabs 12 hourly
  Ciprofloxacin 500 mg 12 hourly
  Amoxicillin 500 mg 8 hourly
  Levofloxacin 500 mg once a day

Parenteral antibiotics
  Cetriaxone 1 g 12 hourly
  Ampicillin 500 mg 6 hourly
  Ciprofloxacin 400 mg 12 hourly
  Imipenem 500 mg 6 hourly

10.6 Infection Associated with Urinary Catheters

Urinary catheters are associated with an increased risk of UTI and should be avoided if possible. Intermittent catheterization has a lower risk of infection. Bacteriuria and pyuria should not be routinely screened for. Treatment should be instituted only if there are symptoms/signs of infection.

Treatment of urine infection in catheterized patients includes:

- removal of catheter
- intermittent catheterization
- oral or parenteral antibiotics, depending on the comorbidity and clinical status of the patient.

Suggested Reading

Abrahamian FM, Moran GJ, Talan DA. (2008) Urinary tract infections in the emergency department. *Infect Dis Clin North Am* 22:73–87.

Craig WD, Wagner BJ, Travis MD. (2008) Pyelonephritis: radiologic-pathologic review. *Radiographics* 28:255–277.

Jacobsen SM, Stickler DJ, Mobley HL, Shirtliff ME. (2008) Complicated catheter-associated urinary tract infections due to *Escherichia coli* and *Proteus mirabilis*. *Clin Microbiol Rev* 21:26–59.

Neal DE Jr. (2008) Complicated urinary tract infections. *Urol Clin North Am* 35:13–22.

Nicolle LE. (2008) Uncomplicated urinary tract infection in adults including uncomplicated pyelonephritis. *Urol Clin North Am* 35:1–12.

Tenke P, Kovacs B, Bjerklund Johansen TE, *et al.* (2008) European and Asian guidelines on management and prevention of catheter-associated urinary tract infections. *Int J Antimicrob Agents* 31 (Suppl 1): S68–S78.

Part II
Chronic Renal Failure and Dialysis

11

Principle of Management for Patients with Chronic Kidney Disease

Meguid El Nahas and Mohsen El Kossi

11.1 Background

Chronic kidney disease (CKD) is defined as kidney damage or a glomerular filtration rate (GFR) of <60 mL/min/1.73 m² for 3 months or more, irrespective of the cause. The Kidney Disease Outcomes Quality Initiative (K/DOQI) guidelines have classified CKD into five stages (refer to Chapter 1).

CKD stage 5 reflects end-stage renal disease (ESRD). Globally, there is a steady rise in the number of ESRD patients requiring treatment by renal replacement therapy (RRT). It is estimated that by 2010 there will be in excess of 2 million individuals with ESRD patients treated by dialysis or transplantation. This rise has been attributed to aging of the population and an increase in the number of those suffering from diabetes mellitus. Table 11.1 outlines the ESRD prevalence by countries.

Whilst ESRD is on the increase and its treatment is cost-prohibitive for most countries/economies, there is also a perceived global increase in the incidence and prevalence of CKD. In Western/developed countries, there are precise estimates of the incidence and prevalence of ESRD through well-documented renal registries. This is, unfortunately, not the case in many emerging countries. It is also not the case worldwide for CKD, as systematic surveys of the prevalence of CKD are lacking. It has been estimated in the US that in excess of 10% of the population may suffer from some degree of CKD. Based on a number of studies, the prevalence of CKD stage 3 worldwide seems to be around 2%–3% of the general population. Of note, only 0.1% of the population reach ESRD, implying either lack of progression to CKD stage 5, lack of access to a registry or to dialysis treatment, or death before reaching ESRD. The latter may be

Table 11.1 Incidence and prevalence of RRT in different parts of the world.

Country	Incidence (pmp/year)	Prevalence (pmp)
USA total population	333	1446
Caucasians	255	1060
African-Americans	982	4467
Australia	94	658
Europe	129	770
Japan	262	1726
China	~15–100[a]	~33–269[b]
India	30–240[a]	~30

[a] Absence of accurate data collection and renal ESRD registries in these countries make it difficult to have a precise and reliable estimation of ESRD incidence and prevalence. Consequently, the values given in the table are approximations and often historically based on a number of reports and personal communication.
[b] Data from Beijing in 2004 for prevalence.

due to the very high cardiovascular morbidity and mortality associated with CKD. In fact, CKD patients are considered to be at the highest cardiovascular risk: a >25% event rate over a 10-year period. Thus, CKD and cardiovascular disease (CVD) combine to cause one of the highest mortality burdens on Western societies, and contribute considerably to the global burden of noncommunicable disease. Whilst diabetic- and hypertensive-related kidney disease contribute more than half of the total burden of ESRD, other well-established causes include chronic glomerulonephritis (affecting ~20%), chronic pyelonephritis/interstitial nephritis (~15%), and polycystic kidney disease (~8%).

11.2 Detection of CKD

Worldwide, there has been an explosion of CKD detection programs. For a detection program to be effective, CKD has to be highly prevalent and has to have serious consequences, the detection tools must be reliable and reproducible, and the detection program has to be cost-effective. With that in mind, there is little scope for general-population CKD detection programs as they are unlikely to be cost-effective. More appropriate would be targeted screening of individuals at risk (Table 11.2).

Screening should be undertaken relying on urinalysis (dipstick testing for proteinuria and/or hematuria) and measurement of serum

Table 11.2 Susceptibility factors predisposing the initiation and progression of CKD.

Susceptibility factors	Initiation factors	Progression factors
Genetic	Hypertension[a]	Genetic/Race/Ethnicity/Poverty
Familial	Diabetes[a]	Gender
Race	Dyslipidemia	Hypertension[a]
Ethnicity	Obesity	Proteinuria[a]
	Poverty	Dyslipidemia
Age	Smoking	Obesity
Gender	Drugs	Smoking
	Infections	

[a] Factors with strong clinical evidence.

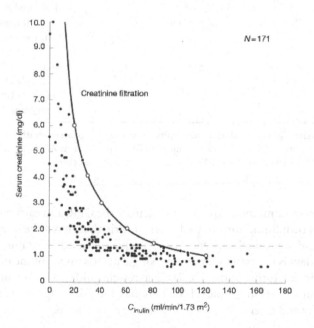

Fig. 11.1 Relationship between serum creatinine and GFR measured by inulin clearance.

creatinine. The latter on its own is not reliable as a sole factor for CKD diagnosis, and this could be explained by the relationship demonstrated in Fig. 11.1 between serum creatinine and glomerular filtration rate (GFR).

Table 11.3 Definition of albuminuria and proteinuria.

Parameter	Level	Equivalent	Management
Albuminuria/ Microalbuminuria	ACR Male: 2.5–30 mg/mmol Female: 3.5–30 mg/mmol	Male:20–200 mg/24 h Female:30–300 mg/24 h	CKD primary care monitoring If isolated (eGFR > 60 and/or no hematuria) Control: DM, BP, smoking ACEIs and ARBs as indicated
Proteinuria	ACR: >30 mg/mmol PCR: >45 mg/mmol	>300 mg/24 h	CKD primary care monitoring If isolated & PCR < 100 mg/mmol Control: DM, BP, smoking ACEIs and ARBs as indicated if PCR > 100 mg/mmol

Abbreviations: ACR, albumin:creatinine ratio; PCR, protein:creatinine ratio; eGFR, estimated GFR; DM, diabetes mellitus; BP, blood pressure; ACEIs, angiotensin-converting enzyme inhibitors; ARBs, angiotensin receptor blockers.

Different methods are used to calculate the GFR, and each method has its own limitations (see Chapter 1). Urinalysis has to be quantitative and reproducible. One of the frequently used laboratory tests nowadays is the estimation, from a single urine sample, of the urinary protein:creatinine ratio (PCR) as a rough guide for 24-h urinary protein excretion (Table 11.3). This has the advantage of avoiding lengthy and often inaccurate 24-h urinary collections.

11.3 Referral of Patients to Nephrology Centers

The management of patients with CKD can be undertaken in either primary or tertiary care. Once detected, CKD management should be optimized in order to slow the progression of the disease as well as to minimize its complications. Patients with stable kidney damage and eGFR > 60 mL/min/1.73 m^2 can be followed up in primary care, as they are unlikely to progress to ESRD and have few systemic complications; these would include patients with isolated microscopic hematuria and those with mild proteinuria (<1 g/24 h; urinary PCR < 100 mg/mmol). These patients warrant regular monitoring of their renal function maybe every 4–6 months, blood pressure, and urinalysis.

On the other hand, patients with eGFR < 60 mL/min/1.73 m², declining renal function (loss of >4 mL/min/year), or moderate-to-heavy proteinuria (>1 g/24 h) should be referred for a nephrological opinion. Table 11.4 outlines the referral guidelines in the United Kingdom.

11.4 Interventions Aimed at Slowing the Progression of CKD

The progression of CKD, regardless of its underlying cause, is associated with poorly controlled hypertension. Consequently, the control of hypertension is considered the single most important intervention to slow the progression of CKD. Target levels of BP have been set by different organizations and societies at <130/80 mmHg; lower targets have been advocated in those with moderate-to-heavy proteinuria (>1 g/24 h) and in those with diabetic nephropathy. In these diabetic and proteinuric patients, with a faster rate of decline in GFR, the use of inhibitors of the angiotensin system such as ACEIs and ARBs has been recommended. In the others, i.e. those with nondiabetic and nonproteinuric nephropathies, there is little evidence that these agents have a therapeutic advantage and national BP control recommendations should be followed. In the United Kingdom, the initial combination of a diuretic and calcium antagonist is thought to have the best risk-benefit profile and be the most cost-effective for nondiabetic and nonproteinuric nephropathies.

Besides the control of hypertension, it is important to reduce proteinuria — hence, the use of ACEIs and ARBs alone or in combination in proteinuric CKD patients with or without diabetic nephropathy. The addition of a diuretic or dietary salt restriction (<60 mmol/day) enhances the antiproteinuric effect of angiotensin inhibition. CKD patients should be advised to reduce their dietary salt intake. It is also important to closely monitor CKD patients started on ACEIs or ARBs, as these agents can seriously compromise kidney function in susceptible individuals (those with renal artery stenosis) as well as induce hyperkalemia. It is therefore advised that renal function test

Table 11.4   Referral guidelines for CKD.

Parameter	Definition	Need for nephrology referral
eGFR CKD stage 3	30–59 mL/min/1.73 m^2	Routine nephrology referral for assessment; if progressive CKD, hypertension, proteinuria, and/or hematuria as detailed below
CKD stage 4	15–29 mL/min/1.73 m^2	Urgent referral
CKD stage 5	<15 mL/min/1.73 m^2	Immediate referral to consider RRT
Hypertension	Malignant hypertension	Immediate nephrology referral
	Refractory hypertension (on 3 drugs)	Urgent nephrology referral
Proteinuria	PCR <100 mg/mmol (<1 g/24 h) without hematuria and with normal eGFR	CKD primary care monitoring
	PCR <100 mg/mmol + hematuria or impaired eGFR <60 mL/min/1.73 m^2	Refer to nephrologist for assessment
	PCR >100 mg/mmol	Refer to nephrologist for assessment
	Nephrotic syndrome	Urgent referral to nephrologist
Hematuria	Macroscopic	Fast-track urology referral
	Microscopic (nonglomerular): age >50 years	Refer to urology
	Microscopic isolated after exclusion of urological cause	CKD primary care program
	Hematuria + proteinuria or eGFR <60 mL/min/1.73 m^2	Refer to nephrologist

should be repeated within 1 week of treatment initiation and again at 4 weeks. An increase in serum creatinine value exceeding 25% of the baseline value should lead to immediate discontinuation of the treatment.

11.5 Slowing the Progression of CKD

The management guidelines are summarized in Table 11.5.

- Try to exclude and treat any reversible causes such as obstruction with early ultrasound imaging, particularly in the elderly.
- Establish the rate of progression by calculating the rate of fall of eGFR (mL/min/1.73 m^2/year).
- Optimize BP control: <130/80 mmHg and possibly lower in diabetic nephropathy and proteinuric nephropathies (>1 g/24 h).
- Start with ACEIs or ARBs in proteinuric and diabetic nephropathies (with proteinuria).
- If BP is uncontrolled and/or if proteinuria > 1 g/24 h, increase the dose of ACEI or ARB and add diuretic (loop diuretic if GFR < 30 mL/min) and dietary salt restriction (<60 mmol/day). ACEIs and ARBs can be administered in combination.

Table 11.5 Management guidelines for CKD.

Parameter	Target	Agent used
Blood pressure	<130/80 mmHg <125/75 mmHg in diabetics and in those with proteinuria >100 mg/mmol (1g/24 h)	Preferably start with ACEIs or ARBs in proteinuric CKD; otherwise, a combination of calcium antagonist and a diuretic is an alternative (caution with ACEIs and ARBs in the elderly and in those with atherosclerosis) Close monitoring of eGFR
Proteinuria	PCR < 100 mg/mmol (<1g/24 h)	To reduce proteinuria use: ACEIs/ARBs + low-salt diet + diuretics
Serum Cholesterol	<5 mmol/L	Statins
Smoking	None	Stop smoking
Alcohol	<2 units/day	Reduce drinking if excessive
Avoid		NSAIDs, COX inhibitors, RCM (particular avoidance of RCM in patients with diabetes, multiple myeloma, and congestive heart failure as well as in the elderly and volume-depleted)

NSAIDs, non-steroidal anti-inflammatory drugs; COX, cyclooxygenase; RCM, radio-contrast material.

- Closely monitor changes in serum creatinine/GFR. Stop ACEI or ARB if the GFR falls by more than 25% at 1–4 weeks after initiation or change of regimen.
- In nonproteinuric, nondiabetic CKD, calcium antagonist + diuretic are an alternative antihypertensive treatment.
- Third-line therapy could consist of alpha- or beta-blockade, depending on associated comorbidities; a cardioselective beta-blocker would be preferred in patients with a history of CVD.
- If BP remains uncontrolled, consider the underlying diagnosis of renovascular hypertension and atherosclerotic renal artery stenosis/ischemic nephropathy.
- Avoid acute decline of GFR precipitated by intercurrent illnesses such as volume depletion in diarrhoeal states or vomiting as well as by the use of NSAIDs, aminoglycosides, and contrast agents in diagnostic imaging. The latter should be avoided if there is any alternative approach for diagnosis; otherwise, use precautions judiciously in these circumstances (refer to Chapter 9).

11.6 Interventions Aimed at Reducing CKD Complications

As mentioned earlier, the major cause of morbidity and mortality in CKD patients is CVD. CKD patients are at the highest CVD risk. This is due to a variety of factors, some conventional (hypertension, smoking, and dyslipidemia) and others CKD-specific (anemia as well as changes in calcium-phosphorus-parathyroid hormone balance oxidant-antioxidant balance, and nitric oxide homeostasis). Consequently, in order to minimize CVD complications in CKD, hypertension and dyslipidemia have to be corrected and smoking has to stop. Also, early management of anemia and calcium-phosphorus homeostasis have to be initiated.

Among the routine investigations for these patients is estimation of serum hematinics including serum ferritin and transferrin saturation. To treat anemia in these patients, we usually start iron-repleting these patients with oral iron at a higher GFR (probably >30 mL/min) and then with intravenous iron at a lower GFR as they do not tolerate oral iron well and iron absorption is affected. After correction of iron depletion by aiming for a serum ferritin target of 500–800 μmol/L and a transferrin saturation more than 20%, the next step is administration of recombinant human erythropoietin. Try to correct metabolic acidosis by adding sodium bicarbonate cautiously, particularly among patients with fluid overload.

Table 11.6   Management guidelines for reducing CKD complications.

Complication	Management	Target
CVD	Hypertension, dyslipidemia, smoking, anemia, renal osteodystrophy (mineral and bone metabolism)	
Hypertension	As discussed above	<130/80 mmHg
Hypercholesterolemia	Statins	Total cholesterol: < 5 mmol/L LDL cholesterol: < 2.1 mmol/L
Smoking	Cessation	Cessation
Anemia	Correct deficiencies: Iron Folate Administer erythropoietin	Hemoglobin: 11–12 g/dL Serum ferritin: 500–800 µmol/L Serum folic acid: 2–5 mg/mL 4000–10,000/units/ week (maintenance dosage according to hemoglobin level)
Calcium (Ca)	Correct hypocalcemia: administer Vitamin D	2.1–2.3 mmol/L
Phosphorus (Pi)	Correct hyperphosphatemia: use phosphate binders	1.2–1.7 mmol/L
Parathyroid hormone (PTH)	Same as for Ca and Pi	2–3 times upper limit of normal (150–300 pg/mL)
Nutrition	Avoid malnutrition Protein intake: 0.8 g/kg/day (CKD stages 3–5) Calories: 35 kcal/kg/day	Serum albumin >40 g/L
Infections	Chest infections HepatitisB	Immunization: influenza and pneumococcus Vaccination (CKD stages 4–5)

Secondary hyperparathyroidism is one of the frequent complications in CKD patients. Advice from a renal dietitian is needed for these patients about a low-phosphate diet; phosphate binders are required if dietary restrictions fail. Vitamin D supplementation, along with the correction of hypocalcemia, hyperphosphatemia, and hyperparathyroidism, will have the advantage of minimizing the severity of renal osteodystrophy. Patients with advanced kidney failure (CKD stages 4 and 5) have some degree of malnutrition due to anorexia and hypercatabolism, as well as many dietary restrictions like low-phosphate and low-potassium diets. It is imperative that adequate nutrition is maintained with the help of a renal dietian to avoid the associated increased morbidity and mortality. Attention should be given to fluid overload by salt and water restriction and high doses of loop diuretics.

11.7 Preparation of Patients for Renal Replacement Therapy (RRT)

Timely referral of CKD patients will allow enough time for proper preparation of these patients for RRT in the form of dialysis or transplantation. This will help avoiding dialysing patients as an emergency with temporary lines and the potential problems of infections and central venous stenosis. At a GFR of 15 mL/min, patients with CKD should be prepared for RRT.

11.8 Conclusion

CKD is a common, detectable, and preventable condition. It is imperative that increased awareness of CKD leads to earlier detection and better management. Care of CKD has to be integrated, involving primary and tertiary care teams. Patient education is also important to raise awareness within communities and to improve compliance and outcomes.

Suggested Reading

Coresh J, Wei GL, McQuillan G, *et al.* (2001) Prevalence of high blood pressure and elevated serum creatinine level in the United States: findings from the third National Health and Nutrition Examination Survey (1988–1994). *Arch Intern Med* 161:1207–1216.
Lysaght MJ. (2002) Maintenance dialysis population dynamics: current trends and long-term implications. *J Am Soc Nephrol* 13(Suppl 1):S37–S40.

National Kidney Foundation. (2002) K/DOQI clinical practice guidelines for chronic kidney disease: evaluation, classification, and stratification. *Am J Kidney Dis* 39(Suppl 1):S1–S266.

Weiner E, Tighiouart H, Elsayed F, *et al.* (2008) The relationship between nontraditional risk factors and outcomes in individuals with stage 3 to 4 CKD. *Am J Kidney Dis* 51:212–223.

Williams B, Poulter R, Brown J, *et al*; British Hypertension Society. (2004) Guidelines for management of hypertension: report of the fourth working party of the British Hypertension Society, 2004-BHS IV. *J Hum Hypertens* 18:139–185.

12

Acceptance into the Chronic Dialysis Program

Dae-Suk Han

The Kidney Disease Outcomes Quality Initiative (K/DOQI) guidelines recommend that patients with chronic kidney disease (CKD) who reach an estimated glomerular filtration rate (GFR) of 15–30 mL/min/ 1.73 m^2 (i.e. stage 4) need to be prepared for kidney replacement therapy. Before commencing dialysis, subjective symptoms and signs of the patient, objective parameters assessed by a nephrologist, and other medical and social considerations should be evaluated in a multidisciplinary approach to provide the optimal therapy.

12.1 Criteria for Acceptance into the Chronic Dialysis Program

There are a number of factors that should be taken into account before accepting a patient into the chronic dialysis program and initiating dialysis:

- Subjective symptoms
- Objective parameters
- Evaluation and management of comorbidity
- Choice of modality
- Timing of dialysis initiation
- Socioeconomic status
- Cultural influences

12.1.1 *Subjective Symptoms*

- Patients with CKD do not feel "well" as kidney function deteriorates.
- In general, they complain of nausea, vomiting, anorexia, general weakness, etc.

- Inadequate food intake due to uremia may lead to malnutrition.
- However, some patients are adapted to such conditions chronically and these symptoms may not be evident even in advanced stage.
- In addition, many medications such as oral iron often have side effects that mimic uremic symptoms.

12.1.2 *Objective Parameters*

- The two most widely used parameters in deciding whether or not to initiate dialysis are estimation of GFR and assessment of nutritional status.
- The Modification of Diet in Renal Disease (MDRD) formula was derived from patients with renal failure and has been used to estimate GFR (see Chapter 1). K/DOQI guidelines suggest that patients with stage 4 CKD should be prepared for kidney replacement therapy, and that dialysis should be considered in those with an estimated GFR (eGFR) less than 15 mL/min/1.73 m^2.
- Malnutrition is another indication for dialysis commencement. Many studies of patients on maintenance dialysis have shown an increased mortality risk associated with malnutrition at the time of initiation. Nutritional status can be easily monitored by assessing daily protein intake. Normalized protein nitrogen appearance (nPNA) is a useful measurement for protein metabolism, and an nPNA below 0.8 g/kg/day is indicative of a malnourished state. Other nutritional markers include plasma concentrations of albumin, prealbumin, creatinine, cholesterol, etc.
- In addition, intractable volume overload, hypertension, and biochemical disturbances unresponsive to medical treatment (i.e. hyperkalemia, metabolic acidosis, hyperphosphatemia, and anemia) warrant prompt dialysis initiation.

12.1.3 *Evaluation and Management of Comorbidity*

- Comorbid conditions at the start of dialysis are important in determining patient outcomes.
- K/DOQI guidelines suggest that the common abnormalities which are found as CKD progresses, such as anemia, renal osteodystrophy, and malnutrition, should be properly treated to reduce comorbidity in end-stage renal disease (ESRD) patients.
- Particularly, traditional as well as nontraditional risk factors associated with cardiovascular disease should be evaluated thoroughly

and managed aggressively because most patients die of cardio-vascular complications.

12.1.4 *Choice of Modality*

- The selection of dialysis modality is influenced by a number of considerations such as patient education about treatment modalities, availability of dialysis facilities, comorbid conditions, socioeconomic status, center experience, method of physician reimbursement, etc.
- Generally, most ESRD patients are suitable for either peritoneal dialysis (PD) or hemodialysis (HD). However, physicians should be aware of the limitations of each modality in specific clinical situations. Absolute and relative contraindications for HD and PD are listed in Table 12.1.
- There have been many studies concerning the relative effect on mortality of PD versus HD. To date, the long-term outcome of PD compared to HD remains uncertain. It has been suggested that PD might confer a survival advantage over HD until 2 years of dialysis initiation. This could be attributable to the more preserved residual renal function in PD patients. Several studies,

Table 12.1 Absolute and relative contraindications for hemodialysis (HD) and peritoneal dialysis (PD).

Absolute contraindications	Relative contraindications
Peritoneal dialysis	
Loss of peritoneal function	Recent aortic graft
Adhesions blocking dialysate flow	Ventriculoperitoneal shunt
Surgically uncorrectable abdominal hernia	Intolerance of intra-abdominal fluid
Abdominal wall stoma	Large muscle mass
Diaphragmatic fluid leak	Morbid obesity
Inability to perform exchanges in absence of suitable assistant	Severe malnutrition
	Skin infection
	Bowel disease
Hemodialysis	
No vascular access possible	Difficult vascular access
	Needle phobia
	Cardiac failure
	Coagulopathy

however, have reported that this survival benefit of PD disappeared after 2 years of dialysis initiation and that the survival rate of PD patients started to decline afterwards compared to HD patients.

- In specific groups such as younger or nondiabetic patients, PD may offer a slight advantage. In addition, PD is often favored in elderly patients with severe cardiovascular disease and unstable hemodynamics.

12.1.5 Timing of Dialysis Initiation

- Timely initiation of dialysis is important because delaying the initiation of dialysis until one or more uremic complications is present may jeopardize the patient's life.
- Whether an early start improves patient outcome remains an open question. Several studies have reported that early initiation of dialysis did not provide a survival benefit and was associated with increased mortality. Although there have been some reports favoring improved survival among timely starters, this survival benefit might result from lead time bias.
- Nevertheless, early initiation appears to have additional advantages in terms of improving nutritional status and allowing better control of hypertension or volume overload.
- No truly randomized trial regarding this issue has been conducted yet. The Initiating Dialysis Early and Late (IDEAL) study is an ongoing trial to determine the impact of early start versus late start on patient outcomes. This study may provide an answer to the question of whether the timing of dialysis initiation has an effect on survival.

12.1.6 Socioeconomic Status

- Patients in advanced CKD with low socioeconomic status often hesitate to seek physicians, thus resulting in delayed dialysis initiation.
- It also has an impact on the quality of life, morbidity and mortality. For example, in patients with PD, low socioeconomic status and low education level are associated with the increased incidence of peritonitis.
- It is suggested that the highly educated and socially active patients tend to prefer self-care dialysis such as PD or home HD.

12.1.7 *Cultural Influences*

- Diverse cultural backgrounds may affect decision making on starting dialysis. Some ethnic minorities tend to operate within a more family-centered model of decision making than Europeans and Americans. In this regard, PD may be particularly suitable for patients who prefer that care be delivered by family.
- On the other hand, there are patients who feel that it is not appropriate for medical treatment to be done at home. For example, in Japan, PD utilization rate is less than 4%, which is less than half the world average because of reluctance to take responsibility for delivering their own care and a desire to avoid complicated procedures.

12.2 Clinical Indications for Commencing Dialysis

- In summary, clinical conditions that may prompt the initiation of dialysis, which are adopted from K/DOQI guidelines, are listed in Table 12.2.
- However, such indications are potentially life-threatening. Therefore, dialysis should be started well before these complications occur

Table 12.2 Clinical indication of the initiation of dialysis.

Nonurgent indications

    Intractable extracellular volume overload and/or hypertension
    Hyperkalemia refractory to dietary restriction and pharmacologic treatment
    Metabolic acidosis refractory to bicarbonate treatment
    Hyperphosphatemia refractory to dietary counseling and to treatment with phosphorus binders
    Anemia refractory to erythropoietin and iron treatment
    Otherwise unexplained decline in functioning or well-being
    Recent weight loss or deterioration of nutritional status, especially if accompanied by persistent nausea and vomiting

Urgent indications

    Progressive uremic encephalopathy or neuropathy, with signs such as confusion, asterixis, myoclonus, wrist or foot drop, or (in severe cases) seizures
    Pericarditis or pleuritis without other explanation
    A clinically significant bleeding diathesis attributable to uremia

---

and patients with CKD should be closely followed up with the eGFR monitored.

- Besides these clinical indications, initiation of dialysis should be strongly considered when the GFR is below 10–15 mL/min/1.73 m², especially in elderly patients and diabetics.

Suggested Reading

Dombros N, Dratwa M, Feriani M, et al. (2005) European best practice guidelines for peritoneal dialysis. 2. The initiation of dialysis. Nephrol Dial Transplant 20(Suppl 9):ix3–ix7.

Hakim RM, Lazarus JM. (1995) Initiation of dialysis. J Am Soc Nephrol 6:1319–1328.

Heaf JG, Lokkegaard H, Madsen M. (2002) Initial survival advantage of peritoneal dialysis relative to haemodialysis. Nephrol Dial Transplant 17:112–117.

Hemodialysis Adequacy 2006 Work Group. (2006) Clinical practice guidelines for hemodialysis adequacy, update 2006. Am J Kidney Dis 48(Suppl 1): S2–S90.

Korevaar JC, Jansen MA, Dekker RW, et al. (2001) When to initiate dialysis: effect of proposed US guidelines on survival. Lancet 358:1046–1050.

Maroni BJ, Steinman TI, Mitch WE. (1985) A method for estimating nitrogen intake of patients with chronic renal failure. Kidney Int 27:58–65.

National Kidney Foundation. (2002) K/DOQI clinical practice guidelines for chronic kidney disease: evaluation, classification, and stratification. Am J Kidney Dis 39(Suppl 1):S1–S266.

Peritoneal Dialysis Adequacy Work Group. (2006) Clinical practice guidelines for peritoneal dialysis adequacy. Am J Kidney Dis 48(Suppl 1):S98–S129.

Tang SC, Ho YW, Tang AW, et al. (2007) Delaying initiation of dialysis till symptomatic uraemia — is it too late? Nephrol Dial Transplant 22:1926–1932.

Traynor JP, Simpson K, Geddes CC, et al. (2002) Early initiation of dialysis fails to prolong survival in patients with end-stage renal failure. J Am Soc Nephrol 13:2125–2132.

Vonesh EF, Snyder JJ, Foley RN, Collins AJ. (2006) Mortality studies comparing peritoneal dialysis and hemodialysis: what do they tell us? Kidney Int 70(Suppl):S3–S11.

13

Peritoneal Dialysis — Management of Tenckhoff Catheter and Ultrafiltration Problems

Wai-Kei Lo

13.1 Introduction

Peritoneal dialysis is a well-established long-term renal replacement therapy for patients with end-stage renal failure. It is basically a home dialysis therapy. There are several forms of peritoneal dialysis, of which continuous ambulatory peritoneal dialysis (CAPD) and automated peritoneal dialysis (APD) are most commonly used. CAPD is performed manually with several exchanges a day. APD refers to peritoneal dialysis conducted with a machine with multiple exchanges at night and a long dwell in day time (continuous cyclic peritoneal dialysis), or multiple nocturnal exchanges with empty peritoneal cavity in day time (nocturnal intermittent peritoneal dialysis).

13.2 Peritoneal Dialysis Catheter — Tenckhoff Catheter

The peritoneal dialysis catheter is the lifeline of patients. The standard peritoneal dialysis catheter is a double-cuffed flexible silicone catheter (Tenckhoff catheter). There are many different configurations in the catheter design. The classical design is a straight catheter with two Dacron cuffs for fixation in the abdominal wall. The commonest variations are swan neck (a fixed bend between the two cuffs) and curled tip. Data suggest that the implantation technique is more important than the catheter configuration.

13.2.1 Specification for Catheter Implantation

For good functioning of the catheter, there are several specifications on the implantation:

- the catheter is best implanted in the lower paramedian abdomen through the anterior rectus muscle;
- the catheter tip should be placed in the pelvic cavity;
- the catheter should exit through a subcutaneous tunnel with a downward direction; and
- the external cuff should be around 1–2 cm beneath the exit site.

13.2.2 Tenckhoff Catheter Implantation Technique under Local Anesthesia

There are four main approaches: — trocar, surgical mini-laparotomy, Seldinger technique (transcutaneous approach) with or without laparoscopic assistance, and peritoneoscopic implantation. All of them can be performed under local anesthesia, although laparoscopy is usually performed under general anesthesia.

13.2.2.1 Implantation with Trocar

This method is a very old technique and is rarely used now. It requires blunt introduction of a trocar through the abdominal wall at the linea alba, and then the catheter is inserted through the trocar towards the pelvis. Acute complications like bleeding, leakage of peritoneal fluid, and visceral organ trauma and dislocation, as well as late complications like incisional hernia, are quite common.

13.2.2.2 Surgical Mini-laparotomy

This is the standard method for Tenckhoff catheter implantation. It can be performed by nephrologists after training. The surgical steps are as follows:

- Make a lower paramedian incision in the skin.
- Dissect the subcutaneous tissue and the anterior rectus sheath.
- Split the rectus muscles to expose the posterior rectus sheath.
- Cut open the posterior rectus sheath and the peritoneum.
- Tie a purse string around the peritoneum opening.

- Insert the Tenckhoff catheter with a stylet or stiff guidewire into the pelvic cavity, and then remove the stylet or guidewire.
- Close the peritoneum tightly by the purse string.
- Embed the inner cuff of the catheter inside the rectus muscle.
- Suture the anterior rectus sheath tightly.
- Create a subcutaneous tunnel so that the catheter exits through the subcutaneous tunnel at a downward direction laterally.
- Suture the skin with absorbable sutures.
- Fix the catheter at the exit with some sterile tapes or immobilizer, but not with stitches.

This technique is best conducted in a proper operating room setting. Though a delayed break-in period of 2–3 weeks is preferred, peritoneal dialysis of small-volume hourly cycles may be started immediately if needed.

13.2.2.3 *Seldinger Technique — With or Without Laparoscopic Assistance*

After a small incison of the skin, a guidewire is inserted through the rectus muscles into the pelvic cavity with an introducer. The catheter is then inserted along the guidewire while the sheath of the introducer is gradually peeled away. A subcutaneous tunnel is created in the usual manner. This method can be performed at the patient's bedside or in an operating room. Laparoscopy through another incision can be used to help locate the catheter tip in the pelvic cavity.

13.2.2.4 *Peritoneoscopic Approach*

This approach uses a peritoneoscope to visualize the pelvis, and the catheter is then inserted through the same track with a modified Seldinger technique. The results of Seldinger technique with or without laparoscopic assistance and peritoneoscopic implantation have been reported as good as, or even better than, surgical mini-laparotomy. Preoperative antibiotics such as 1 g of cephazolin is commonly given intravenously to reduce the chance of wound infection.

13.2.3 *Postoperative Care*

Postoperatively, the exit site should be covered by occlusive dressing. The dressing is usually changed once a week for the first 2–3 weeks, and more frequently if there is oozing or leakage. Thereafter, more frequent changes of dressing are needed until the exit-site wound is completely healed and mature at around 6 weeks.

13.2.4 Common Complications of Implantation

- Hemorrhage — Wound bleeding, exit-site bleeding, subcutaneous or intramuscular hematoma, and intra-abdominal hemorrhage may occur. Intravenous desmopressin (DDAVP) or local injection of subcutaneous adrenaline may help stop the bleeding (refer to Chapter 20 for the dosage).
- Leakage of dialyzate — This can be managed by reducing the dwell volume of peritoneal dialyzate or by stopping peritoneal dialysis temporarily for a few days.
- Visceral organ damage — Bowel or bladder wall perforation during implantation have been reported. Bladder wall perforation can be prevented by prior emptying of the bladder immediately before implantation.
- Dislocation or migration of catheter tip — This may lead to poor ultrafiltration. Various techniques have been developed to reduce the chance of dislocation or subsequent migration of the catheter tip, including catheter designs, fixation of catheter to the anterior abdominal wall, alignment of catheter, and routine omentectomy.
- Wound infection — This can be minimized by preoperative antibiotic prophylaxis (usually an intravenous injection of cephazolin), fixation of the external portion of the catheter, and proper postoperative care.

13.3 Tenckhoff Catheter Exit-Site Infection

Tenckhoff catheter exit-site infection (ESI) is quite common, and may lead to tunnel tract infection or even peritonitis. Signs of ESI include purulent discharge, erythema, swelling, granuloma, and maceration of the sinus tract (the tract between skin and external Dacron cuff). Swelling and erythema over the subcutaneous tunnel tract indicate tunnel tract infection. Sometimes, tunnel tract infection is subclinical and may be diagnosed by ultrasound examination showing a layer of thin film of fluid along the catheter in the tunnel tract.

13.3.1 Prevention

ESI can be prevented or minimized by proper exit-site care. Patients should be taught how to perform daily exit-site cleansing. In addition, daily local antibiotic application prophylaxis has been demonstrated to reduce ESI, including:

(i) mūpirocin cream application

- intranasally for nasal *Staphylococcus aureus* (methicillin-sensitive or methicillin-resistant) carriers or
- to exit site routinely; or

(ii) 0.1% gentamicin cream application to exit site.

Mupirocin is active against Gram-positive organisms. A marked reduction in staphylococcal ESI and peritonitis rate is well documented with routine mupirocin application, but it does not have an effect on Gram-negative organism infections. Gentamicin cream application has been reported to further reduce ESI by both Gram-positive and Gram-negative organisms.

13.3.2 *Management*

When ESI occurs, antibiotics are needed to treat the infection. As ESI is commonly caused by *Staphylococcus aureus*, oral cloxacillin or first-generation cephalosporins are commonly given as first-line antibiotics. Antibiotic therapy should be modified according to the sensitivity of the causative organism identified, and prolonged courses of antibiotic therapy may be needed for eradication of the ESI. When there is granuloma formation, silver nitrate cauterization of the granuloma once every 5–7 days may help.

Catheter removal is indicated for:

- refractory infection after a few weeks of antibiotics
- tunnel infection
- ESI associated with peritonitis.

Simultaneous removal and re-implantation of catheter — thus, avoiding the need for temporary hemodialysis — can be performed if the ESI is not associated with peritonitis or the tunnel tract infection is not too serious.

13.4 Ultrafiltration Problems

Fluid removed across the semipermeable peritoneal membrane is called ultrafiltration. It is essentially determined by the osmotic gradient across the peritoneum contributed by the glucose content in the peritoneal dialyzate. Ultrafiltration problems may arise from mechanical or medical causes.

13.4.1 Causes and Management

13.4.1.1 Mechanical Causes

Tenchoff catheter tip migration or dislocation

Dislocation out of the pelvic cavity leads to incomplete drainage of dialyzate and therefore reduction in ultrafiltration volume. This is easily diagnosed by taking a plain X-ray of the lower abdomen. Predisposing factors for migration of catheter tip include poor alignment of the catheter, constipation, distended bladder, and omental wrapping. Migrated catheters can be repositioned by

- Fleet enema to stimulate peristalsis in order to bring the cavity tip back to the pelvis
- manipulation with a stiff guidewire/stylet under fluoroscopy for straight catheters (it is difficult to pass the stylet through the fixed bend of a swan-neck catheter)
- laparoscopic repositioning ± fixation to pelvis.

Omental wrapping

The omentum may wrap around the catheter tip and cause obstruction to flow and/or migration. Classically, the outflow of dialyzate is affected much more than the inflow. Occasionally, unwrapping can be achieved by manipulating the catheter under fluoroscopy. The majority of cases require laparoscopic omentectomy or catheter removal followed by replacement of a new catheter.

Intraluminal fibrin or blood clots

Fibrin may be formed during peritoneal dialysis and may obstruct the flow of the catheter. Blood clot formation may follow intraperitoneal hemorrhage and obstruct the catheter. Both inflow and outflow are affected. The fibrin or blood clots may sometimes be seen inside the Tenckhoff catheter or the tubings. They may be flushed out of the catheter by normal saline. Intraluminal urokinase can be used to dissolve the clots and restore flow.

Peritoneopleural communication

Occasionally, peritoneal dialyzate may enter the pleural cavity via a communication developed through a congenital weak point in the diaphragm, usually on the right side. This often occurs suddenly and with sudden reduction of ultrafiltration volume followed by shortness of breath. Chest X-ray shows massive right pleural effusion. Diagnosis can be established by:

- paracentesis of pleural fluid demonstrating a glucose level higher than the serum glucose level and a very low protein level. The elevated pleural fluid glucose content may be more obvious when paracentesis is performed after instillation of 4.25% dialyzate into the peritoneal cavity;
- addition of methylene blue into peritoneal dialyzate to demonstrate the blue-colored pleural fluid by paracentesis; or
- computed tomography (CT) peritoneogram and thoracic CT after instillation of contrast-added peritoneal dialyzate, showing the contrast inside the pleural cavity.

The communication may be closed spontaneously with conversion to supine intermittent peritoneal dialysis or hemodialysis for several weeks. If it does not close, medical or surgical pleurodesis or thoracoscopic repair of the diaphragmatic defect may help.

Internal leakage, including retroperitoneal leakage

Internal leakage into extraperitoneal space will lead to reduction of ultrafiltration volume. Common sites of internal leakage are:

- anterior abdominal wall around the incision scars and umbilicus
- inguinal canal with or without hernia
- pelvic cavity.

In contrast to external leakage, no external fluid sipping is seen. Localized edema at the anterior abdominal wall, inguinal canal, or genital area is suggestive of internal leakage. If fluid is leaked into retroperitoneal space, no localized edema is seen. An unexplained reduction in ultrafiltration may be the only sign.

Diagnosis of internal leakage can be confirmed with CT peritoneogram demonstrating the contrast localized in extraperitoneal areas. Magnetic resonance imaging (MRI) may be used to demonstrate the localized water collection in the extraperitoneal space. Internal leakage may subside after a period of conversion to intermittent peritoneal dialysis or hemodialysis.

13.4.1.2 Medical Causes

This is often called ultrafiltration failure. Ultrafiltration failure is defined objectively by less than 400 mL of fluid removed after a 4-hour 2-L dwell of 4.25% dialyzate. The causes are:

- high peritoneal transport (or fast peritoneal transport)
- reduction in the effective peritoneal area
- high lymphatic absorption rate
- deficient aquaporin function.

Of these, high peritoneal transport is the commonest cause. Peritoneal equilibration test (PET) is the most commonly used method to define high peritoneal transport.

13.4.2 Mechanism

During a peritoneal dialysis cycle, which usually lasts for 4–8 h, fluid is removed from the body across the peritoneal membrane by osmosis contributed by the high concentration of glucose in the dialyzate. With time, the osmotic pressure gradient progressively falls as a result of glucose absorption, and the fluid removal rate gradually reduces. When equilibrium is reached, there is no fluid movement across the peritoneum and the intraperitoneal volume plateaus. Thereafter, the intraperitoneal volume gradually reduces due to lymphatic absorption and it will ultimately fall below the initial instillation volume. Fluid drained out at this stage will be less than the instilled volume. A higher concentration of glucose in the dialyzate will increase the peak intraperitoneal volume and delay the onset of equilibrium, thus taking a longer time for the intraperitoneal volume to fall below the initial volume (Fig. 13.1).

The higher the peritoneal transport rate, the faster the glucose is absorbed and hence the faster the osmotic pressure is dissipated and the faster the equilibrium is reached. Therefore, in patients with high peritoneal transport, the peak intraperitoneal volume is smaller and it takes less time for intraperitoneal volume to fall below the initial volume (Fig. 13.2), resulting in poorer ultrafiltration. To achieve

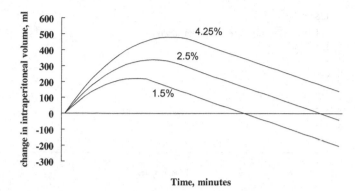

Fig. 13.1 The change in intraperitoneal volume during a peritoneal dialysis cycle using dialyzates with different concentrations of glucose.

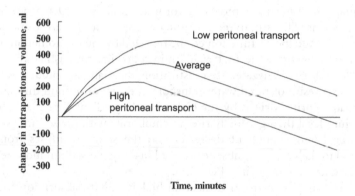

Fig. 13.2 The change in intraperitoneal volume during a peritoneal dialysis cycle in patients with different peritoneal transport rates.

more fluid removal, the dwell cycle has to be shortened by increasing the frequency of exchange, or a higher-glucose-concentration dialyzate has to be used.

Ultrafiltration due to high lymphatic absorption is less common and is difficult to diagnose. Definite diagnosis requires demonstration of the rate of fall of large molecules like radioactive-labeled serum albumin or dextran 70 added into the instilled dialyzate.

Water movement across the mesothelial layer of peritoneum by osmosis passes through both the tight intercellular gap (small pores)

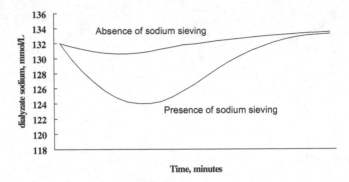

Fig. 13.3 Dialyzate sodium during a peritoneal dialysis cycle in patients with normal sodium sieving and in the absence of sodium sieving.

and intracellular channels or aquaporins (ultra-small pores). Aquaporins only allow movement of water molecules. Deficiency in aquaporins will result in reduced water transport at the same osmotic gradient. Aquaporin function can be reflected by the phenomenon of sodium sieving in the first 30–60 min following the instillation of 3.9% or 4.25% dialyzate. After instillation, the dialyzate sodium level falls as a result of rapid water transport in excess of sodium through the aquaporins, driven by the high osmotic gradient. The dialyzate sodium level then gradually rises to equilibrate with the serum level as the osmotic gradient decreases and the sodium diffuses from blood to dialyzate. The absence of a fall in dialyzate sodium indicates deficiency of aquaporins (Fig. 13.3).

There is no effective treatment for high lymphatic absorption and aquaporin deficiency other than using a higher-glucose-concentration dialyzate.

13.5 Peritoneal Equilibration Test (PET)

PET is a widely used, simple test for assessment of peritoneal function. It provides information on the peritoneal property in terms of peritoneal transport rate and ultrafiltration capacity.

A standard PET is performed in the morning after an overnight dwell with 1.5% dialyzate. After the peritoneal fluid is drained out, the PET is performed via the following steps:

- 2 L of 2.5% dialyzate is instilled into the peritoneal cavity. This takes around 10 min. The patient is asked to change his/her position during instillation to facilitate mixing of the dialyzate with any residual fluid inside the peritoneal cavity. The completion of instillation is regarded as zero time.

- 200 mL of dialyzate is then immediately drained back into the dialyzate bag, and 5–10 mL of fluid is aspirated and sent for creatinine and glucose level assay. The rest is re-instilled back to the peritoneal cavity. The patient is ambulatory after re-instillation is completed.
- At 120 min (2 h), step 2 is repeated. In addition, a blood sample is taken for serum creatinine level.
- At 240 min (4 h), peritoneal dialyzate is completely drained out. A sample of fluid is sent for creatinine and glucose level assay.
- The total volume of the effluent is measured.
- It should be noted that glucose in the dialyzate may interfere with the creatinine assay; therefore, a corrective factor should be determined in each laboratory.

The following data can be generated from the PET:

- dialyzate-to-plasma (D/P) ratio of creatinine at 0 time, 2 h, and 4 h
- dialyzate glucose at 2 h and 4 h against 0 time (D2/D0, D4/D0)
- ultrafiltration volume at 4 h.

A simplified PET has been developed with the dialyzate sample collection at 2 h omitted; the blood sample is still taken at 2 h. This is referred to as the Fast PET. With the Fast PET, only D/P creatinine at 0 and 4 h and D/D0 at 4 h are available.

13.5.1 *Interpretation*

Theoretically, D/P creatinine at zero time is close to zero as there is no creatinine in the instilled dialyzate. It increases with time, but the rate of increase gradually slows down until it reaches equilibrium (D/P creatinine = 1). At 4 h, high D/P creatinine indicates high peritoneal transport (Fig. 13.4).

For D/D0 at zero hour, it will be equal to 1.0. D/D0 progressively falls with glucose absorption, but the rate of decline gradually slows down when the dialyzate glucose concentration approaches the plasma glucose level (equilibrium). For high peritoneal transport, D/D0 at 4 h will be lower in patients with high peritoneal transport

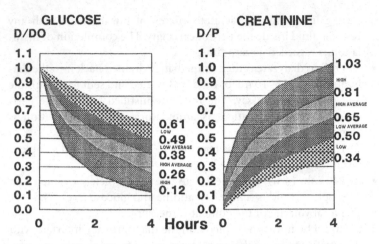

Fig. 13.4 PET result plot in patients with different peritoneal transport rates. [Adapted from Twardowski ZT *et al. Perit Dial Bull* 1987; 7: 137–148.]

Table 13.1 Classification of peritoneal transport rate in PET.

Peritoneal transport types	D/P creatinine at 4 h	D/D0 glucose at 4 h
High	>0.81	<0.26
High average	>0.65–0.81	0.26–<0.38
Low average	0.5–0.65	0.38–0.49
Low	<0.5	>0.49

than in those with low peritoneal transport (Fig. 13.4). D/P creatinine and D/D0 glucose are highly, but inversely, correlated.

As ultrafiltration in peritoneal dialysis is basically driven by the osmotic gradient contributed by the high-glucose content in dialyzate, the higher the peritoneal transport is, the faster the dissipation of the osmotic gradient will be. As a result, ultrafiltration volume is negatively correlated with peritoneal transport rate, i.e. the ultrafiltration volume is lower in patients with high peritoneal transport than in patients with low peritoneal transport.

The peritoneal transport rate is classified into four categories, according to the mean of the original set of data ± 1 standard deviation, as published by Twardowski *et al.* (1987). Table 13.1 shows the definition of peritoneal transport rates according to D/P creatinine and D/D0.

13.5.2 *Application*

PET can be used to:

(i)   identify the cause of ultrafiltration problems due to

   • high peritoneal transport or
   • other causes if peritoneal transport is not high

(ii) adjust dialysis prescription to modify the ultrafiltration volume
(iii) monitor changes in the peritoneal function longitudinally.

13.5.3 *Dialysis Prescription Modification to Increase Ultrafiltration in High Peritoneal Transport*

(i)   Use a higher-glucose-concentration dialyzate.
(ii) Shorten the dwell time and increase the frequency of exchange.

   • Increase the number of cycles per day.
   • Use multiple cycles in the day time but empty peritoneal cavity at night time to avoid negative ultrafiltration with the long nocturnal dwell (day ambulatory peritoneal dialysis or DAPD).
   • Use multiple cycles at night time during sleep performed by a machine with empty peritoneal cavity in day time (APD, nocturnal intermittent peritoneal dialysis or NIPD).
   • Use 7.5% icodextrin peritoneal dialyzate in the long nocturnal dwell of CAPD or the long day dwell of APD.

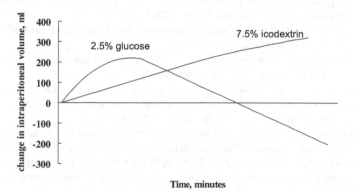

Fig. 13.5 The change in intraperitoneal volume in patients with high peritoneal transport using glucose-containing and icodextrin-containing dialyzate.

Icodextrin is a glucose polymer of variable length, with a molecular weight averaging at around 15 000. It is not osmotically active, but exerts colloid oncotic pressure for fluid removal across the peritoneum (Fig. 13.5). Because of its large size, it is not absorbed across the peritoneum and therefore the oncotic pressure can be maintained for many hours. Fluid removal by icodextrin dialyzate is slow but consistent, compared to that achieved by glucose-containing dialyzate. For optimal fluid removal, the dwell time of icodextrin dialyzate should be around 10–12 h; thus, it is often used in the overnight dwell of CAPD or the long day dwell of APD. Only one 2-L bag of icodextrin dialyzate can be used per day. The ultrafiltration achieved is usually between 300–600 mL. Ultrafiltration less than this amount should alert the possibility of ultrafiltration problems not arising from high peritoneal transport.

Suggested Reading

Bernardini J, Bender F, Florio T, et al. (2005) Randomized, double-blind trial of antibiotic exit site cream for prevention of exit site infection in peritoneal dialysis patients. *J Am Soc Nephrol* 16:539–545.

Chow KM, Szeto CC, Li PK. (2003) Management options for hydrothorax complicating peritoneal dialysis. *Semin Dial* 16:389–394.

Crabtree JH. (2006) Rescue and salvage procedures for mechanical and infectious complications of peritoneal dialysis. *Int J Artif Organs* 29:67–84.

Gadallah MF, Pervez A, El-Shahawy MA, et al. (1999) Peritoneoscopic versus surgical placement of peritoneal dialysis catheters: a prospective randomized study on outcome. *Am J Kidney Dis* 33:118–122.

Krediet R, Mujais S. (2002) Use of icodextrin in high transport ultrafiltration failure. *Kidney Int* 62(S81):S53–S61.

Lam MF, Lo WK, Chu FSK, et al. (2004) Retroperitoneal leakage as a cause of ultrafiltration failure. *Perit Dial Int* 24:466–470.

Lui SL, Yip T, Tse KC, et al. (2005) Treatment of refractory *Pseudomonas aeruginosa* exit-site infection by simultaneous removal and reinsertion of peritoneal dialysis catheter. *Perit Dial Int* 25:560–563.

Majkowski NL, Mendley SR. (1997) Simultaneous removal and replacement of infected peritoneal dialysis catheters. *Am J Kidney Dis* 29:706–711.

Ozener C, Bihorac A, Akoglu E. (2001) Technical survival of CAPD catheters: comparison between percutaneous and conventional surgical placement techniques. *Nephrol Dial Transplant* 16:1893–1899.

Peers E, Gokal R. (1998) Icodextrin provides long dwell peritoneal dialysis and maintenance of intraperitoneal volume. *Artif Organs* 22:8–12.

Piraino B, Bailie GR, Bernardini J, *et al.*; ISPD Ad Hoc Advisory Committee. (2005) Peritoneal dialysis-related infections recommendations: 2005 update. *Perit Dial Int* 25:107–131

Rodrigues AS, Silva S, Bravo F, *et al.* (2007) Peritoneal membrane evaluation in routine clinical practice. *Blood Purif* 25:497–504.

Schmidt SC, Pohle C, Langrehr JM, *et al.* (2007) Laparoscopic-assisted placement of peritoneal dialysis catheters: implantation technique and results. *J Laparoendosc Adv Surg Tech A* 17:596–599.

Tacconelli E, Carmeli Y, Aizer A, *et al.* (2003) Mupirocin prophylaxis to prevent *Staphylococcus aureus* infection in patients undergoing dialysis: a meta-analysis. *Clin Infect Dis* 37:1629–1638.

Twardowski Z, Nolph K, Prowant B, *et al.* (1987) Peritoneal equilibration test. *Perit Dial Bull* 7:138–148.

Twardowski ZJ. (1989) Clinical value of standardized equilibration tests in CAPD patients. *Blood Purif* 7:95–108.

Vychytil A, Lilaj T, Lorenz M, *et al.* (1999) Ultrasonography of the catheter tunnel in peritoneal dialysis patients: what are the indications? *Am J Kidney Dis* 33:722–727.

14

Management of CAPD-Related Peritonitis

Philip K. T. Li and Kai-Ming Chow

This chapter discusses principally the management of peritonitis, one of the most common infective complications of peritoneal dialysis. Peritonitis remains one of the major causes of morbidity, hospitalization, and mortality in patients undergoing continuous ambulatory peritoneal dialysis (CAPD). In a recent local analysis of the cause of death of 296 PD patients, about 17% of the deaths were related to peritonitis.

14.1 Diagnosis

Although cloudy dialysate occurs in over 95% of infective peritonitis, not all instances of cloudy peritoneal dialysate reflect infectious peritonitis. The diagnostic criteria (Table 14.1) are followed, although acute onset of cloudy fluid with abdominal pain should trigger empiric initiation of antimicrobial therapy. Any potential break in the peritoneal dialysis exchange technique and contamination should be enquired (in a non-blaming manner) following any peritonitis.

14.2 Peritonitis Rate

In 1976, when Popovich and Moncrief first started peritoneal dialysis (PD) using two 1-L glass bottles with a long disposable transfer set, the peritonitis rate was 1 in 2.5 patient-months. In 1978, when Oreopoulos used a plastic collapsible dialysate bag for PD, the peritonitis rate was 1 in 10.5 patient-months. Throughout the years of development of the connectology using the technique of "flush before

Table 14.1 Diagnostic criteria of peritonitis complicating peritoneal dialysis.

Two out of three criteria

Cloudy peritoneal dialysis effluent with >100 white blood cells/mm^3 and at least 50% polymorphonuclear cells.
Abdominal pain.
Positive Gram stain or culture from dialysate.

Additional comments

Fluid drained after a prolonged dwell period could appear cloudy in the absence of peritonitis; peritoneal fluid cell count should be obtained whenever feasible.
Patients on automated peritoneal dialysis (APD) might present with peritonitis despite an absolute number of cell counts <100 cells/mm^3 because of the relatively short dwell; a proportion of polymorphonuclear cells > 50% is strong evidence for peritonitis.

---

fill" in the Y-set disconnect system and, later on, the double-bag disconnect system, the peritonitis rate has significantly improved. Recently, peritonitis rates of one episode per 25 patient-months to 46.8 patient-months have been achieved.

14.3 Organisms for Peritonitis

Several routes leading to peritonitis in PD are known: intraluminal (mainly through touch contamination), periluminal (through exit-site or tunnel infections), intestinal, systemic (through the bloodstream), and rarely ascending (through the vagina).

Back in the 1980s when the standard straight set spike system was the most common method for CAPD, Gram-positive organisms accounted for about 60% of all the peritonitis infections (*Staphylococcus aureus*: 10%; *Staphylococcus epidermidis*: 40%; and *Streptococcus species*: 10%) while Gram-negative enteric organisms accounted for about 20%. Our recent data in 2007 showed that Gram-positive and Gram-negative organisms accounted for about 47% and 38% of all peritonitis episodes, respectively. Acid-fast bacilli and fungus accounted for 3% and 2%, respectively, while the remaining 10% grew no organism. This is mainly as a result of the use of technology of "flush before fill" and the double-bag disconnect system, leading to a reduction in Gram-positive organisms while

Gram-negative organisms did not decrease or even proportionately increase.

Peritonitis, particularly in patients with multiple episodes of infection, is not uncommonly caused by the release of planktonic bacteria from biofilm on the walls of catheters. Bacteria can form biofilm on the walls of catheters within 48 h of their placement. These bacteria within the slime layer are resistant to both host defenses and many antibiotics, and may be the cause of recurrent peritonitis. This hypothesis is supported by the observation that catheter exchange, after dialysis effluent clears up, is effective in preventing the relapse of peritonitis. Peritoneal immune defenses are important in preventing peritonitis related to biofilm.

14.4 Management

After obtaining dialysate for analysis and culture, empiric (intraperitoneal) antibiotics should be administered without delay to cover both Gram-positive and Gram-negative organisms.

- Gram-positive organisms may be covered by vancomycin or a first-generation cephalosporin (e.g. cefazolin 1 g loading followed by 250 mg/bag).
- Gram-negative organisms may be covered by a third-generation cephalosporin (e.g. ceftazidime 1 g loading followed by 250 mg/bag) or aminoglycoside.
- Patients might benefit from adjunctive measures:

  (a) Heparin (500 units/L) intraperitoneally (in particular with extremely cloudy effluent) to prevent occlusion of the catheter by fibrinous clots, until signs and symptoms of peritonitis have resolved.
  (b) Intravenous antibiotics if patient appears septic.
  (c) Concomitant prophylactic oral nystatin (to reduce the risk of superimposed fungal peritonitis) — one tablet (500 000 units) three to four times daily.

- The choice of antimicrobial therapy is modified after knowing the culture results and sensitivities (Table 14.2).
- Administer adjuvant oral rifampicin (600 mg daily for 5–7 days) if *Staphylococcus aureus* peritonitis occurs.

Table 14.2 Intraperitoneal antibiotic dosing recommendations for CAPD patients.[a]

	Intermittent (per exchange, once daily)	Continuous (mg/2 L, all exchanges)
Aminoglycoside		
Amikacin	2 mg/kg	LD 50, MD 24
Gentamicin	0.6 mg/kg	LD 16, MD 8
Cephalosporin		
Cefazolin	15 mg/kg	LD 1000, MD 250
Cefepime	1 g	LD 1000–2000, MD 250
Ceftazidime	1000–1500 mg	LD 1000, MD 250
Cefotaxime	ND	LD 1000, MD 500
Cefoperazone	ND	LD 2000, MD 400–1000
Penicillin		
Ampicillin	ND	MD 250
Cloxacillin	ND	MD 250
Amoxicillin	ND	LD 500–1000, MD 100
Penicillin G	ND	LD 50 000 units, MD 25 000 units
Piperacillin[b]	4000 mg iv b.i.d.	LD 4000 iv, MD 500
Others		
Vancomycin	15–30 mg/kg every 5–7 days	LD 2000, MD 50
Aztreonam	ND	LD 2000, MD 500
Combination		
Ampicillin/sulbactam	2 g every 12 h	LD 2000, MD 200
Imipenem/cilastatin	1 g b.i.d.	LD 1000, MD 100

[a] Adopted and modified from the ISPD Ad Hoc Advisory Committee.
[b] Intraperitoneal combination of piperacillin and an aminoglycoside may be incompatible, and mandates the provision of piperacillin by the intravenous route in this setting.
LD, loading dose (in mg), MD, maintenance dose (in mg), ND, not reported.

- Repeat the cell count and culture if there is no improvement after 48 h; a persistently high PD cell count (>1000 cells/mm^3 on day 3) signifies poor prognosis.
- Intraperitoneal instillation of thrombolytic agents (up to 7500–30 000 units of urokinase left in the Tenckhoff catheter for 2 h and then drained) can be considered to facilitate antibiotic penetration into biofilm.

- Tenckhoff catheter removal should be considered if there is no improvement after 5 days of appropriate antibiotics (in order to preserve the peritoneum, and to prevent morbidity and mortality), and for relapsing peritonitis, fungal peritonitis, and refractory exit-site and tunnel infections as well as for peritonitis caused by mycobacteria and multiple enteric organisms not responding to therapy.
- A minimum period of 2–3 weeks is recommended between catheter removal (for infection) and the re-insertion of a new Tenckhoff catheter.
- Consider surgical evaluation and/or computerized tomography (CT) if multiple enteric organisms are grown or intra-abdominal pathology is suspected; metronidazole combined with ampicillin and ceftazidime (or an aminoglycoside) should also be considered.
- A high index of suspicion for *Mycobacterium tuberculosis* peritonitis is needed for diagnosis (polymorphonuclear white cell predominance in dialysate is not uncommon). No consensus has been developed on the optimal drug treatment regimen (Table 14.3) and duration, but Tenckhoff catheter removal is not considered mandatory if the patient responds to the antituberculous drug treatment.
- Treatment of fungal peritonitis should include Tenckhoff catheter removal and antifungal therapy (Table 14.4).

Table 14.3 Suggested treatment for tuberculous peritonitis complicating peritoneal dialysis.

First 2–3 months of quadruple therapy

    Isoniazid 200–300 mg daily
    Rifampicin 450–600 mg daily
    Pyrazinamide 1.5–2.0 g daily
    Levofloxacin 200 mg daily

Total duration of treatment (12 months)

    Isoniazid and rifampicin

Additional comments

    Supplement oral pyridoxine 50–100 mg daily
    Streptomycin not routinely used (ototoxicity and adverse effect on residual renal function)
    Ethambutol not recommended (increased risk of optic neuritis in renal failure subjects).

Table 14.4 Treatment for fungal peritonitis complicating peritoneal dialysis.

Tenckhoff catheter removal immediately (in view of biofilm formation around
    dialysis catheter, rendering eradication of infection difficult)

Antifungal therapy

Oral fluconazole 200 mg daily for 3–4 weeks (recommended, in general,
    to be continued for an additional 10 days after catheter removal) or
Intravenous amphotericin B 30 mg daily for 21 days (for those who fail to
    respond to oral fluconazole)
Oral flucytosine 1000 mg daily can be added

Additional comments

Choice of antifungal agents needs to be individualized, depending on the
    species isolated.

- Elective Tenckhoff catheter exchange (after the dialysis effluent
  clears) can be considered in patients with relapsed peritonitis
  (which is often caused by the persistence of bacterial biofilm, such
  as *Pseudomonas aeruginosa*, on the indwelling Tenckhoff catheter).

14.5 Complications

Peritonitis results in a marked increase in effluent protein losses,
which may contribute to the protein malnutrition of PD patients.
More importantly, ultrafiltration problems are common during
acute peritonitis because peritoneal permeability is increased
during an episode of peritonitis. After an episode of severe peritonitis, an increase in solute transport and loss of ultrafiltration
may occur, resulting in a hyperpermeable membrane and permanent loss of ultrafiltration capability. This process is probably
proportional to the extent of inflammation and the number of
peritonitis episodes.

The final stage of this process is peritoneal fibrosis, sometimes
referred to as sclerosing encapsulating peritonitis (SEP). SEP is possibly more common in Japan, and the condition is present in 0.9% of
patients undergoing PD. The peritonitis rate among patients who experienced SEP was 3.3 times higher than that among the rest of the patients.
Peritoneal fibrosis is a severe complication of PD. In addition to ultrafiltration failure, the patient becomes progressively malnourished because

of recurrent partial intestinal obstruction from encasement of the bowel. PD cannot be continued, and this complication is frequently lethal despite conversion to long-term hemodialysis.

14.6 Prevention

14.6.1 *Contamination Protocols*

Contamination at the time of peritoneal exchange procedure should be recognized and followed by seeking advice from the dialysis center.

- If the clamp on the transfer set remains closed at the time of contamination (prior to infusion of dialysate), only change of the sterile tubing (transfer set) by the nurse is needed.
- If there is disconnection of the sterile system during a PD treatment or there is an equipment failure (such as a hole in the solution bag) that is noticed after infusion, it must be treated with both sterile transfer set changes and antibiotic prophylaxis (after collecting the effluent for cell count and culture) as soon as possible.
- Prophylactic antibiotics (such as quinolones) should cover both Gram-positive and Gram-negative organisms.
- If the culture is positive (even if the cell count is normal), the patient should be treated with further antibiotic therapy.

14.6.2 *Iatrogenic Peritonitis*

Emptying of the abdomen and prophylactic intravenous antibiotics should be given just prior to high-risk procedures:

- Uterine procedure such as endometrial biopsy or hysteroscopy
- Colonoscopy, especially with polypectomy
- Renal transplantation

14.6.3 *Continuous Quality Improvement*

Monitoring of peritonitis (and exit-site infection) rates is strongly recommended, at a minimum, on a yearly basis (Table 14.5). The culture-negative peritonitis rate should be below 20% of all episodes. Monitoring of cultured organisms should also be performed, in addition to the overall peritonitis rates.

Table 14.5 Calculation of the peritonitis rate.

Expressed as

Interval in months between episodes (months of peritoneal dialysis at risk divided by number of episodes): "1 episode every *n* months"

Episodes per year (number of infections within a given time period divided by dialysis-years at risk): "*n* episodes per patient-year at risk"

Standard

The peritonitis rates should be monitored in each peritoneal dialysis program; the peritonitis rate should be no more than 1 episode every 18 months (0.67 episodes per patient-year at risk).

Suggested Reading

Bernardini J, Price V, Figueiredo A. (2006) Peritoneal dialysis patient training, 2006. *Perit Dial Int* 26:625–632.

Caring for Australians with Renal Impairment (CARI). (2004) The CARI guidelines. Evidence for peritonitis treatment and prophylaxis: treatment of peritoneal dialysis-associated peritonitis in adults. *Nephrology (Carlton)* 9(Suppl 3):S91–S106.

Chow KM, Szeto CC, Cheung KK, *et al.* (2006) Predictive value of dialysate cell counts in peritonitis complicating peritoneal dialysis. *Clin J Am Soc Nephrol* 1:768–773.

Dasgupta MK. (2002) Biofilms and infection in dialysis patients. *Semin Dial* 15:338–346.

Li PK, Law MC, Chow KM, *et al.* (2002) Comparison of clinical outcome and ease of handling in two double-bag systems in continuous ambulatory peritoneal dialysis — a prospective randomized controlled multi-center study. *Am J Kidney Dis* 40:373–380.

Li PK, Leung CB, Szeto CC. (2007) Peritonitis in peritoneal dialysis patients. In: Nissenson AR, Fine R (eds.), *Handbook of Dialysis Therapy*, 4th ed. Elsevier, Philadelphia, pp. 396–413.

Lui SL, Chan TM, Lai KN, Lo WK. (2007) Tuberculous and fungal peritonitis in patients undergoing continuous ambulatory peritoneal dialysis. *Perit Dial Int* 27(Suppl 2):S263–S266.

Oreopoulos DG, Robson M, Izatt S, Clayton S, de Veber GA. (1978) A simple and safe technique for continuous ambulatory peritoneal dialysis. *Trans Am Soc Artif Intern Organs* 24:484–489.

Piraino B, Bailie GR, Bernardini J, *et al.* ISPD Ad Hoc Advisory Committee. (2005) Peritoneal dialysis-related infections recommendations: 2005 update. *Perit Dial Int* 25:107–131.

Popovich RP, Moncrief JW, Decherd JB, Bomar JB, Pyle WF. (1976) The definition of a novel portable/wearable equilibrium peritoneal dialysis technique. *Trans Am Soc Artif Intern Organs* 5:64 (abstract).

Prasad N, Gupta A. (2005) Fungal peritonitis in peritoneal dialysis patients. *Perit Dial Int* 25:207–222.

Szeto CC, Chow KM. (2007) Gram-negative peritonitis — the Achilles heel of peritoneal dialysis? *Perit Dial Int* 27(Suppl 2):S267–S271.

Wiggins KJ, Craig JC, Johnson DW, Strippoli GF. (2008) Treatment for peritoneal dialysis-associated peritonitis. *Cochrane Database Syst Rev* (1):CD005284.

15

Hemodialysis

Bharathi Reddy and Alfred K. H. Cheung

15.1 Mechanisms of Solute Transport

Solute removal during extracorporeal renal replacement therapy occurs by three mechanisms: diffusion, convection, and adsorption.

15.1.1 *Diffusion*

- Hemodialysis removes solutes primarily by diffusion.
- Solutes pass through the semipermeable membrane based on differences in the concentration of solutes between the blood and the dialysate.
- It is particularly effective in the transport of small solutes such as urea, potassium, calcium, and bicarbonate.
- Diffusive clearance of solutes by hemodialysis decreases rapidly with increasing molecular size.

15.1.2 *Convection*

- Hemofiltration removes solutes by convection.
- Filtration of plasma water across the membrane of the hemofilter occurs as a result of hydrostatic pressure gradient across the membrane. Solutes that are dissolved in the water are transported passively with the water movement, a process known as solvent drag. The amount of solute removed by convection is therefore dependent on the amount of plasma water transported across the membrane and the size of the solute relative to the pore size of the membrane.
- A crucial distinction between hemodialysis and hemofiltration is that fluid removal, but not a concentration gradient of the solute, is required for solute removal in hemofiltration;

while fluid transport is not required for solute removal in hemodialysis.

- Although convection is accompanied by the loss of total body mass of a solute, there is no change in its plasma concentration if there is no restriction in the transport of the solute across the hemofiltration membrane (i.e. sieving coefficient = 1). A large amount of replacement fluid that is devoid of particular solutes is given to replace the fluid removed by the hemofilter. This process decreases the plasma concentration of solutes by dilution, in a manner that is quite similar to the tubules of the native kidney.
- Convection is effective in the removal of both small and large solutes.
- Hemodiafiltration refers to the combination of hemodialysis and hemofiltration that requires both dialysate and replacement fluid.
- Protein-bound substances (e.g. those bound to serum albumin) are usually not cleared by either hemodialysis or hemofiltration.

15.1.3 *Adsorption*

- Adsorption (binding) of solutes to the hemodialysis membrane or hemofiltration membrane occurs to various extents, depending on the physicochemical properties of the solute and the membrane.
- Hemoperfusion is the removal of solutes from blood by adsorption onto materials, such as charcoal or resins, in the extracorporeal circuit that is purposely designed for this mechanism of solute removal.
- Charcoal hemoperfusion is effective in clearing protein-bound compounds. It is primarily used for the removal of drugs in acute poisoning, although it has also been used to a limited extent for the treatment of end-stage renal disease.

15.2 Hemodialysis Membranes

15.2.1 *Composition of Membrane*

- The type of membrane material used may determine the performance and biocompatibility of the membrane. There are two broad categories of membranes based on the material used for manufacturing: cellulose-based membranes and synthetic membranes.
- Cellulose membranes are further classified into unsubstituted cellulose and substituted cellulose membranes.

- Unsubstituted cellulose membranes: Cellulose is obtained from processed cotton. Regenerated cellulose and cuprammonium cellulose (or Cuprophan®) are examples of unsubstituted cellulose membranes. There are a large number of free hydroxyl groups on the cellulose polymer that are thought to be responsible for the activation of serum complement proteins and, consequently, the activation of leukocytes, causing bioincompatibility.
- Substituted cellulose membranes: Chemical substitution of free hydroxyl groups on cellulose membranes results in modified cellulose membranes. The free hydroxyl groups can be substituted by acetate (cellulose acetate, cellulose diacetate, or cellulose triacetate), tertiary amino compounds (Hemophan®), and other moieties.
- Synthetic membranes are manufactured from non-cellulose synthetic polymers. Synthetic membranes in clinical use include polyacrylonitrile (PAN), polyamide, polymethylmethacrylate (PMMA), polysulfone, polycarbonate, or a combination of some of these polymers. Synthetic membranes tend to be more biocompatible than unsubstituted cellulose membranes, by most criteria used in the nephrology literature.

15.2.2 *Membrane Efficiency and Membrane Flux (Table 15.1)*

- Mass transfer coefficient × surface area product (K_0A): K_0A is the calculated product of the mass transfer coefficient (K_0) and membrane surface area (A), with its unit in mL/min. K_0A is specific for any particular dialysis membrane and any particular solute, although it is most often used to characterize urea. It is largely independent of blood solute concentration, blood flow rate, and dialysate flow rate. Conceptually, K_0A is the theoretical maximum

Table 15.1   Membrane efficiency vs. membrane flux.

Membrane efficiency	Determined largely by membrane surface area
	Determines the ability of a dialyzer to remove small molecules (e.g. urea)
Membrane flux	Determined largely by membrane pore size
	Determines the ability of a dialyzer to remove middle molecules (e.g. β_2-microglobulin) and water

clearance of a particular solute for a given dialyzer when blood and dialysate flow rates are infinite.

- Membrane efficiency: The ability of a dialyzer to remove the small molecule urea is arbitrarily defined as its efficiency. The efficiency of a dialyzer is largely determined by the surface area. High-efficiency dialyzers have large surface areas and K_0A values for urea >600 mL/min, while low-efficiency dialyzers have low surface area and K_0A values for urea <450 mL/min. High-efficiency dialyzers can be high flux or low flux.

- The K_0A of a dialysis membrane only provides a rough estimation of what might be achieved clinically. The actual solute clearance also depends on the blood flow rate that presents the solute to the dialyzer, the dialysate flow rate that provides the diffusion gradient, and the rate of fluid removal that supplements the diffusion by convective loss of the solute.

- Ultrafiltration coefficient (K_{UF}): The permeability of a dialysis membrane to water is measured as the ultrafiltration coefficient. K_{UF} is defined as the volume of water transferred across the membrane per hour, for each mmHg of transmembrane hydrostatic pressure gradient.

- Membrane flux: The flux of a dialyzer is defined by the US Food and Drug Administration according to its K_{UF}. Water flux is largely determined by pore sizes, but membrane surface area is also a determinant. Dialyzers with K_{UF} values >12 mL/h/mmHg are classified as high flux and require an ultrafiltration control device in the dialysis machine to use. Low-flux hemodialysis membranes usually have K_{UF} values 2–5 mL/h/mmHg.

- Clinical definition of membrane flux: Clinically, the flux of the dialysis membrane is more frequently defined by its ability to remove middle molecules (often using β_2-microglobulin as the marker). Low-flux dialyzers have small pores, which severely restrict the transport of β_2-microglobulin; while high-flux dialyzers permit the transport of β_2-microglobulin to various extents. Modified cellulosic membranes and synthetic membranes can both be configured into either high-flux or low-flux dialyzers.

15.2.3 Biocompatibility

- Bioincompatibility refers to a variety of biologic responses that occur in a patient induced by contact of blood with the dialysis membrane and other components of the extracorporeal circuit. The biologic responses elicited by blood–membrane interactions include activation of the complement system, coagulation system, other plasma proteins and lipids, platelets, leukocytes, and erythrocytes.

- It is generally accepted that unsubstituted cellulose is the most bioincompatible membrane, while modified cellulose membranes and synthetic membranes are considered to be more biocompatible. However, depending on the specific criteria, unsubstituted cellulose membranes may be more biocompatible than certain synthetic membranes (e.g. interactions between the plasma kallikrein system and the AN69® polyacrylonitrile membrane).
- Epidemiologic studies suggest that the chronic use of unmodified low-flux membranes is associated with higher patient mortality, compared to synthetic membranes and modified cellulose membranes. However, many of the dialyzers that are made of more biocompatible membranes are also high-flux dialyzers. Therefore, it is difficult to distinguish the effects of biocompatibility from flux on clinical outcomes in these studies.

15.3 Dialysate

Dialysate is prepared by blending properly purified water with concentrates of electrolytes and other solutes. The typical solutes and their concentrations in dialysates are listed in Table 15.2.

Table 15.2   Typical concentrations of solutes present in dialysate.

Component	Concentration
Sodium	135–145 mmol/L
Potassium	0–4 mmol/L
Calcium	0–1.5 mmol/L
Chloride	102–106 mmol/L
Bicarbonate	30–39 mmol/L
Magnesium	0.25–0.5 mmol/L
Acetate	2.0–4.0 mmol/L (higher in acetate dialysates)
Dextrose	11 mmol/L
pH	7.1–7.3

15.3.1 Sodium

- The dialysate sodium concentration is usually 140 mmol/L ± 10 mmol/L. Sodium is removed from the blood primarily by convection instead of diffusion during hemodialysis, so that there is little change in plasma sodium concentration. This is necessary to prevent hyponatremia or hypernatremia.
- The concentration of sodium in the dialysate can be varied during the course of individual treatments, a process called sodium profiling or sodium modeling. During this process, the dialysate sodium concentration at the beginning of the dialysis session is set at a higher value (e.g. 160 mmol/L) with subsequent falls to a lower value (e.g. 140 mmol/L) at the end of the session. Sodium profiling is designed to reduce intradialytic intravascular hypovolemia and symptomatic hypotension as well as the postdialysis washed-out feeling; however, increasing the sodium concentration in the dialysate may also produce postdialysis hypernatremia and increase interdialytic thirst, intradiaytic fluid weight gain, and hypertension.

15.3.2 Potassium

- The dialysate potassium concentration is 0–4 mmol/L, depending on the patient's predialysis plasma potassium concentration. The commonly used dialysate potassium concentrations are 2–3 mmol/L.
- If the patient is prone to cardiac arrhythmias or is on digitalis therapy, or if the predialysis plasma potassium concentration is <4.0 mmol/L, the use of a higher dialysate potassium concentration (≥3 mmol/L) is recommended.
- The use of 1 mmol/L potassium or potassium-free dialysates is associated with higher incidence of arrhythmias and should generally be avoided.

15.3.3 Calcium

- Calcium concentrations in the dialysate should be individualized, based on the serum calcium, phosphorus, and parathormone (PTH) levels; the oral intake of calcium; and the use of active vitamin D analogs.
- In patients who are taking calcium-containing binders or active vitamin D analog, dialysates containing 1.25 mmol/L of calcium

(which is all ionized because there are no proteins in the dialysate) are usually used to avoid hypercalcemia or high plasma calcium × phosphate product.

- A low dialysate calcium concentration may predispose the patient to intradialytic hypotension. Calcium-free dialysate has been used for the treatment of severe hypercalcemia or calciphylaxis; however, it is associated with cardiac arrhythmias and should be largely avoided, especially without intradialytic cardiac monitoring.

15.3.4 *Base*

- One of the main complications of chronic kidney disease is metabolic acidosis. A goal of hemodialysis is to provide base supplement in the form of acetate or bicarbonate to correct the metabolic acidosis.
- Acetate is converted into bicarbonate in many tissues in the body. Acetate-containing dialysates are less expensive than bicarbonate-containing dialysates. However, it is associated with untoward effects, including hypoxemia, intradialytic hypotension, and an ill sensation in some patients.
- Technical developments in modern dialysis machines have made the delivery of bicarbonate dialysate an easy task. Bicarbonate-containing dialysate is most commonly used in the USA, Europe, and some other countries.
- Bicarbonate levels in the dialysate are usually 32–39 mmol/L, in order to generate a positive bicarbonate balance and to keep the predialysis serum bicarbonate >22 mmol/L.

15.3.5 *Magnesium*

- Magnesium levels in the dialysate are 0.25–0.50 mmol/L.
- Hypomagnesemia and severe muscle cramps can occur with the use of magnesium-free dialysate.

15.3.6 *Dextrose*

- Dialysates containing dextrose concentrations of 100–200 mg/dL (5–10 mmol/L) are used routinely.
- Use of glucose-free dialysate may induce hypoglycemia in patients who are prone to developing hypoglycemia, such as those taking

anti-diabetic medications. In addition, glucose-free dialysates promote the loss of glucose and calories and, therefore, catabolism.

- High-glucose dialysate may impair the removal of potassium and phosphorus.

15.4 Hemodialysis Apparatus

Hemodialysis equipment has blood circuit components and dialysate circuit components that converge at the dialyzer. The hemodialysis machine has safety and monitoring devices to ensure safe operation.

15.4.1 *Blood Circuit*

The blood circuit has the following components (Fig. 15.1):

- Arterial portion of blood circuit: Blood is pumped from the vascular access into the dialyzer through an arterial blood tubing.
- Blood pump: The blood in the arterial blood circuit is pumped by a peristaltic roller pump in most machines that sequentially compresses different segments of the tubing. The elastic tubing recoils after compression by the roller and refills with blood.
- Pre-pump arterial pressure monitor: The hydrostatic pressure is negative between the vascular access and the blood pump. When the upper or lower pre-set pressure limit is exceeded, the system will trigger alarms, stop the blood pump, and clamp the venous tubing. Causes of high and low arterial pressure alarms are listed in Table 15.3.
- Heparin is infused in the post-pump, pre-dialyzer segment of the blood circuit.
- Venous portion of blood circuit: Blood is returned from the dialyzer to the patient through the venous blood tubing.
- Post-pump venous pressure monitor: The hydrostatic pressure in this segment is positive. When the upper or lower pre-set pressure limit is exceeded, the system will trigger alarms, stop the blood pump, and clamp the venous tubing. Causes of high and low venous pressure alarms are listed in Table 15.4.
- Venous bubble trap and air detector are important safety devices located in the venous blood segment. When the air detector senses the presence of air, it triggers alarms, stops the blood pump, and clamps the venous tubing. This feature is critical in preventing air embolism.

BLOOD CIRCUIT

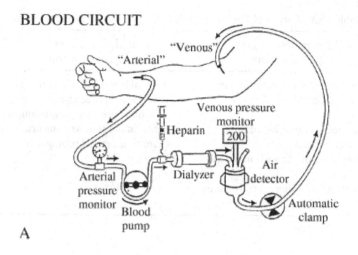

A

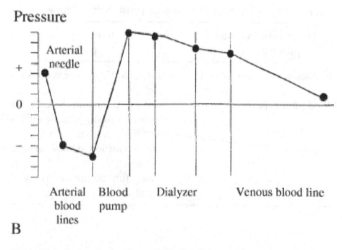

B

Fig. 15.1 Blood circuit for hemodialysis. (A) Extracorporeal blood circuit for hemodialysis. (B) Pressure profile in the blood circuit with an arteriovenous fistula. [From Misra M. *Hemodial Int* 2005; 9: 30–36].

15.4.2 *Dialysate Circuit*

The dialysate delivery system is as follows:

- Dialysate is made by mixing the electrolyte concentrate with a proportionate volume of purified water. The mixing can be performed centrally or by individual dialysis machines.

Table 15.3 Causes of low and high arterial (pre-pump) pressure alarms.

Low (more negative) arterial pressure alarm	High (less negative) arterial pressure alarm
Kinks in the arterial blood line	Arterial blood line disconnection
Hypotension	Blood leak between the patient and the pressure monitoring site
Improper positioning of the arterial needle	Infusion of saline and medications into the arterial tubing
Arterial inflow stenosis in vascular access	
Poorly functioning central venous catheter	

Table 15.4 Causes of low and high venous (post-dialyzer) pressure alarms.

Low (less positive) venous pressure	High (more positive) venous pressure
Venous blood line disconnection	Blood clotting in the venous drip chamber
Low blood pump speed	Kinks in the venous blood tubing
	Improper positioning or infiltration of the venous needles
	Venous outflow stenosis in vascular access
	Poorly functioning central venous catheter

- In central dialysis delivery systems, the premixed dialysate is distributed to the individual machines. Central dialysate systems have the advantage of lower costs; however, they do not permit modifications in the dialysate concentration according to individual patient needs.
- The dialysate flows countercurrent to the blood flow in order to maximize the diffusion gradient for solutes.
- A single-pass dialysate delivery system is commonly used. In this system, the dialysate is discarded after a single passage through the dialyzer.

The dialysate circuit has the following components:

- Heating and deaeration: The purified water is heated to physiologic temperatures (35°C–38°C). The heated water is subjected to negative pressure to remove its air content. Air in the dialysate can impair flow in the dialyzer and cause the malfunctioning of blood-leak and conductivity monitors.
- Proportioning: The heated and deaerated water is mixed with the dialysate concentrate in correct proportions. To prevent the precipitation of calcium and magnesium salts with bicarbonate, the dialysate is mixed from two separate concentrates: the bicarbonate concentrate and an acid concentrate. The acid concentrate contains sodium, potassium, calcium, magnesium, chloride, and dextrose; it also contains a small amount of acetic acid. The final dialysate is made by mixing the two concentrates sequentially with purified water.
- A conductivity monitor ensures proper proportioning of the dialysate with water. Conductivity is determined by the total ionic concentration of the dialysate. The normal range for conductivity is 12–16 ms/cm (millisiemens per centimeter). Severe electrolyte disturbances can occur if the proportioning system malfunctions.
- The temperature monitor in the dialysate circuit monitors the temperature of the dialysate before it reaches the dialyzer. The dialysate temperature is usually maintained at 36°C–37°C. Cool dialysate, defined as a dialysate with a temperature lower than the patient's core temperature, is sometimes used to prevent intradialytic hypotension by inducing vasoconstriction. A major side-effect of cool dialysate is shivering. An excessively warm dialysate produced by error can cause protein denaturation (>42°C) and hemolysis (>45°C).
- If the dialysis solution conductivity or temperature is out of range, the bypass valve is activated and the dialysate is diverted to the drain instead of entering the dialyzer.
- The blood-leak detector at the dialysate outflow segment detects blood in the dialysate. The presence of blood in the dialysate indicates rupture of the dialyzer membrane. When this occurs, the patient may experience major blood loss and the blood can be contaminated by the nonsterile dialysate. When blood leak is detected, alarms are triggered and the blood pump is deactivated.
- Ultrafiltration is controlled by transmembrane pressure (TMP), which is the hydrostatic pressure difference between the blood and dialysate compartments. Older dialysis machines used pressure-controlled

ultrafiltration, in which the dialysis personnel calculates the necessary TMP (based on the ultrafiltration coefficient (K_{UF}) of the dialyzer membrane and the desired amount of fluid removed), monitors the filtration, and readjusts the TMP as needed. Modern dialysis machines use volume-controlled ultrafiltration, which is much more precise in controlling the amount of fluid removed during dialysis. Volume-controlled ultrafiltration devices are mandatory for high-flux dialyzers in order to prevent excessive fluid removal.

15.4.3 *Advanced Control Options*

Some modern dialysis machines also incorporate more sophisticated features:

- Intravascular volume monitors — These devices estimate changes in the patient's intravascular volume based on intradialytic changes in the hematocrit as a result of hemoconcentration induced by ultrafiltration. Intravascular volume monitoring is used in some dialysis units to prevent excessive fluid removal resulting in hypovolemic symptoms, or to prevent inadequate fluid removal resulting in hypervolemia. The usefulness of these devices has not been well established.
- Computer software programs for modeling — These can be pre-set to automatically alter the ultrafiltration rate and dialysate sodium concentration during the dialysis session, according to individual patient needs, in order to maintain the intravascular volume and prevent symptomatic hypotension. The technique of altering ultrafiltration rates during hemodialysis is known as ultrafiltration modeling or ultrafiltration profiling.
- Sodium clearance and urea removal monitors — Sodium clearance is a convenient method to provide instantaneous online determination of small-solute clearance for the assessment of dialyzer performance. Total urea removal can be estimated by measuring dialysate urea concentrations at various time points during hemodialysis.

15.5 Vascular Access

- Creating and maintaining an adequate vascular access is essential for delivering the necessary blood flow rates and, hence, the appropriate dialysis dose in chronic hemodialysis.

Table 15.5   Comparison of vascular accesses.

Feature	Native fistula	Synthetic graft	Catheter
Primary failure rate	20–60%	10–20%	<5%
Time to first use	4–16 weeks	2–4 weeks	Same day
Blood pump speed allowed	200–500 mL/min	400–500 mL/min	150–350 mL/min
Frequency of thrombosis	Low	Moderate	High
Frequency of infection	Very low	Moderate (~0.08 per patient-year)	Very high (~2 per patient-year)
Longevity (after in use)	Longest (~5 yr)	Intermediate (~2 yr)	Shortest (<1 yr)

Modified from Maya ID, Allon M. *Am J Kidney Dis* 2008; 51: 702–708.

- An ideal vascular access is one that can be readily used without a waiting period upon creation, provides adequate blood flow rates, has no complications, and has prolonged patency without interventions.
- There are three common forms of vascular access: native arteriovenous fistulas (AVFs), arteriovenous grafts (AVGs), and central venous catheters which can be cuffed or non-cuffed (temporary catheters). The subcutaneous cuff helps to anchor the catheter and maintains its position in the central vein.
- The native AVF is usually considered the best form of vascular access for chronic dialysis, but the relatively high rate of primary failure as a result of inability to mature has recently raised concerns. Comparisons of different vascular accesses are presented in Table 15.5.

15.5.1 *Non-cuffed Catheters (Temporary Catheters)*

- Temporary catheters are placed in patients requiring emergent hemodialysis. Acute hemodialysis is provided to patients with acute kidney injury, for the removal of ingested toxins or treatment of drug overdose, and to patients with end-stage renal disease who require dialysis but do not have a mature permanent vascular access.
- These catheters can be inserted into the femoral vein, internal jugular vein, or subclavian vein. The advantages and disadvantages

Table 15.6 Advantages and disadvantages of various sites for temporary hemodialysis catheters.

Femoral catheters	Few life-threatening complications
	More prone to infections
	Patients should remain recumbent
	Considered only when the need for dialysis is expected to be short (<72 h)
Internal-jugular catheters	Complications include carotid arterial puncture, pneumothorax, hemothorax, and air embolism
	Less prone to infections than femoral catheters
	Chest radiograph should be obtained before use to exclude pneumothorax and to confirm catheter position
Subclavian catheters	Complications include carotid arterial puncture, pneumothorax, hemothorax, and air embolism
	Less prone to infections than femoral catheters
	Chest radiograph should be obtained before use
	High incidence of central venous stenosis; should be avoided in patients who may need chronic dialysis

of inserting catheters at the various sites are presented in Table 15.6.

15.5.2 *Cuffed Dialysis Catheters*

- Cuffed dialysis catheters are most suitable in the setting of acute kidney injury or as an intermediate measure while waiting for the maturation of a permanent arteriovenous access for chronic dialysis, and rarely in patients who have exhausted all other vascular sites for AVF or AVG.
- Advantages of cuffed catheters are easy placement and no waiting time before they can be used.
- Cuffed catheters are placed under ultrasound guidance and positioned using fluoroscopy with the tip adjusted to the level of the caval-atrial junction. The right internal jugular site is preferential since it is a more direct route to the caval-atrial junction, compared to the left side. Insertion at the subclavian vein appears to be

associated with a greater risk of venous stenosis and ipsilateral arm swelling, and should therefore be avoided if possible.

- The major problem with cuffed catheters is a much greater risk of infection of the vascular access and subsequent sepsis, compared to AVF and AVG. Unfortunately, cuffed catheters are often used as a form of permanent vascular access nowadays in the USA because of convenience or the preference of patients who refuse repeated needle puncture of the arteriovenous access.

15.5.3 *Arteriovenous Fistula (AVF)*

- AVF is constructed by surgical anastomosis between an artery and a vein, which often involves connecting the end of the vein to the side of an artery (end-to-side anastomosis). The anastomosis leads to dilatation of the venous lumen and thickening of the venous wall, which allow the vein to become suitable for repeated needle puncture and provide high blood flow rates for dialysis — a process known as maturation.
- Three major types of AVF are commonly created (Fig. 15.2): radiocephalic (wrist), brachiocephalic (elbow), and transposed brachiobasilic (upper arm). The brachiobasilic transposition surgery is more extensive than the placement of radiocephalic or brachiocephalic AVF.
- The artery and vein used for AVF placement should be determined by the availability of suitable blood vessels in a particular patient. This assessment can be facilitated by the preoperative vascular mapping using duplex ultrasound.
- A limitation of native AVF is the requirement for sufficiently large native vessels, which may be lacking in elderly and diabetic patients.
- A disadvantage of native AVF is that it requires 4–16 weeks for maturation before it can be used. Hand exercises (e.g. squeezing a rubber ball) are believed to accelerate AVF maturation. Sometimes, AVFs never mature sufficiently to become usable — a condition known as primary failure.
- Common causes of maturation failure and unusability of AVF as well as interventions are presented in Table 15.7.
- A major advantage of native AVF is that once it becomes mature, it requires fewer interventions to maintain long-term patency and is less prone to infections, compared to AVG and catheters.
- Planning and placement of a permanent native AVF before the patient requires chronic dialysis should ideally take place early

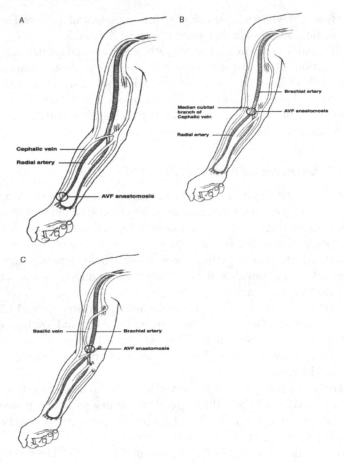

Fig. 15.2 Anatomy of arteriovenous fistulas (AVFs). (A) A radiocephalic fistula is created by anastomosis of the end of the cephalic vein to the side of the radial artery near the wrist. (B) A brachiocephalic fistula is created by anastomosis of the end of the cephalic vein to the side of the brachial artery near the antecubital fossa. (C) A transposed brachiobasilic fistula is created by anastomosis of the end of the basilic vein to the side of the brachial artery near the antecubital fossa. Because the basilic vein is deep and medial, super-ficialization of the fistula is necessary for frequent needle puncture for dislysis. This is accomplished by a longitudinal incision from the antecubital fossa to the shoulder. The basilic vein is then freed from its native bed and tunneled superficially and laterally either before its anastomosis to the artery (one-stage procedure) or after demonstration of the maturation of the deep fistula (two-stage procedure). [From Maya ID, Allon M. *Am J Kidney Dis* 2008; 51: 702–708].

Table 15.7   Causes and interventions for primary unusability of native AVFs.

Cause of maturation failure	Intervention to enhance maturity
Juxta-anastomotic stenosis	Balloon angioplasty or surgical revision of stenosis
Presence of accessory veins that decrease the blood flow through the main draining vein	Coil embolization or surgical ligation of the accessory veins
Presence of a deep fistula	Surgical superficialization of the mature fistula

when the patient reaches stage 4 or 5 chronic kidney disease, depending on the rate of deterioration of the kidney function. Early AVF placement avoids the emergency placement of catheters when the patient becomes frankly uremic.

15.5.4 *Arteriovenous Graft (AVG)*

- If a native AVF cannot be constructed, another option is to place a graft between the artery and the vein. Most grafts used for chronic dialysis are made of synthetic materials such as polytetrafluoroethylene (PTFE) or its derivative expanded PTFE (ePTFE), or, less frequently, polyurethaneurea (PUU).
- Advantages of AVG are that it can be cannulated earlier (at 2–4 weeks) than AVF and its primary failure rate is also lower. It is relatively easy to cannulate because it has a pre-existing wide lumen.
- The major disadvantages of AVG are that it is prone to stenosis at the anastomosis, requires more salvage interventions, and has an inferior long-term patency rate compared to that of a functioning AVF.

15.5.5 *Complications of Arteriovenous Access*

Complications of arteriovenous access are summarized in Table 15.8.

15.5.5.1 *Arteriovenous Access Stenosis and Thrombosis*

- Stenosis is the most common cause of access thrombosis. Nonanatomic factors causing access thrombosis include hypotension, hypovolemia, elevated hemoglobin levels, hypercoagulable states, and excessive access compression postdialysis.

Table 15.8   Complications and interventions of arteriovenous access.

Complication	Intervention
Access stenosis	Percutaneous balloon angioplasty with or without stent placement
Access thrombosis	Surgical thrombectomy or percutaneous thrombolysis
Access infection	Antibiotics
	Excision if infection is severe or cannot be eradicated by antibiotics
Distal ischemia	Access ligation
	Access banding to decrease the luminal diameter
	Distal revascularization-interval ligation (DRIL)
High-output heart failure	Banding or ligation of access
Aneurysm and pseudoaneurysm	Avoid needle puncture at the aneurysm site
	Resection of aneurysm and insertion of an interposition graft to avoid rupture if the aneurysm is rapidly expanding or if the overlying skin becomes thin

- Arteriovenous access stenosis occurs most frequently at the juxta-anastomotic area, and is more common at the outflow (venous) tract than the inflow (arterial) tract. It is less common in native AVF than in synthetic AVG.
- Arteriovenous access stenosis is almost invariably due to neointimal hyperplasia, which is comprised of proliferating myofibroblasts, neovasculature, and extracellular matrices.
- Development of stenosis at the venous anastomosis results in an increased intra-access pressure and resistance. This results in decreased access blood flow rate and, if severe, diminished efficiency of dialysis.
- There are several approaches to monitoring access stenosis. A rapid change in the nature and intensity of the thrill or bruit along the length of the access and the presence of distal swelling in the arm suggest the presence of stenosis. Other clues are prolonged bleeding from needle sites after needle withdrawal because of the high intra-access pressure, difficult cannulation, or an unexplained decrease in the dose of dialysis (Kt/V, see below). Several objective surveillance techniques have been used to detect graft stenosis, including measurement of static and dynamic outflow (venous)

pressures, or measurement of the access blood flow rate intradia-lytically by ultrasound dilution techniques. The gradual decrease in blood flow rate through the AVF or AVG over time provides a useful clue. Stenosis suggested by these surveillance techniques can be confirmed using duplex ultrasound.

- AVGs suspected to have stenosis are often referred for contrast-enhanced angiography and angioplasty. However, recent randomized trials failed to show any benefit of stenosis surveil-lance with pre-emptive angioplasty in terms of thrombosis-free survival or overall graft survival.
- No therapy has been shown to decrease neointimal hyperplasia formation and stenosis associated with AVF or AVG in dialysis patients.
- In a large randomized clinical trial, oral clopidogrel administered immediately after native AVF placement for 6 weeks increased the short-term patency rate, but did not increase their maturation rate.
- In another large randomized trial, the daily administration of combined aspirin and dipyridamole immediately after AVG place-ment resulted in a modest increase in the primary unassisted patency rate, with no effect on cumulative graft survival.

15.5.5.2 *Distal Ischemia*

- Steal syndrome is a complication that occurs occasionally after the placement of either AVF or AVG. It is due to the shunting of blood to the arteriovenous access, resulting in reduced perfusion to the distal extremity.
- The elderly and patients with diabetes or peripheral vascular disease are at increased risk for developing the steal syndrome.
- Common symptoms include coldness, paresthesia, numbness, impaired motor function, non-healing ulcers, pain during exer-cise, and muscle wasting of the distal extremity. Physical findings include a decrease in skin temperature, motor function, and distal arterial pulses, as well as discoloration and diminution of sensation.
- Mild symptoms can be managed symptomatically, such as wear-ing gloves and tactile stimulation. Severe ischemia with nerve damage, ulcer, or gangrene may require abandonment of the vas-cular access in order to restore blood flow to the distal extremity. For severe ischemia such as digital necrosis, amputation may be necessary.

15.5.5.3 *Arteriovenous Access Infection*

- Infections are rare in AVFs compared to AVGs. Infections in AVFs are usually caused by *Staphylococcus* and can often be treated successfully with antibiotics.
- Infections occur in 5%–20% of AVGs. Infections in old thrombosed AVGs are typically silent and often missed. The majority of infections are due to *Staphylococcus* and rarely Gram-negative organisms and enterococci. AVG infection can sometimes be treated successfully with antibiotics alone. Excision of the AVG is necessary if the infection is severe or if the infection is resistant to prolonged antibiotic treatment.

15.5.5.4 *Heart Failure*

- High-output heart failure is a rare complication of arteriovenous access.
- It occurs in patients with pre-existing cardiomyopathy or when the AVF has grown extraordinarily large, allowing very high blood flow rates (e.g. >2 L/min). It occurs more commonly with upper-arm accesses than lower-arm accesses.

15.5.5.5 *Aneurysm and Pseudoaneurysm*

- Aneurysms and pseudoaneurysms (skin pouch covered by skin without a true vascular wall) are formed by vascular trauma from needle punctures.
- Large aneurysms may limit needle puncture sites. More importantly, when the overlying skin is significantly compromised, the risks of rupture of the aneurysm or pseudoaneurysm constitute a surgical emergency.

15.6 Anticoagulation

- Exposure of blood to the extracorporeal circuit activates the coagulation pathways in the blood. Risk factors for clotting in the extracorporeal circuit include inadequate anticoagulation, slow blood flow, high hemoglobin levels, and intradialytic blood transfusions.
- Partial clotting in the dialyzer interferes with solute clearances. Complete clotting results in the loss of blood (approximately

120–150 mL in the entire hemodialysis circuit) and loss of the dialyzer.

- Unfractionated heparin is the main anticoagulant used for intermittent hemodialysis. It is often administered as an intravenous bolus of 2000–5000 units or 30–100 units/kg at the beginning of the session, followed by continuous infusion at 500–2000 units/h until 30–60 min before the end of dialysis. Alternatively, the continuous infusion is replaced by a repeated bolus method. Higher doses of heparin are usually employed to prevent clotting in fibers if the dialyzers are reused.
- Monitoring of the activated clotting time or partial thromboplastin time is seldom performed or necessary in the chronic dialysis setting because of the short duration of dialysis sessions.
- A single dose of low-molecular-weight heparin (LMWH) given as a bolus at the beginning of the session without further supplementation has been used successfully for anticoagulation in hemodialysis.

15.6.1 *Anticoagulation in Hemodialysis Patients at Risk for Bleeding*

- Some patients are at high risk for bleeding because of anatomical abnormalities (e.g. gastrointestinal ulcers) or bleeding diathesis (e.g. thrombocytopenia or chronic warfarin therapy).
- Under these circumstances, low-dose (tight) heparin regimens or heparin-free dialysis can be instituted. Careful visual monitoring of the extracorporeal circuit and monitoring of the pressure in the venous tubing for impending clotting, and sometimes periodic flushing of the extracorporeal circuit with boluses (50 mL) of saline, are necessary to prevent clotting.
- Other techniques that are employed for hemodialysis in patients with high bleeding risks are regional heparinization and regional citrate anticoagulation. In regional heparinization, heparin is infused into the inflow (arterial) tubing and the anticoagulation in the dialyzer is reversed in the outflow (venous) tubing by the infusion of protamine sulfate. In the regional citrate technique, citrate is infused into the arterial tubing as the anticoagulant, while calcium is infused into the venous tubing to reverse the anticoagulation. These anticoagulation techniques are presented in Table 15.9. Regional anticoagulation is cumbersome and the dosages are not simple to titrate; therefore, it is seldom used in chronic dialysis.

Table 15.9 Anticoagulation in hemodialysis patients at risk for bleeding.

Heparin-free dialysis	Recommended for patients who are actively bleeding, who are at high risk for bleeding, or who have heparin-induced thrombocytopenia.
	Performed by pre-rinsing the extracorporeal circuit with heparin (avoid in heparin-induced thrombocytopenia), using high blood flow rates and periodic flushing of the dialyzer with 50 mL of normal saline every 15–30 min.
Tight or low-dose heparin	Recommended in patients with a modest risk of bleeding or when heparin-free dialysis has been unsuccessful.
Regional heparinization	Heparin is infused into the arterial tubing before the blood reaches the dialyzer, and protamine sulfate is infused into the circuit distal to the dialyzer to neutralize the heparin before the blood is returned to the patient.
	Disadvantages: dissociation of the heparin–protamine complex in the body; the intrinsic anticoagulant property of protamine may also cause bleeding diathesis.
Regional citrate	The citrate solution infused into the arterial tubing chelates plasma calcium, thus inhibiting activation of the coagulation cascade. Calcium-free dialysis solution should be used. Calcium infused into the venous tubing restores the plasma ionized calcium concentration before the blood is returned to the patient.
	Disadvantages: imbalance between citrate and calcium may lead to increased or decreased plasma ionized calcium concentrations, which should be monitored frequently; the citrate may also cause severe metabolic alkalosis.

15.6.2 *Heparin-Induced Thrombocytopenia (HIT)*

- HIT is a complication of heparin therapy. The pathogenesis is the development of antibodies against the heparin–platelet factor 4 complex, leading to systemic platelet activation and consumption.

Table 15.10   Alternative anticoagulants.

Low-molecular-weight heparin (LMWH)	LMWH has a longer half-life in end-stage renal disease. A single loading dose predialysis is sufficient to provide adequate anticoagulation for the entire dialysis session.
Danaproid	Mixture of heparin sulfate, dermatan sulfate, and chondroitin sulfate. It is usually given as a bolus predialysis. Half-life is prolonged in kidney failure. Anti-Xa activity should be monitored and the dose should be adjusted accordingly.
Prostacyclin	Associated with side effects including hypotension.
Lepirudin (recombinant hirudin)	A direct thrombin inhibitor. Metabolized by the kidney; therefore, half-life is prolonged in kidney failure. There is no antidote for lepirudin in case of bleeding complications.
Argatroban	A direct thrombin inhibitor. Metabolized by the liver; half-life is not affected by kidney failure. The high cost can be prohibitive for long-term use.

- The clinical manifestations are thrombocytopenia and paradoxical systemic arterial and venous thrombosis.
- Heparin should be stopped as soon as HIT is confirmed. In patients with HIT, heparin-free dialysis can be attempted. If unsuccessful, regional anticoagulation with citrate or alternative anticoagulants, such as prostacyclin and direct thrombin inhibitors (lepirudin and argatroban), can also be used (Table 15.10). LMWH and danaproid cross-react with HIT antibodies, and should not be used in these patients.

15.7 Chronic Hemodialysis Prescription

- The major goal of hemodialysis is to normalize electrolytes and to remove toxins and excessive fluids.
- The amount of fluids that needs to be removed during each hemodialysis session is quite empirical, since the fluid volume

status in chronic intermittent hemodialysis patients is practically never in steady state. Second, the intravascular and total body fluid volumes that are associated with the best long-term clinical outcomes are unknown. Third, the fluid volume that can be removed depends greatly on the tolerability of the patient. The general objectives are prevention of pulmonary edema and maintenance of normal blood pressure at all times.

- The amount of toxins that should be removed is somewhat better defined. The marker that is commonly used is blood urea nitrogen (BUN). The parameter that is commonly used to guide chronic hemodialysis therapy is the urea reduction ratio (URR), which is defined as: (predialysis BUN minus postdialysis BUN) divided by predialysis BUN.

- An index related to URR that is also commonly used is the single-pool Kt/V (spKt/V) of urea, where K = dialyzer clearance of urea, t = duration of the dialysis session, and V = volume of distribution of urea in the body. In a single-pool kinetic model, urea is assumed to be evenly distributed in the body and there is no barrier to transport within its distribution volume.

- For patients treated three times per week, the US National Kidney Foundation K/DOQI practice guidelines (2006) recommend that the minimum dialysis dose per session be a spKt/V of 1.2 or a URR of 65%. To allow for imprecision in delivery, the recommended prescribed dose is a spKt/V of 1.4 or a URR of 70%.

- A large randomized trial (HEMO Study) did not show that a higher spKt/V (approximately 1.65) is associated with better survival than an spKt/V of 1.25, although the higher spKt/V was associated with better survival in the female subgroup in that trial and other observational studies. Thus, the K/DOQI guidelines recommend a higher Kt/V target for women and smaller patients in whom the distribution volumes of urea are low.

- The following steps can be used for the initial prescription to achieve a desired spKt/V:

  o Estimate the patient's urea distribution volume (V) using the anthropometric equations devised by Watson or Hume and Weyers.

  o Calculate ($K \times t$) by dividing the target spKt/V by V.

  o Set a desired dialysis treatment time (t), with a minimum of 3 h for patients who are dialyzing three times per week and have little residual kidney function. It should be noted that the treatment time is important not only for urea removal, but also for fluid and phosphate removal.

o Divide $(K \times t)$ by the desired t to obtain the dialyzer clearance (K).

o K is a function of the dialyzer mass transfer coefficient–surface area product (K_0A), blood flow rate (Q_B), and dialysate flow rate (Q_D). Next, choose a Q_B that can be reliably achieved and a Q_D that the hemodialysis machine can deliver and the dialysis unit policy permits. The necessary K_0A can then be derived from a nomogram, using the K, Q_B, and Q_D values. Dialyzers with the K_0A or greater K_0As are then selected.

o Alternatively, instead of deciding the dialysis treatment time (t) first, all of the other necessary variables (dialyzer, Q_B, and Q_D) are obtained and then the dialysis treatment time can be calculated.

o The URR or spKt/V is then measured monthly, and the prescription is adjusted accordingly.

o If there are changes in any of the variables that may change the spKt/V, such as changing from an arteriovenous access to a catheter, the dialysis prescription should be re-assessed and altered accordingly and the achieved URR or spKt/V measured again.

• Use of high-flux vs. low-flux membranes:

o The primary results of both the US HEMO Study and the European Membrane Permeability Outcome Study did not show a survival benefit using high-flux membranes, although secondary analyses suggested that survival benefits could be observed by the use of high-flux membranes in certain subgroups.

o In the HEMO Study, assignment to the high-flux arm was associated with improved mortality in patients who had been on long-term (>3.7 years) dialysis. Furthermore, there was a 20% reduction in cardiac deaths in the entire high-flux arm, compared to the low-flux arm.

o High-flux membranes are recommended for chronic hemodialysis if the quality of the dialysate water is high, so that the transfer of bacterial products (such as endotoxin fragments) into the blood can be minimized.

• To the extent that high-flux dialysis (which removes serum β_2-microglobulin effectively) may be beneficial and serum β_2-microglobulin levels have been shown to inversely correlate with mortality in chronic dialysis patients, serum β_2-microglobulin may be useful as a middle-molecule marker to guide hemodialysis therapy, in addition to using urea as a small-molecule marker.

Suggested Reading

Allon M. (2007) Current management of vascular access. *Clin J Am Soc Nephrol* 2:786–800.

Chang JJ, Parikh CR. (2006) When heparin causes thrombosis: significance, recognition, and management of heparin-induced thrombocytopenia in dialysis patients. *Semin Dial* 19:297–304.

Clark WR, Hamburger RJ, Lysaght MJ. (1999) Effect of membrane composition and structure on solute removal and biocompatibility in hemodialysis. *Kidney Int* 56:2005–2015.

Daugirdas JT. (2008) Prescribing and monitoring hemodialysis in a 3–4 ×/week setting. *Hemodial Int* 12:215–220.

Eknoyan G, Beck GJ, Cheung AK, *et al.*; Hemodialysis (HEMO) Study Group. (2002) Effect of dialysis dose and membrane flux in maintenance hemodialysis. *N Engl J Med* 347:2010–2019.

Fischer KG. (2007) Essentials of anticoagulation in hemodialysis. *Hemodial Int* 11:178–189.

Hayashi R, Huang E, Nissenson AR. (2006) Vascular access for hemodialysis. *Nat Clin Pract Nephrol* 2:504–513.

Hoenich N, Thijssen S, Kitzler T, *et al.* (2008) Impact of water quality and dialysis fluid composition on dialysis practice. *Blood Purif* 26: 6–11.

Leypoldt JK, Cheung AK. (2006) Revisiting the hemodialysis dose. *Semin Dial* 19:96–101.

Maya ID, Allon M. (2008) Vascular access: core curriculum 2008. *Am J Kidney Dis* 51:702–708.

Misra M. (2005) The basics of hemodialysis equipment. *Hemodial Int* 9:30–36.

National Kidney Foundation. (2006) KDOQI clinical practice guidelines and clinical practice recommendations for 2006. Updates: hemodialysis adequacy, peritoneal dialysis adequacy and vascular access. *Am J Kidney Dis* 48(Suppl 1):S1–S322.

Opatrný K Jr. (2003) Clinical importance of biocompatibility and its effect on hemodialysis treatment. *Nephrol Dial Transplant* 18(Suppl 5):v41–v44.

Sam R, Vaseemuddin M, Leong WH, *et al.* (2006) Composition and clinical use of hemodialysates. *Hemodial Int* 10:15–28.

16

Hemofiltration and Hemodiafiltration

Matthew K. L. Tong

16.1 Introduction

Hemofiltration is primarily a dialytic technique by which solutes are removed by a convective transport imitating the filtration process in the glomerulus of natural kidneys within the limits of the pore size. All solutes pass the filters with the same velocity and in the same amount, depending on the solute concentration of the blood compartment and the transmembrane pressure difference. Ultrafiltrate is either partially or completely replaced with sterile solution, infused either prefilter (predilution) or postfilter (postdilution).

Both hemofiltration and hemodiafiltration make use of the process of convection to remove solutes. Hemodiafiltration is a hybrid between hemofiltration and hemodialysis and, as such, incorporates a countercurrent dialysate solution within the hemofiltration circuit. With this procedure, low molecular substances are predominantly cleared by diffusion, while larger molecules [e.g. beta-2 microglobulin (β_2M), an amyloidogenic factor] are cleared mainly by convection (Fig. 16.1). These highly efficient methods are similar to, but distinct from, other continuous renal replacement therapies.

16.2 Hemofiltration versus Hemodialysis

Long-term hemofiltration treatment of patients with terminal renal failure has become less popular since the 1980s because:

- hemofiltration is more expensive than hemodialysis due to higher costs for filters and substitution fluid;
- the experience encountered in hemofiltration has brought about an improvement in hemodialysis, making use of a controlled ultrafiltration process with bicarbonate as the dialysis buffer; and

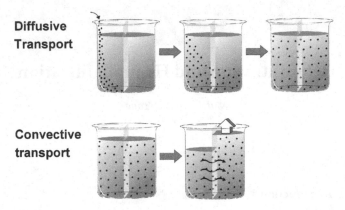

Fig. 16.1 Removal of uremic toxins.

- the emergence of hemodiafiltration has provided a more efficient method of removing low molecular substances.

16.3 Technical Requirements for Hemofiltration and Hemodiafiltration

- A hemofilter with a membrane that is highly permeable to fluid and solutes.
- A dialysis machine with accurate control of fluid removal and fluid replacement.
- Large volumes of sterile and physiological substitution fluid.
- In hemodiafiltration, a countercurrent dialysate solution within the hemofiltration circuit (Fig. 16.2).

16.4 Evolution for Hemodiafiltration

The evolution for hemodiafiltration has become possible due to advances in the construction of dialysis membranes. The high-flux membrane, partially hydrophilic with high sieving coefficients, and a reduced wall thickness have made it possible to combine diffusion and convection conveniently for blood purification. The second important step has been the development of accurate ultrafiltration control systems. The third step involves the production of large amounts of ultrapure dialysate and replacement fluid. This online production of substitution fluid has enabled high volume exchanges

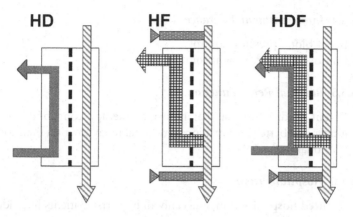

Fig. 16.2 Fluid route determines the mode of therapy. HD, hemodialysis; HF, hemofiltration; HDF, hemodiafiltration.

in hemodiafiltration. This is a major breakthrough in reducing the treatment cost.

16.5 Evidence for Clinical Efficacy in Hemofiltration and Hemodiafiltration

16.5.1 *Blood Purification*

- Excellent removal of small- and middle-sized molecules, including the amyloidogenic factor of β_2M
- Lower incidence of carpal tunnel syndrome

16.5.2 *Management of Anemia*

- Improved anemia management
- Studies have shown a reduced need for erythropoietin. This may be related to an excellent treatment biocompatibility and/or to a superior solute removal.

16.5.3 *Intratreatment Tolerance*

- Fewer hypotensive episodes
- Lower incidence of muscle cramps and posttreatment fatigue
- Suggested mechanisms include removal of the vasodepressor, less cytokine production, improved heat balance, and better blood volume preservation.

16.5.4 *Intertreatment Tolerance*

- Better blood pressure control
- Improved intertreatment comfort

16.5.5 *Residual Renal Function*

- Recent studies suggest that high-flux therapy contributes to a longer and better preservation of residual renal function than conventional hemodialysis.

16.5.6 *Hospitalization*

- Reduced hospitalization, especially in high-risk patients like elder patients and diabetics

16.5.7 *Mortality*

- No large-scale studies to demonstrate improved survival of patients on long-term convective dialysis therapies

16.6 Potential Complications and Drawbacks

- Pyrogenic reaction — There is a potential risk of passage into the circulation of bacteria-derived products either by direct infusion of contaminated on-line substitution fluid or by backfiltration of dialysate. This can be manifested as acute pyrogenic reactions with fever, hypotension, tachycardia, dyspnea, and cyanosis. Chronic exposure to low-grade pyrogen creates a chronic microinflammatory state that may contribute to long-term dialysis-related complications.
- Deficiency syndromes — There is a risk of enhanced loss of nutrients, including soluble vitamins and trace elements. Peptides and proteins may be lost during high-flux treatments. The total amount of nutrients lost per session, however, is usually negligible.
- Expensive treatment — Compared with hemodialysis, on-line hemofiltration or hemodiafiltration is more expensive due to the higher costs of hemofilters and ultrafilters for the preparation of ultrapure dialysate and substitution fluid.

16.7 Indications for Hemofiltration/Hemodiafiltration

- Patients with cardiovascular disease and blood pressure instability during hemodialysis

- Patients who are expected to remain on dialysis for a long time in order to reduce the risk of dialysis-related amyloidosis
- Patients who are experiencing symptoms related to the long-term accumulation of middle- and large-sized solutes like $\beta_2 M$.

16.8 Prescription

16.8.1 *Predilution versus Postdilution Mode*

Postdilution high-flux therapy offers greater clearance of both small solutes (like urea) and middle-sized to large solutes (like β_2-M). Hemodiafiltration is more efficient in removing small solutes. Predilution mode may be chosen when the achievable total ultrafiltration rate in postdilution mode is considered too low, which may be the case when blood hematocrit is high and/or the blood flow rate is low (Table 16.1).

16.8.2 *On-line Preparation of Sterile Nonpyrogenic Replacement Solution and Dialysis Solution*

Other than the USA, most countries allow the use of dialysis machines with direct on-line production of virtually unlimited amounts of sterile, nonpyrogenic substitution fluid at a relatively low cost (Table 16.2). Water should comply with the stringent criteria of purity with the concept of "ultrapure water". Apart from a proper pre-treatment system (microfiltration, softeners, and activated carbon) and reverse osmosis machines in series, water and dialysis fluid have to be filtered by a series of ultrafilters.

The ultrapure dialysis fluid should be checked regularly for quality control with bacteria count <0.1 CFU/mL and endotoxin <0.03 EU/mL before infusion into the patient's circulation. The ultrafilters

Table 16.1 Solute removal in optimized hemodiafiltration and hemofiltration.

	Urea	Kt/V-urea	Phosphate	$\beta_2 M$	Ultrafiltration volume
Post-HDF	75	1.70	55	74	40.3
Post-HF	52	0.91	46	74	43.3
Pre-HDF	70	1.45	49	74	86.7
Pre-HF	56	1.00	46	74	87.5

Note: [From Wingren K, Alquist M, Hegbrant J. *J Am Soc Nephrol* 1999; 10: 271A.]

Table 16.2 The chemical composition of hemodiafiltration fluid.

Type of HDF concentrate	Na^+ (mmol/ L)	K^+ (mmol/ L)	Ca^{++} (mmol/ L)	Mg^{++} (mmol/ L)	Cl^- (mmol/ L)	$Acetate^-$ (mmol/ L)	HCO_3^- (mmol/ L)
Normal Ca	138.00	2.00	1.75	0.50	109.50	3.00	32.00
Low Ca	138.00	2.00	1.25	0.50	108.50	3.00	32.00

should be replaced periodically to prevent supersaturation and release of endotoxins.

16.8.3 *Hemofilter*

The dialyser membrane should have a high hydraulic permeability (K_{uf}, 40–80 mL/h/mmHg), a high solute permeability, and a large membrane surface area of exchange (1.3–2.4 m^2).

16.8.4 *Flow Parameters*

- Blood flow Q_B: 300–400 mL/min
- Dialysate flow Q_D: 500–1000 mL/min
- Treatment time: around 4 h per session, 12 h per week.

16.8.5 *Substitution Volume*

Substitution volume = total ultrafiltration − weight gain.

(i) Hemofiltration

- Target Kt/V per session × patient's water volume (55% of body weight) or urea distribution volume in postdilution mode
- Volume doubled in predilution mode.

(ii) Hemodiafiltration

A simple rule of thumb of setting the substitution fluid rate:

- Postdilution: substitution rate = Q_B × 0.30
  (e.g. if Q_B = 300 mL/min: 300 × 0.30 = 90 mL/min)
- Total substitution volume = substitution rate × treatment time
  (e.g. if time = 240 min: 90 × 240 = 21.6 L)
- Predilution: substitution rate = Q_B × 0.50.

16.8.6 Anticoagulant

Convective dialysis therapy may result in higher blood procoagulatory activity when compared to standard hemodialysis, due to increased sheer forces that activate blood platelets. Administration of unfractionated or low-molecular-weight heparin via the arterial line may result in the convective loss of these middle molecules.

Administration of the initial bolus through the venous line is advisable, and one should allow 3–5 min for mixing of the bolus dose with the patient's blood before initiating extracorporeal blood flow. The dosage of unfractionated or low-molecular-weight heparin varies widely. Dose adjustments are based on body weight, response to therapy, and impact on reuse of dialyser. In general, the heparin dose requirement is comparable to that in hemodialysis.

Suggested Reading

Canaud B, Krieter D. (2007) Hemodiafiltration and hemofiltration. In: *Handbook of Dialysis*, 4th ed., Lippincott Williams & Wilkins, Philadelphia, pp. 265–275.

Ledebo I. (1998) Principles and practice of hemofiltration and hemodiafiltration. *Artif Organs* 22:20–25.

Locatelli F, Di Filippo S, Manzoni C. (2007) Clinical aspects of hemodiafiltration. In: Ronco C, Canaud B, Aljama P (eds.), *Hemodiafiltration*, Contributions to Nephrology, Vol. 158, Karger, Basel, Switzerland, pp. 185–193.

Locatelli F, Marcelli D, Conte F, et al. (1999) Comparison of mortality in ESRD patients on convective and diffusive extracorporeal treatments. The Registro Lombardo Dialisi E Trapianto. *Kidney Int* 55:286–293.

Tang HL, Tsang WK, Fung KS, et al. (2001) On-line hemodiafiltration and high-flux hemodialysis: comparison of efficiency and cost analysis. *Hong Kong J Nephrol* 3:21–26.

Vidi E, Bianco F, Panzetta G. (1993) The contribution of hemofiltration among the treatment modalities of chronic uremia. *Int J Artif Organs* 16:809–815.

17

Adequacy of Dialysis and Dietary Advice

Simon J. Davies and Barbara Engel

17.1 Adequacy of Dialysis

The term "adequacy" has been adopted by the nephrology community to describe that component of dialysis treatment that refers to the amount delivered as it relates to clinical outcomes. It is an attempt to provide clinicians with a common measurement of dialysis dose in order to ensure that a population-derived minimum (adequate) amount is delivered to each patient, as defined by clinical studies, which can then act as a benchmark for the quality of dialysis care. Although dialysis is designed to treat several aspects of kidney failure, including the removal of uremic toxins, correction of acidosis, and maintenance of satisfactory salt and water balance, the term "adequacy" has come to stand for one particular component: small-solute clearance.

Most commonly, the solute concerned is urea, although creatinine clearance is also used, especially in peritoneal dialysis and the quantification of residual renal function (RRF; see below). The reason urea has dominated the field derives from the highly influential National Cooperative Dialysis Study (NCDS) undertaken in the USA in the early 1980s. This study found that the survival of dialysis patients was not directly proportional to the dialysis dose if this was delivered to achieve a target plasma urea. The reason for this is simple: the average urea is a function of both its removal (clearance) and its generation from dietary protein intake or muscle catabolism. A patient may have a low plasma urea due to either a high clearance or a low protein intake, and in the NCDS these two extremes had different clinical outcomes. From this study, the concept of urea kinetic modeling was developed, which enables the separation of the determinant of plasma urea into its two components, urea clearance (Kt/V) and protein catabolic rate (PCR).

17.2 Measuring Small-Solute Clearance

17.2.1 *Hemodialysis: Urea Reduction Ratio (URR) and Kt/V*

- The simplest approach to measuring dialysis dose is to determine the proportional reduction of plasma urea during a midweek dialysis session. Blood samples are taken before and after the treatment, and the reduction ratio is calculated. A minimum reduction of 67% is considered as adequate.
- The main limitation of the URR is that it takes no account of the actual amount of urea removed and its appropriateness to the size of a patient.
- Kt/V_{urea} is the universal term used to describe the clearance of urea that takes patient size into account. K is the solute clearance across the dialysis membrane; t, the treatment length; and V, the volume of urea distribution in the body, generally considered to be equivalent to the body water.
- Kt/V is a dimensionless ratio, which can be estimated using Daugirdas' formula as follows:

$$\frac{K \cdot t}{V} = -\ln(R - 0.008 \cdot t) + (4 - 3.5 \cdot R)\frac{\Delta BW}{BW},$$

where R is the ratio of postdialysis urea to predialysis urea, t is the treatment time in hours, BW is the body weight, and ΔBW is the intradialytic weight change.

- Kt/V can be formally measured if either the dialysis membrane urea clearance characteristics are known or on-line measurement of dialysate solute concentration is possible, enabling direct quantification of urea removal. V is estimated from the Watson formula (see Appendix).
- There is a rebound increase in the blood urea during the first 30 min after completion of dialysis. This should be taken into account if the $[urea_{Post}]$ is measured immediately after dialysis (unequilibrated Kt/V); typically, this will overestimate the fully equilibrated Kt/V by 0.15 per session.

17.2.2 *Peritoneal Dialysis: Kt/V and Creatinine Clearance*

The measurement of peritoneal dialysis (PD) dose differs from hemodialysis (HD) dose in two important respects: first, it is a steady state treatment; and second, the measurement of actual solute removed is much simpler, whereas the volume of solute distribution (V) can only be estimated (Watson formula). Creatinine clearances are normalized to the body surface area (BSA).

- Solute removal is calculated from the product of dialysate concentration and the total drained dialysis volume over a 24-h period, typically multiplied by 7 to give the weekly clearance. Aliquots are taken from the dialysate drainage bags.
- Weekly solute clearance is calculated as follows:

$$\text{Urea clearance } (Kt/V) = 7 \times (\text{24-h dialysate urea removal/} \\ (\text{plasma urea} \times V)),$$

$$\text{Creatinine clearance} = 7 \times (\text{24-h dialysate creatinine removal/} \\ (\text{plasma creatinine})) \times (1.73/\text{BSA}).$$

17.2.3 Residual Renal Function (RRF)

- There is ample evidence that, for both PD and HD patients, the presence of RRF is associated with a survival advantage.
- This advantage is proportional to the amount of RRF, whether measured as urine volume or as solute clearance.
- When quantified as solute clearance (either Kt/V_{urea} or creatinine clearance), the survival value per unit of RRF clearance is greater than that associated with the equivalent dialysis clearance in observational studies; when adding RRF and dialysate clearances together, this should be taken into account.
- RRF is calculated as follows:

$$\text{Urea clearance } (Kt/V) = \text{24-h urine urea removal/(plasma} \\ \text{urea} \times V) \times 7,$$

$$\text{Creatinine clearance} = \text{24-h urine creatinine removal/} \\ (\text{plasma creatinine}) \times 7 \times (1.73/\text{BSA}).$$

- Because the renal secretion of creatinine is proportionally large at low levels of function, the overall RRF is the mean of the urea and creatinine clearances.

17.3 Present Strategy for Achieving Adequate Dialysis

As currently practised, for HD an adequate target for an unequilibrated Kt/V is 1.3 per treatment (URR $\equiv$ 67%) when given three times per week. This is based on the failure of the Hemodialysis (HEMO) Study to show any additional survival advantage when the Kt/V was increased to 1.7, likely reflecting the ceiling of what can be achieved in three sessions per week.

For PD, which is a continuous treatment, a minimal weekly peritoneal Kt/V of 1.7 or creatinine clearance of 50 L per week is recommended, based largely upon the ADEMEX study that failed to show a survival advantage of higher dose delivery. The difference between the weekly cumulative Kt/V_{urea} for HD and PD (3.3 vs. 1.7) is entirely a function of the intermittent versus continuous nature of the treatments.

17.3.1 Hemodialysis

The three components of dialysis dose are K (dialyser clearance), t (treatment length), and V (volume of distribution).

17.3.1.1 K (Clearance)

- The clearance of small solutes, e.g. urea, across a dialysis membrane is influenced by the surface area in contact with blood, the rate of blood flow, and the rate of dialysate flow.
- For each commercially produced membrane, the optimal dialysate and blood flow characteristics are published; typically, best clearances will be achieved with a blood pump speed of ~300–400 mL/min and a dialysate flow rate of 0.5–1 L/min.
- If blood and dialysate flows are optimal, or as good as can be achieved with current vascular access, then dialysis efficiency can be increased by increasing the membrane area; larger patients will require larger membranes.

17.3.1.2 t (Time)

- The optimal length of a dialysis session is determined by the rate of small-solute equilibration; typically for urea, when achieving optimal dialyser clearance this will be 3–5 h.
- For a larger solute (e.g. phosphate), equilibration is slower, thus taking longer. As discussed above, to obtain substantially larger PO_4 clearances requires more than three sessions per week.
- It must also be remembered that the length of a treatment session may be determined by the need to remove salt and water and by cardiovascular stability.

17.3.1.3 *V (Volume of Distribution)*

- The clinician cannot control this, but its relationship to survival and the limitations in its assessment need to be understood.
- Malnourished patients have a low V, so they will relatively easily obtain an adequate Kt/V; it can be argued that this should be taken into account when patients are below their ideal body weight.
- Secondary analysis of the HEMO Study suggested that women benefit from a higher Kt/V, whereas the opposite is true for men. Estimates of V are gender-dependent (see Watson formulas), and the 95% confidence interval for these estimates is ±20%.

17.3.2 *Peritoneal Dialysis*

The three components of peritoneal clearance are the volume of dialysate used, the membrane function (rate of solute transport), and the volume of solute distribution (V).

17.3.2.1 *Dialysate Volume*

- This is the most important determinant of dialysis dose. Assuming no contribution from RRF, then the daily volume required will range between 6 and 15 L per day depending on patient size.
- Dialysis dose can be increased by using a larger dwell volume (e.g. 2.5 L) and additional exchanges (e.g. 5–7 per day) using automated peritoneal dialysis (APD).
- High-volume, rapid-exchange regimes should not be used as they compromise sodium removal and expose the membrane to excessive glucose.

17.3.2.2 *Membrane Solute Transport Rate*

- The rate at which solute diffuses across the peritoneal membrane is highly variable between individuals. The dialysate: plasma ratio for creatinine at 4 h varies between 0.4 and 1.0, and is used to classify patients into rapid (>0.65) and slow (<0.65) transporters.
- Rapid transporters should avoid long dialysis dwell periods unless using icodextrin, as this will result in overall fluid and solute reabsorption, and are good candidates for APD which can deliver short exchanges overnight.

- Rapid-transport patients will achieve relatively high creatinine clearances compared to slow transporters, whereas urea clearance will be determined by dialysate volume.

17.3.2.3 V (Volume of Distribution)

- As with HD, there are problems in the interpretation of V, made worse by the fact that it is not possible to make an independent assessment from the urea kinetics. V has to be estimated and can be underestimated in malnourished patients or overestimated in the obese, leading to a wrong change in dialysis dose.
- The use of creatinine clearances, normalized for BSA, and dietetic assessment (see below) can be used to make the correct decision.

17.4 Protein Catabolic Rate (PCR) or Normalized Protein Nitrogen Appearance (nPNA) Rate

Another reason for employing urea kinetics is that urea generation rates can be derived. As the nitrogen in urea derives from protein catabolism, this can be converted into a measure of the net breakdown of protein (a small amount is lost via the gastrointestinal route). For a patient in nitrogen balance, the protein intake from the diet will be equivalent to the protein nitrogen appearance (PNA); hence, by measuring PNA, it is possible to estimate the patient's intake.

- PCR/PNA rate may be calculated from the interdialytic urea generation rate in HD patients and the daily measured urea losses in PD patients (see Appendix).
- For both HD and PD, daily urinary urea and protein losses should be added.
- In PD patients, there is a significant daily peritoneal protein loss (0.1–0.2 g/kg/day) which should added to the PNA rate.
- If the patient is catabolic due to sepsis, starvation, inflammation, or trauma, the net generation of urea will overestimate the dietary intake of protein.
- If the patient is anabolic due to exercise training or is regaining body cell mass after an illness or period of starvation, the PNA will be less than the dietary intake.

- For this reason, the normalized PCR (nPCR) measurement should only be used as an indicator of nutritional status and used in conjunction with a nutritional assessment that measures dietary intake as well as changes in body composition.

17.5 Dietary Advice

17.5.1 *Assessing Nutritional Status and Dietary Intake*

The nutritional status of a renal patient is known to decline from stage 4 chronic kidney disease (CKD), often marked by a spontaneous decrease in protein intake to below 0.8 g protein/kg by stage 5. Poor nutritional state at the start of dialysis is correlated with a poor outcome, and therefore it is important that patients with progressive renal disease are reviewed early on in their treatment. Malnutrition is common in renal patients, with the prevalence varying from 30% to 70% of the dialysis population.

Nutritional status is dependent not only on the intake of adequate amounts of nutrients, but also on the ability of the body to utilize these substances and dispose of the excess and waste products created from metabolic processes. The causes are multi-factorial and have been listed in the Kidney Disease Outcomes Quality Initiative (K/DOQI) guidelines, and include:

- dietary restriction
- anorexia (uremia, underdialysis)
- inflammation (contributes to anorexia and tissue catabolism, exacerbated by the dialysis procedure)
- metabolic acidosis
- endocrine disorders (insulin resistance, hyperparathyroidism)
- comorbidity (diabetes, cardiovascular disease)
- dialysis-related causes (inadequate dose, bioincompatible membranes, loss of nutrients, dialysate solutions)
- psychosocial causes (depression, low physical activity, loneliness, poverty).

Marinos Elia states that "*Mal*nutrition is a state in which a deficiency or excess (or imbalance) of energy, protein and other nutrients causes measurable adverse effects on tissue/body form (body shape, size and composition), function and clinical outcome." (*Clinical Nutrition*, 2005) By this definition, a thorough assessment of nutritional status should include measurements from each of the four following categories:

(i)   Adequate intake of nutrients — method: diet history (1-day recall or 3-day history), PCR, biochemistry;
(ii) Ability of body to utilize these nutrients (and dispose of excess/waste products) — method: biochemistry, gastrointestinal function;
(iii) Maintenance of function — method: grip strength, sit-to-stand and shuttle tests, activity questionnaires;
(iv) Renewal of components — method: body shape, size, and composition; distribution and quantity of fat, muscle, and fluid using anthropometrics and bioimpedance.

Tools which have been validated for use in the renal patient include the Subjective Global Assessment (SGA). This combines dietary intake, function (gastrointestinal tract and physical function), and body composition. It is practical, taking only 15 min to perform, and reproducible. It has also been shown to

- be an independent predictor of survival in PD patients,
- identify changing nutritional status in PD patients,
- correlate with measures of body composition.

Both the K/DOQI guidelines and the Renal Association of the UK recommend the use of SGA for assessing renal patients. If the patient is shown to be malnourished, it should be linked to a protocol for intervention (see below).

17.5.2 Recommendations for Daily Intake

These are influenced by metabolic requirements as well as the ability to utilize the nutrients and dispose of waste products. The current recommendations are described in Table 17.1 by nutrient, showing the varying considerations that need to be taken into account according to dialysis modality. Some key points are given below.

17.5.2.1 Dialysis

- In HD (3 times weekly) and PD patients, removal of phosphorus is only 10–14 mmol/day, which is less than 30% of the intake associated with the recommended protein intake.

- Some essential nutrients are also removed as they are water-soluble, e.g. amino acids and vitamins. The Dialysis Outcomes and Practice Patterns Study (DOPPS) showed that water-soluble vitamin supplementation is associated with a 15% decrease in mortality.
- Although water and sodium are removed during dialysis by ultrafiltration, excessive intake will result in large interdialytic weight gain in HD patients and overuse of PD solutions containing the higher glucose concentrations.
- During PD, 70% of the glucose is absorbed from the dialysate. This may be a useful source of energy in an undernourished patient (providing 300–1200 kcal/d). On the other hand, it may contribute to an excessive calorie intake that is converted to increased circulating triglycerides and excess body fat, increasing the risk of cardiovascular disease and diabetes.

17.5.2.2 *Dietary Restrictions: What and How?*

Restrictions of phosphorus, potassium, sodium, and fluid are usually required as indicated in Table 17.1.

Phosphorus

- Absorption of phosphorus from the diet is thought to be between 40% and 60% from grains, dairy, and meat due to competition and binding from phytates and calcium.
- Inorganic phosphates which are used as food additives (preservatives, moisture retention) may be 100% absorbed, and it has been estimated that this could provide up to 33 mmol (1000 mg) phosphorus per day.
- Generally speaking, phosphorus is associated with protein-rich foods such as meat, fish, dairy products, nuts, and pulses, but also with whole-grain foods and even soft drinks (see Table 17.2 for the relative PO_4 content of different foods).

Potassium

- About 50% of potassium intake comes from vegetables, potatoes, and fruit.
- Potassium content of food is also affected by cooking methods: boiling and throwing away cooking water will reduce potassium; whereas steaming, microwaving, and baking will retain potassium.

Table 17.1 Recommendations for dietary intake/restriction in CKD stage 5 patients, including modality-specific interactions.

Nutrient	Effect of dialysis/CKD stage 5	Dietary recommendation
Protein	HD: 6–12 g of amino acids are lost per session. PD: 6–12 g protein in addition to 3 g amino acids are lost per day.	Recommended minimum intake is 0.9 g/kg/day for HD and 1 g/kg/day for PD. K/DOQI guidelines (2000) advise a larger safety margin, aiming for 1–1.2 g/kg/day for HD and 1.2–1.3 g/kg/day for PD.
Energy	HD: a small amount of glucose (23 g) may be absorbed from dialysate. PD: significant glucose is absorbed from dialysate (300–1200 kcal/day), depending on the prescription.	HD: 30–35 kcal/kg IBW or use of Schofield equations with activity factor if weight changes (loss or gain) are desirable. PD: calculate calorie gain from dialysate and reduce dietary requirements by this amount. If the patient is diabetic or overweight, consider the use of icodextrin (a PD solution which contains glucose polymers), which will reduce glucose absorption by 50% compared to a 3.86% exchange.
Fat	Increased risk of cardiovascular disease; triglycerides tend to be raised in PD patients.	< 35% energy: reduce saturated fatty acids, increase polyunsaturated fats and monounsaturated fats.
Carbohydrate	Insulin resistance is common; at least 30% of the dialysis population are diabetic. Glucose absorption in PD may affect diabetic control.	50% of energy: decrease monosaccharides, encourage foods with low glycemic index, and increase sources of soluble and insoluble fiber. Use icodextrin to improve glycemic control in diabetic patients. Insulin requirements may be altered to cope with additional glucose load in PD.

(*Continued*)

Table 17.1 (*Continued*)

Nutrient	Effect of dialysis/CKD stage 5	Dietary recommendation
Phosphorus	Dialysis clears some phosphorus, but not all. Phosphate binders are used to bind phosphate in food present in the gastrointestinal tract.	0.5–0.6 mmol/kg ideal weight or 31–45 mmol/d (1000–1400 mg/d). A dietary restriction is required (see Table 17.2 for the relative PO_4 content of different foods).
Sodium	Sodium intake will stimulate the thirst mechanism, and hence the patient may drink excessively.	80–110 mmol/day (1.8–2.5 g elemental sodium, ≈5–7 g table salt). Dietary restriction is usually required.
Potassium	HD: maximum plasma levels should be less than 6.5 mmol/L. PD: continuous dialysis may remove excessive amounts of potassium.	HD: ≈1.0 mmol/kg IBW per day. PD: potassium restriction may not be necessary, although it is wise to avoid very high sources.
Minerals	HD: loss of iron from blood loss during dialysis. PD: loss of protein-bound trace elements.	PD and HD: calcium, magnesium, iron, zinc, selenium, and chromium supplementation should be considered.
Vitamins	Some water-soluble vitamins may be dialysed, although it is debatable whether this is greater than urine losses. Fat-soluble vitamins may accumulate.	Reported low levels of B1, B6, folate, vitamin C. Active vitamin D is usually required. Vitamin A supplements should be avoided. Water-soluble vitamin supplements recommended in the USA contain mostly 100% RDI, except B6 (500% RDI) and folate (250% RDI).
Fluid	HD: aim for an IDWG of 1.5–2.0 kg. EDTNA/ERCA nutrition guidelines (2002) suggest 4% of dry weight.	HD: the daily allowance is calculated as 500–750 mL plus the average daily urine output. PD: the fluid allowance depends upon the amount of fluid that can be removed using dialysate

(*Continued*)

Table 17.1 (*Continued*)

Nutrient	Effect of dialysis/CKD stage 5	Dietary recommendation
	PD: dry weight should remain stable from day to day (morning weight, drained out).	with the lowest glucose concentrations to avoid excess glucose absorption.

Note: IBW, ideal body weight; RDI, recommended daily intake; IDWG, interdialytic weight gain; EDTNA/ERCA, European Dialysis and Transplant Nurses Association/European Renal Care Association.

Table 17.2 Phosphorus-to-protein ratio of staple foods.

Phosphorus-to-protein ratio	<10 mg/g	10–14 mg/g	15–19 mg/g	>20 mg/g
Food type	Beef, lamb, pork, chicken, turkey	Processed/ Dried meats (sausage, bacon, meat paste), salmon, herring, mackerel, white bread, white pasta, vermicelli, rice noodles, tofu	Offal (liver, kidney), soya beans (boiled), pulses, soya milk, white rice, egg	Dairy (milk, yogurt, hard cheese), bony fish, dried fish, seafood, nuts (peanuts, pistachios), whole-grain cereals (brown rice, pasta, and flour)

Asian and Chinese diets, which use rice rather than potato as the staple carbohydrate food, reduce the intake of potassium. However, these diets traditionally have a greater intake of vegetables and pulses, and the cooking methods (steaming, stir-frying) tend to retain potassium.

Foods such as lotus root, taro, and yam have similar potassium content as potato.

Sodium

- About 80% of salt intake in Western diets comes from processed foods, including staple food items such as bread and breakfast cereals.
- Convenience foods, i.e. ready-made and take-away meals, have high sodium content. Tinned, smoked, and cured meat and fish are high in sodium, as are sauces (soy sauce, black bean sauce, oyster sauce), chutneys, pickles, and flavorings such as monosodium glutamate.
- Sodium intake can be reduced by using fresh ingredients, and using herbs and spices to flavor food rather than salt.

Fluid

The best way to control thirst is to avoid excess salt intake. Fluid allowance includes all drinks, but should also take into account the fluid content of gravies, sauces, curries, and soups as well as ice cream, jelly, and yogurt. Tips to help the patient control their fluid intake include:

- Use a small cup or glass and divide the fluid allowance throughout the day.
- Ice cubes or frozen fruit segments may be more thirst-quenching (but each cube contains 30 mL fluid).
- Stimulate saliva production by sucking a piece of lemon or grapefruit or by chewing gum.
- Try artificial saliva sprays.

17.5.2.3 *Dietary Supplements: What and When?*

Malnutrition increases morbidity (increased infection, electrolyte imbalance, length of hospital stay, and lethargy, and decreased physical function) and ultimately increases mortality. Macronutrient (fat, protein, carbohydrate) as well as individual micronutrient (electrolytes, trace elements) deficiency can result in malnutrition. It should not be assumed that an adequate macronutrient intake automatically ensures sufficient micronutrient intake. It is thus important when using modular supplements to increase macronutrient intake that there is attention to micronutrients. Electrolyte supplementation may be required in very malnourished patients, as refeeding may cause severe electrolyte imbalance ("refeeding syndrome").

After a thorough assessment of the patient has been carried out (Sec. 17.5.1), an appropriate plan of nutrition support can be implemented (NICE 2006). This includes the type, route, and rate of supplementation. The use of these methods requires calculation of their impact on phosphate, potassium, and fluid intake. It is also important to assess the impact of the nutrition support plan on the family/main carer.

The methods used include:

(i) *Increasing oral intake*. For patients who are able to eat and drink, encourage:

- foods with a high nutrient content.
- modified consistency if necessary.
- fortified foods (additional fat, protein, or sugar) — ordinary household foods (oil/butter, milk powder, table sugar) or modular nutritional supplements (protein powder, lipid emulsions, carbohydrate powders and liquids, carbohydrate and lipid mixtures) can be used.
- sip feeds (but soups, desserts, and bars are also available); these usually contain macronutrients as well as micronutrients. Various flavors include savory, sweet, and neutral.
- support and encouragement with eating.

(ii) *Nasogastric (NG) or gastrostomy feeding (PEG/RIG tubes)*. National Institute for Health and Clinical Excellence (NICE) guidelines (2006) recommend PEG placement if NG tube feeding is not appropriate or if feeding is likely to be required for more than 4 weeks. Renal formulas are more concentrated than regular formulas (to reduce the fluid intake), but also have lower electrolyte content. Tube feeding can take place overnight, to encourage eating during the day.

(iii) *Intraperitoneal amino acids (IPAAs) with PD*. Dialysate containing 1.1% amino acid solution seems to be well tolerated. It will provide a net gain of 18 g amino acids in 2 L. However, as with all modular supplements, it is important to ensure that energy and micronutrient requirements (e.g. vitamin B6) are also being met. Studies have shown an improvement in nitrogen balance, but the benefit is limited in catabolic patients.

(iv) *Intradialytic parenteral nutrition (IDPN)*. Parenteral formulas containing 50–70 g amino acids as well as 1000–1200 kcal from fat and carbohydrate are delivered via the venous return during hemodialysis. This is well tolerated, although glucose monitoring is necessary (even in non-diabetics) and fluid balance should be adjusted accordingly. Micronutrients (multivitamin and mineral supplements) should be supplied to ensure efficient use of the protein and calories. A meta-analysis has shown that IDPN improves outcome in very malnourished patients.

(v) *Total parenteral nutrition (TPN)*. This should only be used in patients whose gastrointestinal tract is not functioning sufficiently, e.g. in cases of sclerosing encapsulating peritonitis, as a preparation for surgery.

Finally, physical activity and physiotherapy can improve muscle mass and should be an integral part of nutrition support. In renal patients, exercise training can improve muscular atrophy and exercise endurance, and has a synergistic effect when applied alongside nutritional supplementation.

Appendix

Body surface area (Dubois equation):

$$\text{BSA (m}^2) = 0.20247 \times \text{height (m)}^{0.725} \times \text{weight (kg)}^{0.425}.$$

Watson formulae for estimation of total body water (volume of distribution of urea):

Males: $V = 2.447 - 0.09156 \times \text{age (years)} + 0.1074 \times \text{height (cm)} + 0.3362 \times \text{weight (kg)}$

Females: $V = -2.097 + 0.1069 \times \text{age (years)} + 0.2466 \times \text{weight (kg)}$.

Calculation of protein nitrogen appearence (mathematically the same as protein catabolic rate):

$$\text{PNA (g/day)} = \text{total nitrogen appearance (g/day)} \times 6.25.$$

Most simply, in HD patients the nitrogen appearance rate is determined from the urea generation rate between two dialysis sessions, i.e. the rate of increase of the blood urea nitrogen × V urea distribution (taken from Watson formula). In PD patients, it is directly calculated from the daily dialysate urea removal.

Suggested Reading

[Anonymous]. (2000) Clinical practice guidelines for nutrition in chronic renal failure. K/DOQI, National Kidney Foundation. *Am J Kidney Dis* 35: S1–S140.

Eknoyan G, Beck GJ, Cheung AK, *et al.*; Hemodialysis (HEMO) Study Group. (2002) Effect of dialysis dose and membrane flux in maintenance hemodialysis. *N Engl J Med* 347: 2010–2019.

Elia M. (2005) Chapter 1: Principles of Clinical Nutrition. In: Gibney MJ, Elia M, Ljungqvist O, Dowsett J. (eds.), *Clinical Nutrition*, The Nutrition Society. Blackwell Science, Oxford, pp. 1–14.

K/DOQI Workgroup. (2005) K/DOQI clinical practice guidelines for cardiovascular disease in dialysis patients. *Am J Kidney Dis* 45: S1–S153.

National Institute for Health and Clinical Excellence (NICE). (2006) Nutrition support in adults: oral nutrition support, enteral tube feeding and parenteral nutrition. http://www.nice.org.uk/CG32/.

Paniagua R, Amato D, Vonesh E, *et al.*; Mexican Nephrology Collaborative Study Group. (2002) Effects of increased peritoneal clearances on mortality rates in peritoneal dialysis: ADEMEX, a prospective, randomized, controlled trial. *J Am Soc Nephrol* 13: 1307–1320.

Toigo G, Aparicio M, Attman PO, *et al.* (2000) Expert Working Group report on nutrition in adult patients with renal insufficiency (Parts 1 and 2). *Clin Nutr* 19: 197–207, 281–291.

18

Prevention and Management of Renal Osteodystrophy

David B. N. Lee

18.1 Introduction

This chapter focuses on renal osteodystrophy, i.e. bone disease associated with chronic kidney disease (CKD). Renal osteodystrophy is now considered as one component of the CKD mineral-bone disorder (CKD-MBD), defined as a systemic syndrome that includes, in addition, abnormalities of calcium (Ca), phosphorus (P), parathyroid hormone (PTH), and vitamin D metabolism as well as vascular and soft tissue calcification. Frequent reference will be made to the K/DOQI[a] Clinical Practice Guidelines for Bone Metabolism and Disease in Chronic Kidney Disease (from hereon referred to as "K/DOQI"). A list of abbreviations used throughout the text is tabulated (Table 18.1). Similar issues in renal transplant patients are discussed in Chapter 25.

18.2 Renal Osteodystrophy: Classification

18.2.1 *Histological*

A recent classification (the TMV system) is summarized in Table 18.2, and the different types of renal osteodystropy based on this classification are depicted in Fig. 18.1. Bone turnover (T), mineralization (M), and volume (V) are assessed by a combination of static quantitative histomorphometric parameters and dynamic double-tetracycline-based label measurement of bone formation. Abnormal bone histology

---

[a] Kidney Disease Outcomes Quality Initiative of the National Kidney Foundation; see www.kidney.org/professionals/kdoqi/guidelines.cfm/.

Table 18.1 List of abbreviations.

1,25D	1,25-dihydroxyvitamin D	D sterol(s)	Active vitamin D
25D	25-hydroxyvitamin D		sterol(s)
ABD	Adynamic bone disease	FGF23	Fibroblast growth
Al	Aluminum		factor 23
AP	Alkaline phosphatase	GFR	Glomerular
BMD	Bone mineral density		filtration rate
Ca	Calcium	Non-CaPB	Non-calcium-
CaPB	Calcium-based phosphate		based phosphate
	binders		binders
Cbfa1	Core-binding factor	P	Phosphorus
	alpha-1	PTH	Parathyroid
CKD	Chronic kidney disease		hormone
CKD 3	CKD stage 3	qCT	Quantitative
CKD 4	CKD stage 4		computerized
CKD 5	CKD stage 5		tomography
CKD-MBD	CKD–Mineral and bone	SERM	Selective estrogen
	disorder		receptor
D_2	Vitamin D_2		modulator
D_3	Vitamin D_3	TMV	Turnover/
DAA	Dialysis-associated		mineralization/
	amyloidosis		volume
DEXA	Dual energy X-ray	VDR	Vitamin D receptor
	absorptiometry	[X]	Concentration of X
DFO	Deferoxamine		

becomes perceptible in CKD patients as the glomerular filtration rate (GFR) dips below 50–60 mL/min/1.73 m^2, a level at which an elevation in PTH and a reduction in 1,25-dihydroxyvitamin D (1,25D) also become detectable.

18.2.2 *Clinical*

In day-to-day clinical practice, the diagnosis of the type of bone disease associated with CKD is based on clinical and laboratory evaluation.

18.2.2.1 *Predialysis Patients*

Patients with serum intact [PTH] greater than 70 pg/mL (7.7 pmol/L) in CKD 3, greater than 110 pg/mL (12.1 pmol/L) in CKD 4, and greater than 300 pg/mL (33.0 pmol/L) in CKD 5 patients are likely to either have or develop hyperparathyroid-related bone disease. Some

Table 18.2   Bone biopsy: *TMV classification* and *Indications for bone biopsy*.[a]

TMV classification		
Histological descriptors	Categories	Implications/Comments
Turnover (T)	Low Normal High	Reflects bone remodeling rate, normally the coupled process of bone resorption and formation Assess by static histomorphometric parameters and dynamic measurement of bone formation using double-tetracycline labeling Influenced by hormones, cytokines, mechanical stimuli, and factors that affect the recruitment, differentiation, and activity of bone cells
Mineralization (M)	Normal Abnormal	Reflects bone formation through calcification/mineralization of bone collagen (osteoid) Assess by osteoid volume and thickness (histomorphometric measurements) as well as by mineralization lag time and osteoid maturation time (tetracycline labels) Influenced by vitamin D and mineral status, acid-base homeostasis, and toxic agents (e.g. Al)
Volume (V)	Low Normal High	Reflects amount of bone per unit volume of the biopsy sample Assess by histomorphometric measurement of bone volume in cancellous bone (sometimes also in cortical bone) Influenced by age, gender, race, genetic factors, nutrition, endocrine disorders, mechanical stimuli, toxic agents, neurological function, vascular supply, growth factors, and cytokines ·

(Continued)

Table 18.2 (*Continued*)

Indications for bone biopsy

Inconsistencies among biochemical parameters that preclude a definitive
  interpretation
Unexplained skeletal fracture or bone pain
Severe progressive vascular calcification
Unexplained hypercalcemia
Suspicion of overload or toxicity from Al, and possibly other metals
Before parathyroidectomy (in patients with history of significant Al
  exposure, or with biochemical parameters not fully consistent with severe
  secondary or tertiary hyperparathyroidism)
Prior to decision on long-term bisphosphonate treatment

---

[a] Based on the position statement of KDIGO. (Moe S, Drüeke T, Cunningham J, *et al.*,
Kidney Int 2006; 69: 1945–1953).

also use, in addition, total or bone-specific serum alkaline phosphatase (AP) as an index for bone turnover activities. Bone-specific
AP is more costly and its possible advantage is marginal. Early therapy directed towards attaining the target range recommended for
PTH and other mineral metabolic abnormalities (Table 18.3) is likely
to reduce the risk of extraskeletal calcifications and the subsequent
development of refractory secondary hyperparathyroidism.

18.2.2.2 *Dialysis Patients*

Most of the available bone histological data in CKD patients are based
on bone biopsy in dialysis patients.

High-turnover hyperparathyroid-related bone
disease and mixed uremic osteodystrophy

Patients with serum intact PTH > 300 pg/mL (33.0 pmol/L) and high
AP are more likely to have these forms of bone lesion.

Osteomalacia

Osteomalacia is diagnosed by typical clinical, laboratory, and imaging
evaluation (see Table 18.5). Causes include aluminum (Al) toxicity,
vitamin D deficiency (nutritional or drug-associated, such as anticonvulsants that upregulate cytochrome P450 activities), alcohol
abuse, and Ca and P deficiency.

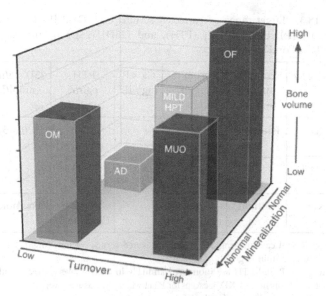

Fig. 18.1 Classification of renal osteodystrophy based on the TMV system. Bone turnover (T), mineralization (M), and volume (V) are represented by x-, y-, and z-axes, respectively. Osteomalacia (OM, red bar) is categorized as low-turnover bone with abnormal mineralization; the bone volume may be low to medium, depending on the severity and duration of the process and other factors that affect bone metabolism. Adynamic bone disease (AD, green bar) is described as low-turnover bone with normal mineralization and low bone volume; other patients may have normal bone volume. Mild hyperparathyroid-related bone disease (mild HPT, yellow bar) and osteitis fibrosa or advanced hyperparathyroid-related bone disease (OF, purple bar) represent a range of abnormalities along a continuum of medium- to high-turnover bone with variable bone volume, depending on the duration of the disease process. Mixed uremic osteodystrophy (MUO, blue bar) is characterized as high-turnover bone with abnormal mineralization and normal bone volume; consensus on the definition of this disorder is not unanimous. Reproduced with permission from: Moe S, Drüeke T, Cunningham J, *et al. Kidney Int* 2006; 69: 1945–1953. Macmillan Publishers Ltd, copyright 2006.

Adynamic bone disease (ABD)

ABD is more likely in patients with low intact PTH (<100 pg/mL or <11.0 pmol/L) in association with conditions known to oversuppress the parathyroid gland, such as excessive use of active vitamin D sterols

Table 18.3 Target range of corrected serum [Ca] (Ca),[a] [P] (P), [Ca] × [P] (Ca × P), intact [PTH] (PTH), and [25D] (25D) by the stage of CKD[b] based on K/DOQI.

CKD stage	Serum Ca, mg/dL (mmol/L)	Serum P, mg/dL (mmol/L)	Ca × P, mg²/dL²	PTH, pg/mL (pmol/L)	25D, ng/mL (nmol/L)
CKD 3	Footnote[c]	2.7–4.6 (0.87–1.49)		35–70 (3.9–7.7)	≥30 (75)[e]
CKD 4			<55	70–110 (7.7–12.1)	
CKD 5	Footnote[d]	3.5–5.5 (1.13–1.78)		150–300 (16.5–33.0)	Footnote[f]

[a] Corrected total calcium (mg/dL) = total measured serum calcium (mg/dL) + 0.8 × (4 − serum albumin in g/dL).
[b] Ca, albumin, P, and PTH are monitored annually in CKD 3; every three months in CKD 4; and monthly in CKD 5, except for PTH which is measured every three months.
[c] Within the "normal" range for the laboratory used.
[d] As for CKD 3 and 4, but preferably toward the lower end of 8.4–9.5 mg/dL (2.10–2.37 mmol/L).
[e] As recommended by K/DOQI. Currently no guidelines for the upper limit of 25D level for CKD patients. Ergocalciferol repletion (Table 18.7), if serum level of 25D < 30 ng/mL (75 nmol/L).
[f] Many follow the recommendation for CKD 3 and 4 (see footnote "e", above). K/DOQI recommends active vitamin D sterols if 25D < 30 ng/mL (75 nmol/L).

(D sterols), chronic Ca overload, or parathyroidectomy. Aging and diabetes mellitus are other risk factors.

- [PTH] > 400 pg/mL (44.0 pmol/L) does not exclude ABD (see Sec. 18.4.2). Definitive diagnosis is by bone biopsy.
- The low bone buffering capacity is reflected by a relatively low serum [P], a proneness to develop hypercalcemia with minimal (or no apparent) Ca loading, and the propensity for metastatic calcifications.

18.2.3 *Factors Which Can Modify CKD Bone Disease*

18.2.3.1 *CKD-related Factors*

These include therapeutic agents (e.g. glucocorticoids, vitamin D metabolites, phosphate binders); associated medical conditions

Table 18.4   Deferoxamine (DFO) test.[a]

Indications	In patients with elevated serum Al levels (60–200 µg/L) associated with clinical manifestations of Al toxicity (see Sec. 18.7.2.1). Prior to parathyroid surgery in patients with a significant history of Al exposure.
Procedure	*Hemodialysis*

1. After obtaining a baseline serum sample for [Al], administer intravenously 5 mg/kg DFO in 150 mL of 5% glucose water,[b] during the last hour of a dialysis session.
2. Repeat serum [Al] in 2 days (44 h after DFO administration), prior to the initiation of the next dialysis session.
3. Because DFO can further increase serum [Al], in patients with baseline serum [Al] > 200 µg/L, the test is delayed until a course of intensive dialysis is completed.[c]

Peritoneal dialysis

1. Following a baseline serum sample for [Al], administer intravenously 5 mg/kg DFO in 150 mL of 5% glucose water during the last hour of a CAPD[d] exchange. Alternatively, DFO is added to the overnight exchange in CAPD patients or to the long-dwell daytime exchange in CCPD[e] patients.
2. Repeat serum [Al] 44 h after intravenous DFO infusion or intraperitoneal DFO administration.

Monitoring

Abort DFO administration if hypotension occurs. Give volume expanders and other appropriate management.

Interpretation	An increment in serum [Al] ≥ 50 µg/L constitutes a positive test. In a dialysis patient with the combination of clinical features of (and risk factors for) Al toxicity, an elevated baseline serum [Al] > 60–200 µg/L, and an intact PTH < 150 pg/mL (16.5 pmol/L), a positive DFO test constitutes strong evidence for Al overload as a cause of Al bone disease.

(Continued)

Table 18.4 (*Continued*)

Definitive diagnosis requires a bone biopsy demonstrating increased Al staining of the bone surface (>15% to 25%), usually associated with osteomalacia or ABD.

---

[a] Based on K/DOQI and Delmez and Kaye (2001).
[b] Use of low-dose DFO based on prior reports of ophthalmological damage with permanent visual loss from single, high-dose (20–40 mg/kg) DFO.
[c] See Table 18.13 (hemodialysis patients in DFO treatment).
[d] CAPD: continuous ambulatory peritoneal dialysis.
[e] CCPD: continuous cycling peritoneal dialysis.

Table 18.5 Imaging techniques in renal osteodystrophy.

Technique	Comments
X-ray	Skeletal X-ray is not indicated in the routine management of renal osteodystrophy.
	May be useful in:
	(a) advanced osteitis fibrosa (e.g. subperiosteal resorption)
	(b) severe osteomalacia (e.g. Looser zone)
	(c) β_2-microglobulin amyloidosis.
	Extraskeletal calcifications:
	(a) May find evidence in patient's imaging library.
	(b) Lateral abdominal X-ray has been proposed for demonstration of aortic calcification.
	(c) Computed tomography scans have been used as a research tool, not for screening purposes.
DEXA[a]	BMD[b] measured at the distal radius is reported to be predictive of fracture risks and correlates with PTH levels.
	Consider in patients with fractures and in those with risk factors for osteoporosis.
qCT[c]	Distinguishes cortical BMD from trabecular BMD.
	(a) Hyperparathyroid-related bone disease
	(i) Sclerotic trabecular bone with increased BMD
	(ii) Resorption of cortical bone with decreased BMD
	(b) Low-turnover ABD: reduction in trabecular BMD

[a] Dual energy X-ray absorptiometry.
[b] Bone mineral density.
[c] Quantitative computed tomography.

(e.g. diabetes mellitus, postparathyroidectomy state); and other factors including toxic exposure to Al, metabolic acidosis, and β_2-microglobulinemic amyloidosis.

18.2.3.2 *General Factors*

Factors that affect bone morphology and function in the general population can cause additional bone changes in CKD patients and may exacerbate renal osteodystrophy. These include demographic factors (e.g. age, race, postmenopausal state); abnormal vitamin D metabolism (e.g. nutritional deficiency); medications (e.g. anticonvulsants); and other factors including neoplasia, physical inactivity, and immobilization.

18.2.3.3 *Osteoporosis and β_2-Microglobulin Amyloidosis*

See Sec. 18.7 for more details.

18.3 Renal Osteodystrophy: Diagnostic Tests

18.3.1 *Bone Biopsy*

See Table 18.2.

18.3.2 *Deferoxamine (DFO) Test*

DFO test is used in CKD patients for the diagnosis of Al overload and toxicity. See Table 18.4.

18.3.3 *Imaging Techniques*

These are summarized in Table 18.5.

18.4 Treatment of Hyperparathyroidism

18.4.1 *General Schematic*

This is summarized in Table 18.6.

Table 18.6 Basic principles in the management of hyperparathyroidism in CKD patients.

Secondary hyperparathyroidism
  Goals: to bring serum [25D], [Ca], [P], [Ca] × [P], and [PTH] to their
    respective target ranges as recommended by K/DOQI (Table 18.3).
  Strategy:
        Step I: correction of vitamin D deficiency, if present
        Step II: control of P retention and hyperphosphatemia[a]
        Step III: optimal use of D sterols and calcimimetics
In CKD patients with hypercalcemia
  If PTH is high, rule out primary hyperparathyroidism in predialysis
    CKD patients, and tertiary (refractory) hyperparathyroidism in dialysis
    patients.
  If PTH is relatively "low", consider low-turnover bone disease, malignancy,
    and other causes of hypercalcemia.

---

[a] In CKD 3 and 4 patients who present with [25D], [Ca], and [P] within goals, but [PTH] above target, some advocate a trial of phosphate binders and monitoring of serum PTH response prior to progressing to step III. This is based on the rationale that: (1) [P] may be within the population "normal" range, but high for an individual patient; or (2) a patient may be in a P-retaining state, and a normal [P] is maintained at the expense of increased PTH secretion. The relief of P-retention with phosphate binders could reverse such a sequence of events, with reduction in PTH secretion to (or towards) normal.

18.4.2 *Note on Intact PTH Measurement*

K/DOQI-recommended PTH levels are based on intact PTH measurements using first-generation assays. Most of the biological activities of the PTH molecule, which consists of 84 amino acids, reside in the N-terminal, largely in the first seven amino acid residues. PTH measurements by the first-generation assays also include the biologically inactive fragments, i.e. fragments without amino acid residues 1–7. Thus, some patients may not have significant hyperparathyroid-related bone disease (or may even have low-turnover bone disease), even though their serum [PTH] may be elevated; while in others, aggressive treatment to attain the lower end of the PTH target range may expose them to the risk of developing low-turnover bone disease. Second-generation immunoradiometric two-site sandwich assays, which purportedly measure biologically active PTH only (providing values of about 50%–60% of those based on the current intact PTH assays), are not readily available in clinical practice at this time.

18.4.3 *Management Strategy*

18.4.3.1 *Step 1: Vitamin D Insufficiency and Deficiency*

In addition to the traditional focus on vitamin D resistance, recent observations have also stressed the importance of vitamin D deficiency in CKD. Arguments for maintaining adequate 25-hydroxy-vitamin D (25D) store include (a) supplying substrate for 1,25D synthesis in nonrenal tissues that express 1α-hydroxylase and (b) that 25D may mediate bone effects different from those of 1,25D. A recent study reported that vitamin D deficiency is common in CKD patients at initiation of hemodialysis and is associated with early (within 90 days) mortality (Wolf *et al.* 2007). A rigorous cause-and-effect relationship, however, remains to be established.

Indication for repletion

K/DOQI recommends ergocalciferol repletion in CKD 3 and 4 patients, if serum [PTH] is above the respective target range (Table 18.3) and serum [25D] is <30 ng/mL or <75 nmol/L. A similar repletion strategy has also been advocated in dialysis patients (Saab *et al.* 2007).

The question of correcting vitamin D deficiency in patients with normal or "low" serum [PTH] is not resolved. In a survey of about 1000 incident hemodialysis patients, 79% of patients with serum [PTH] <150 pg/mL or <16.5. pmol/L had 25D levels <30 ng/mL or <75 nmol/L (Wolf *et al.* 2007). Current practice favors raising serum 25D to 30 ng/mL, even in patients with [PTH] below the recommended target ranges.

Diagnosis and management

This is summarized in Table 18.7. If PTH remains above goal after vitamin D repletion, proceed to steps 2 and 3.

Table 18.7 Ergocalciferol/vitamin D_2 (D_2) management of nutritional vitamin D insufficiency (D_{isf}) or deficiency (D_{def}) in CKD patients[a] based on serum 25D status in ng/mL or [nmol/L].

25D status	D_2 dose	Comments
<5 [<12]: severe D_{def}	Oral 50,000 IU/wk × 12, then monthly × 3[b]	Initiate treatment only in patients with [Ca] and [P] (with or without phosphate binders) within target range (Table 18.3).
5–15 [12–37]: mild D_{def}	Oral 50,000 IU/wk × 4, then monthly × 5	Measure serum [Ca] (corrected) and [P] every three months. Stop vitamin D therapy if patient becomes hypercalcemic or hyperphosphatemic (persists with P-binder treatment).
15–30 [40–75]: D_{isf}	Oral 50,000 IU/ month × 6	Measure 25D at 6 months and determine the need for further treatment based on 25D status.
>30 [>75]: D replete	No treatment	Monitor 25D annually.

[a] See text for additional discussion.
[b] May give 500,000 IU as a single intramuscular dose.

18.4.3.2 *Step 2: Control of P Retention and Hyperphosphatemia*

Rationale for treatment

P retention is an early event that leads to increased production and release of PTH (and other phosphaturic factors, such as fibroblast growth factor 23 (FGF23)). As CKD advances, these compensatory mechanisms are overwhelmed and hyperphosphatemia emerges and exacerbates. Other effects of P retention and hyperphosphatemia include inhibition of vitamin D activation (exacerbated further by the FGF23-mediated inhibition of renal 1α-hydroxylase activity); downregulation of parathyroid vitamin D receptor (VDR); and upregulation of core-binding factor alpha-1 (Cbfa1), which transforms vascular smooth muscle cells into osteoblast-like cells that calcify and mineralize. In addition, there is now persuasive evidence linking hyperphosphatemia to increased morbidity and mortality in end-stage renal disease (ESRD) patients.

Management strategy

A stepwise management strategy is summarized in Table 18.8.

18.4.3.3 *Step 3: Use of Activated Vitamin D Sterols and Calcimimetics (CaM)*

See Tables 18.9 and 18.10.

- If PTH remains high despite adequate 25D levels (step 1) and optimization of serum [Ca] and [P] to within target ranges (Table 18.3) with management of P retention (step 2), initiate treatment with a D sterol. If necessary, and when appropriate, add cinacalcet (Sensipar®) (see Table 18.9 for dosage) to achieve control of the hyperparathyroid state.
- One may reverse the order and consider initiation with cinacalcet if [Ca] is close to the high end of the target range, with subsequent addition of a D sterol, if appropriate. This approach can also be considered if high [PTH] is associated with hyperphosphatemia that is difficult to control, or limits the initiation or optimization of D sterols, or a combination of both.

18.5 Parathyroidectomy

18.5.1 *Indications*

Parathyroidectomy should be considered in patients with sustained elevation in serum PTH (>800 pg/mL or >88.0 pmol/L) — associated with hypercalcemia (reflecting autonomous, nonsuppressible PTH synthesis and secretion) or hyperphosphatemia, or both — who are refractory or intolerant to medical therapy. Clinical improvement has also been reported, following parathyroidectomy, in patients with calciphylaxis, associated with PTH levels >500 pg/mL (>55.0 pmol/L).

18.5.1.1 *Clinical Aspects of Refractory Hyperparathyroidism*

Patients may present with relentless escalation of hyperparathyroid bone disease and features of nonskeletal involvements, which include intractable pruritus; debilitating myopathy; progressive extraskeletal calcification; and debilitating arthritis, periarthritis, and spontaneous tendon ruptures. Because a number of these

Table 18.8　A stepwise management strategy for P retention and hyperphosphatemia.

Modalities	Comments
Dietary P restriction	Reduce P intake to 800–1000 mg/day (adjusted to dietary protein needs).
	Initiate in patients with serum [PTH] and/or [P] above targets.
	Monitor serum [P] monthly.
	Requires dietary counseling/monitoring for avoidance of protein malnutrition.
	Usually needs phosphate binders to allow optimal nutritional intake.
Ca-based phosphate binders (CaPB)[a]	Total Ca intake from CaPB <1.5 g/day OR total Ca intake <2.0 g/day.
	(a) Ca carbonate: CalciChew™ contains 0.5 g Ca/1.25 g tablet (3)[b]; TUMS™ contains 0.2 g Ca/0.5 g tablet (7.5).[b]
	(b) Ca acetate: PhosLo™ contains 0.167 g Ca/0.667 g tablet (9).[b]
	If necessary, add non-CaPB.
Non-Ca-, non-Al-, non-Mg-based phosphate binders (non-CaPB)[a]	Use, in addition to CaPB, in patients whose serum [P] remains elevated with maximum recommended (or tolerable) doses of CaPB.
	(a) Optimize dose of one non-CaPB.
	(b) Follow by a second non-CaPB, if necessary.
	Use in place of CaPB in CKD 5 patients if:
	(a) [Ca] >10.2 mg/dL (2.54 mmol/L).
	(b) PTH <150 pg/mL (16.5 pmol/L).[c]
	(c) Patient has significant vascular/soft tissue calcifications.

(Continued)

Table 18.8 (*Continued*)

Modalities	Comments
	Sevelamer hydrochloride (Renagel®)
	(a) 400 or 800 mg/tablet.
	(b) Initial dose:
	(i) 800 mg orally 3 times/day with meal, if [P] is 5.5–7.4 mg/dL.
	(ii) 1200 mg orally 3 times/day with meal, if [P] is 7.5–8.9 mg/dL.
	(iii) 1600 mg orally 3 times/day with meal, if [P] is ≥9.0 mg/dL.
	(c) Increase by 400 mg/meal at 2-weekly intervals, if [P] > 5.5 mg/dL.
	(d) Decrease by 400 mg/meal at 2-weekly intervals, if [P] < 3.5 mg/dL.
	(e) Maximum daily dose studied: 13 g.
	(f) Side effects: include gastrointestinal disturbances such as constipation and flatulence, exacerbation of metabolic acidosis.[d] Consult drug information for details.
	Lanthanum carbonate (Fosrenal®)
	(a) 250, 500, 750, or 1000 mg/chewable tablet.
	(b) Initial dose: 250 to 500 mg orally 3 times/day, with or immediately after meals.
	(c) Increase by 750 mg/day every 2–3 weeks.
	(d) Usual dose range: 1500–3000 mg/day.
	(e) Maximum daily dose: 3750 mg.
	(f) Side effects: include nausea, vomiting. Long-term safety data in progress. Consult drug information for details.

(*Continued*)

Table 18.8 (*Continued*)

Modalities	Comments
Al-based phosphate binders	Used by some as a one-time, short course (4 weeks) for severe hyperphosphatemia, e.g. >7.0 mg/dL (>2.26 mmol/L).
Niacin	Niacin (nicotinic acid, vitamin B3) and related compounds inhibit NaPi2b cotransporter and reduce intestinal phosphate absorption.
	Several studies reported serum P-lowering effect in dialysis patients.
	Long-term safety not established (Berns 2008).
Increase dialytic P clearance	Increase dialytic time and/or frequency.
	Most effective and "physiological" means of attaining P balance.
	Economically and logistically challenging.

[a] Take with meals (to maximize phosphate binding and, in the case of CaPB, to limit the amount of Ca absorption) and apportion the number of tablets to match the estimated meal P content. For sevelamer, a study reported that thrice-daily and once-daily dosing are equally effective (Fischer *et al.* 2006).

[b] Number in parentheses indicates number of tablets/day that contains 1.5 g elemental Ca.

[c] Likely to have low-turnover bone disease with low Ca buffering capacity. Thus, the Ca load associated with CaPB administration can increase the risk for extraskeletal calcification.

[d] Possibly secondary to bicarbonate binding in the intestine by sevelamer hydrochloride. A new formulation, sevelamer carbonate (Renvela™), is not expected to worsen metabolic acidosis.

Table 18.9   Active vitamin D sterols (D sterols) and cinacalcet (Sensipar®, CaM): combination therapy.[a]

Rationale for combination therapy

(a) D sterols and CaM provide complementary and additive/synergistic mechanisms in the net suppression of PTH secretion, while:
   (i) D sterols cause *increases* in [Ca] and [P]; and
   (ii) CaM causes *decreases* in [Ca] and [P] (in dialysis patients).
(b) Thus, combination therapy:
   (i) suppresses PTH in concert, while balancing out the opposing effects on [Ca] and [P]; and
   (ii) allows reduction in D sterols to low "physiologic" doses,[b] with no loss in PTH suppression and improvement in the control of [Ca] × [P].

D sterols: see Table 18.10.[c]

Cinacalcet

(a) Dose: Initiate at 30 mg/day with stepwise increments to 60, 90, and 180 mg/day at 4-weekly intervals, until goal is achieved. Not to be given if [Ca] < 8.4 mg/dL (< 2.1 mmol/L). Unlike the D sterols, hyperphosphatemia is not a contraindication for cinacalcet treatment.
(b) Side effects:
   (i) Nausea and vomiting: often resolved with continued use.
   (ii) Hypocalcemia: Manage with CaPB, D sterols, or dose reduction. Rigorous monitoring for seizures and QT_c prolongation. If response to corrective measures is suboptimal, discontinue medication.
   (iii) Consult drug information for details.

(c) Notes:

   (i) May increase [P] in predialysis CKD patients (versus decreasing [P] in dialysis patients), probably secondary to reduction in PTH with parallel reduction in urine phosphate excretion.
   (ii) Not yet approved for use in predialysis CKD patients in the USA.
   (iii) Treatment to be monitored by weekly serum [PTH], [Ca], and [P].

[a] See text for additional discussion.
[b] Defined as paricalcitol 2 μg, doxercalciferol 1 μg, or calcitriol 0.5 μg per dialysis session (Chertow *et al.* 2006).
[c] D sterol treatment dosages in Table 18.10 are from K/DOQI and other publications not based on the concept of combination therapy with cinacalcet.

Table 18.10A Active (1-hydroxylated) vitamin D sterols[a]: suggested treatment[b] in CKD 3 & 4 (CKD) and peritoneal dialysis (PD) patients.

Sterols	Oral dose
Rocaltrol® Calcitriol $1,25(OH)_2D_3$	CKD: 0.25 µg/day PD: 0.25 µg/day OR 0.5–1.0 µg 2–3 times/week
Hectorol® Doxercalciferol $1\alpha(OH)D_2$	CKD: 2.5 µg 3 times/week PD: 2.5–5.0 µg 2–3 times/week
Zemplar® Paricalcitol 19-nor-1, $25(OH)_2D_2$	CKD: 1–2 µg/day OR 2–4 µg, 3 times/week (Coyne *et al.* 2006) PD: mean dose, 3.9–7.6 µg 3 times/week (Ross *et al.* 2008)

[a] Alfacalcidol ($1\alpha(OH)D_3$), falecalcitriol (F6-$1,25(OH)_2D_3$, hexaflurinated analog), and maxacalcitriol (22-oxacalcitriol) are not available in the USA.
[b] See K/DOQI and other indicated references for details on dosage optimization and monitoring. Also see footnotes "b" and "c" in Table 18.9.

Table 18.10B Active (1-hydroxylated) vitamin D analogs[a]: suggested treatment,[b] either oral or intravenous, in hemodialysis (HD) patients according to serum [PTH] (PTH) levels.

Analog	PTH (pg/mL/pmol/L)	Dose (µg/HD treatment)	
		Oral	Intravenous
Rocaltrol® Calcitriol $1,25(OH)_2D_3$	300–600/33–66 600–1000/66–110 >1000/>110	0.5–1.5 1.0–4.0 3.0–7.0	0.5–1.5 1.0–3.0 3.0–5.0
Hectorol® Doxercalciferol $1\alpha(OH)D_2$	300–600/33–66 600–1000/66–110 >1000/>110	5 5–10 10–20	2 2–4 4–8
Zemplar® Paricalcitol 19-nor-1, $25(OH)_2D_2$	300–600/33–66 600–1000/66–110 >1000/>110		2.5–5.0 6.0–10.0 10.0–15.0

[a] Alfacalcidol ($1\alpha(OH)D_3$), falecalcitriol (F6-$1,25(OH)_2D_3$, hexaflurinated analog), and maxacalcitriol (22-oxacalcitriol) are not available in the USA.
[b] See K/DOQI and other indicated references for details on dosage optimization and monitoring. Also see footnotes "b" and "c" in Table 18.9.

features, including hypercalcemia and hyperphosphatemia, can develop in dialysis patients with modest or even low serum [PTH], parathyroidectomy is considered only in patients with [PTH] >800 pg/mL or >88.0 pmol/L (see Sec. 18.5.2). High [PTH] as an isolated finding does not constitute an indication for parathyroidectomy.

18.5.2 Relative Contraindication

Bone biopsy is recommended prior to making the decision for parathyroidectomy in patients with a history of Al exposure/toxicity or in patients at risk for the development of ABD (see above and Table 18.2).

18.5.3 Parathyroid Imaging

Parathyroid glands can be scanned using ^{99}Tc-sestamibi scan, ultrasound, computerized tomography (CT) scan, or magnetic resonance imaging (MRI) (see Chapter 28). It is not a routine preoperative test in the surgical management of secondary hyperparathyroidism. It is useful:

- in the diagnosis of primary hyperparathyroidism
- prior to re-exploration for recurrence
- for possible identification of tertiary hyperparathyroidism with adenomatous transformation.

Clinicians need to be aware of the risk of nephrogenic systemic fibrosis associated with the use of gadolinium-based contrast agents.

18.5.4 Operative Options

18.5.4.1 Surgical Parathyroidectomy

This includes subtotal parathyroidectomy, or total parathyroidectomy with or without parathyroid tissue autotransplantation (usually into the brachioradialis muscle of the forearm).

18.5.4.2 *Chemical/Pharmacological Parathyroidectomy*

Percutaneous injection of ethanol or D sterols (e.g. calcitriol) into nodular hyperplastic glands has been used in specialized centers.

18.5.5 *Hungry Bone Syndrome*

This can occur as an early complication following parathyroidectomy and is characterized by profound hypocalcemia. A management protocol is tabulated (Table 18.11).

18.6 Treatment of Hypercalcemia in Dialysis Patients

Some causes for hypercalcemia in dialysis patients are listed in Table 18.12.

18.6.1 *Hypercalcemia Caused by Factors Related to Dialysis*

18.6.1.1 *Calcium Loading and D Sterols*

The most common cause of hypercalcemia in dialysis patients is the excessive administration of CaPB or D sterols, or a combination of

Table 18.11 Management of postparathyroidectomy (PTX) "hungry bone" syndrome.[a]

In postparathyroidectomy patients, blood ionized calcium concentration $[Ca^{2+}]$ should be measured every 4–6 h for 48–72 h, and twice daily thereafter until stable.

   (a) If $[Ca^{2+}] < 3.6$ mg/dL (0.9 mmol/L) or corrected total [Ca] < 7.2 mg/dL (<1.80 mmol/L), start Ca gluconate infusion at 1–2 mg elemental Ca/kg body weight/h and titrate to maintain a normal $[Ca^{2+}]$ (4.6–5.4 mg/dL or 1.15–1.36 mmol/L). A 10-mL ampule of 10% calcium gluconate contains 90 mg of elemental calcium.

   (b) Gradually wean off Ca infusion as $[Ca^{2+}]$ normalizes and exhibits stability.

   (c) If the patient can tolerate oral feeding, administer 1–2 g of Ca carbonate 3 times a day and up to 2 µg/day calcitriol. Tailor therapy to maintain $[Ca^{2+}]$ in the normal range.

   (d) Monitor serum [P], and institute appropriate reduction or elimination of phosphate binders.

[a] Adapted from K/DOQI.

Table 18.12   Some causes of hypercalcemia in dialysis patients.

Causes related to CKD and dialysis
  Excess ingestion of:
  (a) active vitamin D sterols
  (b) calcium-containing phosphate binders
  Severe secondary hyperparathyroidism:
  (a) "massive" parathyroid hyperplasia
  (b) adenomatous transformation (tertiary hyperparathyroidism)
  Low bone-turnover osteodystrophy
Causes not specifically related to CKD and dialysis
  Humoral hypercalcemia of malignancy
  Multiple myeloma
  Granulomatous disease (e.g. tuberculosis)
  Fungal infections (e.g. pulmonary cryptococcosis)
  Sarcoidosis
  Isolated adrenocorticotropic hormone deficiency

---

both. Dialysate [Ca] should be reduced down to 2.5 mEq/L if the patient is being treated at a higher dialysate [Ca] (see Sec. 18.8). CaPB should be reduced or discontinued, with appropriate parallel addition of, or replacement with, non-CaPB. Also consider reduction or discontinuation of D sterols and, if appropriate, initiate cinacalcet for optimal parathyroid suppression (see Table 18.9). In cases with severe hypercalcemia, a temporary course of dialysis using dialysate [Ca] lower than 2.5 mEq/L may be considered (see Sec. 18.8). Recent increase in the use of ergocalciferol for the management of vitamin D insufficiency or deficiency in CKD patients has not yet led to reports of hypercalcemia.

18.6.1.2 *Severe Hyperparathyroidisim*

The development of hypercalcemia in secondary hyperparathyroidism signifies that parathyroid glands have become "autonomous", and is an indication of severe parathyroid hyperplasia or tertiary hyperparathyroidism. In patients refractory to optimal or maximally tolerable medical treatment, parathyroidectomy should be considered (see Sec. 18.5).

18.6.1.3 Low Bone Turnover Osteodystrophy

Hypercalcemia in this disorder may first emerge or become aggravated with the use of CaPB, with or without D sterols. The discontinuation of these treatments constitutes the first step in the management. Other management issues are discussed in Sec. 18.7.1 and Sec. 18.8.2.

18.6.2 Causes for Hypercalcemia Not Specifically Related to CKD

Causes for hypercalcemia in the general population have also been reported in dialysis patients. These include humoral hypercalcemia of malignancy, multiple myeloma (Trimarchi *et al.* 2006), granulomatous disease such as tuberculosis, pulmonary cryptoccocosis (Wang *et al.* 2004), sarcoidosis (Huart *et al.* 2006), and a case report of isolated adrenocorticotropic hormone deficiency (Kato *et al.* 2003). Management is based on etiology.

18.6.3 Other Treatment Modalities

- Both hemodialysis and peritoneal dialysis, using low [Ca] or no [Ca] dialysate, have been used in the management of acute and severe hypercalcemia. Such measures provide clinicians with time to reach a definitive diagnosis and treatment strategy.
- Ca-free peritoneal dialysis solution has been made up by a hospital pharmacy using distilled water, 50% dextrose, sodium chloride, and sodium bicarbonate to yield a 1.5% dextrose solution with the following composition in mEq/L: sodium, 130; chloride, 100; and bicarbonate, 30 (Querfeld *et al.* 1988).
- In a hemodialysis patient with multiple myeloma, hypercalcemia was treated with a combination of low dialysate [Ca] (1.25 mEq/L) and three consecutive days of 30 mg of disodium pamidronate in 300 mL of normal saline, administered intravenously over 20 min (Trimarchi *et al.* 2006).

18.7 Other Components of Renal Osteodystrophy

18.7.1 Adynamic Bone Disease

- Originally described in association with Al toxicity, aplastic bone disease or ABD is now attributed to parathyroid oversuppression, secondary to Ca overloading and excessive administration of

D sterols, or both. Other risk factors include aging, diabetes mellitus, malnutrition, and parathyroidectomy.

- Early reports of calciphylaxis in dialysis patients were associated with hyperparathyroidism and responded to parathyroidectomy. In more recent reports, the condition may be associated with low [PTH] and adynamic changes in bone.
- Diagnosis of ABD is discussed in Sec. 18.2 and Sec. 18.3.
- The rationale for treating ABD is based on the possibility that it is associated with fractures and risks for vascular and soft tissue calcifications.
- K/DOQI recommends decreasing doses of CaPB and vitamin D, or eliminating such therapies. While limiting calcium intake to 1.0–1.4 g/day (or even lower in cases with hypercalcemia) is generally accepted, the consensus on eliminating vitamin D is less unanimous.

(a) Accumulating data support VDR activation as an effective treatment for ABD by stimulating bone formation. VDR activation is required for normal osteoblast formation and bone formation and mineralization. Thus, correction of low circulating 25D and judicious use of D sterols have been proposed in the prevention and treatment of low-turnover bone disease (Andress 2008).

(b) Use of a low [Ca] dialysate in the treatment of low-turnover bone disease is discussed in Sec. 18.8.2.1.

18.7.2 *Aluminum Bone Disease and Osteomalacia*

Osteomalacia in CKD may result from Al toxicity or other causes, including vitamin D deficiency and P depletion.

18.7.2.1 *Aluminum (Al) Toxicity and Al Bone Disease*

History

Al toxicity in CKD patients was first recognized in dialysis patients, but can also occur in CKD 4 and CKD 5 patients prior to the initiation of dialysis. Discontinuation of the practice of using Al-based phosphate binders and the institution of stringent control of Al concentration in dialysate have virtually eliminated this devastating complication in most dialysis units. Sporadic cases, however, continue to occur.

Clinical aspects

Excess Al is deposited in many tissues and organs (including the bone, brain, and parathyroid glands), causing Al-mediated osteomalacia or ABD, dialysis encephalopathy and dementia, acute Al neurotoxicity, and parathyroid suppression. Variations in the manifestation and severity may depend on the rate and magnitude of Al loading.

Diagnosis

Diagnosis is based on clinical and laboratory evaluation (Table 18.4).

Prevention and treatment

See Table 18.13.

Table 18.13   Management of Al toxicity in dialysis patients.[a]

Prevention
  (a) *Minimize Al exposure.*
    (i) Keep dialysate [Al] < 10 µg/L.
    (ii) Avoid Al-containing compounds (e.g. Al-based phosphate binders, other common Al-containing medications such as sucralfate). Note: citrate (e.g. AlkaSeltzer™, Citracal™), enhances Al absorption.
    (iii) Monitor exposure with measurement of serum [Al] annually, and in those receiving Al-containing medications, every three months. Keep serum [Al] < 20 µg/L.

DFO treatment
  (a) *Eliminate exposure.* Identify and eliminate source(s) of Al exposure.
  (b) *Hemodialysis patients*
    (i) In patients with baseline serum [Al] > 200 µg/L, a course of intensive dialysis is recommended prior to conducting DFO test (see Table 18.4) or DFO Al-chelation therapy. This is a prophylactic measure against further rises in serum [Al] with DFO treatment and consequent neurotoxicity. K/DOQI suggests a regimen of daily hemodialysis 6 days a week, using high-flux membranes and dialysate [Al] less than 5 µg/L. This is continued for 4–6 weeks or until predialysis serum [Al] is reduced to less than 200 µg/L.

(Continued)

Table 18.13 (*Continued*)

(ii) If the post-DFO test rise in serum [Al] is 50–300 µg/L, administer DFO 5 mg/kg in 150 mL of 5% glucose water[b] into the venous blood line during the last hour of a dialysis session. This is followed by a high-efficiency hemodialysis 44 h later.

(iii) If post-DFO test rise in serum [Al] is >300 µg/L, administer DFO 5 mg/kg in 150 mL of 5% glucose water,[b] 4–5 h prior to the start of a dialysis session, followed by high-efficiency hemodialysis.

(iv) DFO is administered once a week.

(v) Repeat DFO test (Table 18.4) every three months after a 4-week washout period. If post-DFO test rise in serum Al < 50 µg/L in two successive tests, 1 month apart, no further DFO treatment is recommended.

(c) *Peritoneal dialysis patients*

(i) A similar protocol as suggested for hemodialysis is recommended.

(ii) DFO can also be administered by the peritoneal route (see Table 18.4). The intramuscular route has also been used.

(d) *Monitoring during DFO administration.* See Table 18.4.

(e) *Side effects.* These include *Yersinia* sepsis, mucormycosis, sensorineural hearing loss, and visual acuity reduction and maculopathy.

---

[a] Based on K/DOQI and Delmez and Kaye (2001).
[b] See Table 18.4, footnote "b".

18.7.2.2 *Other Causes of Osteomalacia in CKD*

- Osteomalacia secondary to vitamin D deficiency or P depletion is treated with appropriate repletion.
- If osteomalacia fails to respond to ergocalciferol or cholecalciferol, particularly in CKD 5 dialysis patients, treatment with D sterols should be considered.
- In osteomalacia secondary to P depletion, doses of phosphate supplementation should be adjusted upwards until normal serum [P] is attained.

18.7.3 *Metabolic Acidosis*

In CKD 3–5 patients, K/DOQI recommends keeping serum total [CO_2] at or above 22 mmol/L for improving bone histology and ameliorating excessive protein catabolism. Supplemental alkali administration may be necessary for this purpose, but may be difficult to accomplish in practice. Citrate-based alkali salts are not recommended because of the risk of increasing absorption of dietary Al. Sodium bicarbonate is often poorly tolerated by the patient and may cause sodium overload.

18.7.4 *Osteoporosis*

Although the prevalence of osteopenia and fractures with decreasing GFR has been well reported, the definitive diagnosis and treatment of osteoporosis in CKD patients remain a challenging issue that has so far raised more questions than answers. Dual energy X-ray absorptiometry (DEXA) and quantitative CT (qCT) are the current methods for assessing bone mineral density (BMD). Interpretation of the data obtained in CKD patients is, however, not straightforward (Cunningham *et al.* 2004).

18.7.4.1 *Treatment*

Currently, there is no consensus on the management of osteoporosis in CKD (Table 18.14). Prior to considering the specific treatment for osteoporosis, optimal management of other components of renal osteodystrophy should first be addressed.

18.7.4.2 *Apparent Similarities Between Osteoporosis and Low Bone Volume ABD*

Both conditions share some of the same risk factors and are characterized by low-turnover activities in the bone. Low dialysate [Ca]-mediated increase in PTH with parallel improvement in ABD parameters in dialysis patients is also reminiscent of the recent use of intermittent PTH for stimulating bone formation in osteoporosis in the general population. Thrice-weekly low [Ca] dialysate hemodialysis would be anticipated to mimic intermittent PTH administration in a pulsatile pattern (see Sec. 18.8.2.1).

18.7.5 *β_2-Microglobulin Amyloidosis*

18.7.5.1 *Clinical Aspects*

β_2-microglobulin amyloidosis or dialysis-associated amyloidosis (DAA) is a debilitating musculoskeletal disorder mainly affecting

Table 18.14 Possible treatment considerations for osteoporosis in CKD patients.

Agents	Comments
Bisphosphonates	Consider for use only after bone biopsy to exclude low-turnover ABD, given the lack of efficacy and safety data in CKD patients.
	Some consider the use of bisphosphonates in CKD patients questionable (Ersoy 2007); others are not averse to their use with caution (Miller 2007).
SERM[a]	Evista® (raloxifene) increases BMD and reduces vertebral fractures in postmenopausal women with CKD (Ishani *et al.* 2008).
Estrogen, androgen/ anabolic steroids	Potential use in hypogonadism. Efficacy and safety data in CKD patients not established.
Calcitonin	Uncertain efficacy.
Speculative novel approaches	Manipulate endogenous PTH secretion into a pulsatile pattern.
	(a) Use of low [Ca] dialysate in low turnover bone disease with "low" [PTH] (see Sec. 18.7.4.2). Possible use of calcilytics?
	(b) Use of intermittent calcimimetics in high-turnover bone disease with high [PTH].

[a] Selective estrogen receptor modulator.

long-term (>2 years) hemodialysis patients, but has also been seen in peritoneal dialysis and predialysis patients. Clinical manifestations include joint pain and restriction in mobility, spondyloarthropathies, hemarthrosis, and carpal tunnel syndrome. Pathologically, amyloid deposits (predominantly β_2-microglobulin fibrils) are found in joints and periarticular tissues with the possible presence of cystic lesions in the long bones, which mimic the changes of hyperparathyroidism. Systemic deposits can also occur elsewhere, e.g. the gastrointestinal tract and the heart.

18.7.5.2 *Management*

K/DOQI recommends the use of non-cuprophane high-flux dialyzers in patients with evidence of, or at risk for DAA. Successful kidney transplantation is the current treatment modality that may provide symptomatic relief and halt the progression of the disease.

18.8 Use of Low-Calcium Dialysate

18.8.1 *Historical Vignettes*

In current practice, the most frequently used dialysate [Ca], in both hemodialysis and peritoneal dialysis, is 2.5 mEq/L (1.25 mmol/L).

- This is the concentration first used in the 1960s, when widespread chronic dialysis first began and predated the discovery of D sterols and the use of CaPB. Many patients were found to develop hypocalcemia, hemodynamic instabilities during dialysis, and exacerbations in hyperparathyroid bone disease. This led to the use of a higher dialysate [Ca], usually up to 3.5 mEq/L (1.75 mmol/L).
- A return to the "low" [Ca] dialysate, 2.5 mEq/L (1.25 mmol/L), was precipitated by two main factors. First, with the increasing use of D sterols and CaPB in the 1980s, hypercalcemia emerged with greater frequency. Second, even in patients without hypercalcemia, calcium loading with higher dialysate [Ca] was suspected as a cause for vascular/extraskeletal calcification and the development of ABD.
- The current strategy of using 2.5 mEq/L Ca dialysate, in conjunction with D sterol and CaPB administration, appears to be a reasonable strategy. Further adjustments are expected as the natural history and therapy for hyperparathyroidism of CKD evolve.

18.8.2 *Therapeutic Applications*

18.8.2.1 *Adynamic Bone Disease*

A lower dialysate [Ca], e.g. 1.5–2.0 mEq/L, has been used to increase serum [PTH] and bone turnover in patients with ABD. The goal is to raise serum [PTH] to a range of 100–300 pg/mL (11.0–33.0 pmol/L). Similar beneficial effects have been reported using 2.5 mEq/L (1.25 mmol/L) [Ca] dialysate (Spasovski and Vanholder 2007).

18.8.2.2 *Hypercalcemia*

Both hemodialysis and peritoneal dialysis using dialysate [Ca] of 1.5–2.0 mEq/L or lower have been used in the treatment of hypercalcemia, both in CKD patients and in patients without kidney disease.

18.8.3 *Monitoring*

Careful monitoring for cardiac arrhythmia is mandatory whenever low [Ca] dialysate is used. Prolongation of the QT_c interval, not infrequently seen in patients during regular dialysis, may be exacerbated with lower [Ca] dialysate and can lead to fatal outcomes. Some prefer to use at least 2.5 mEq/L [Ca] in the dialysate to prevent a too-rapid and excessive reduction in serum ionized Ca concentrations, while others have reported the successful use of "zero" [Ca] dialysate in the treatment of severe hypercalcemia. In all cases, close clinical and laboratory monitoring are obligatory.

18.8.4 *Notes on Acute Dialysis*

The recommended dialysate [Ca] for acute dialysis is 3.0–3.5 mEq/L or 1.5–1.75 mmol/L (Delmez and Kaye 2001). There is some evidence that dialysis solution [Ca] < 3.0 mEq/L predisposes to hypotension. In patients with predialysis hypocalcemia, unless an adequate dialysate [Ca] is used, correction of acidosis can result in further lowering of the ionized Ca levels with possible precipitation of seizures. In addition, QT_c dispersion may increase (potentially promoting arrhythmia) with a low dialysate [Ca].

Suggested Reading

Andress D. (2008) Adynamic bone in patients with chronic kidney disease. *Kidney Int* 73:1345–1354.

Berns JS. (2008) Niacin and related compounds for treating hyperphosphatemia in dialysis patients. *Semin Dial* 21:203–205.

Chertow GM, Blumenthal S, Turner S, *et al.* (2006) Cinacalcet hydrochloride (Sensipar) in hemodialysis patients on active vitamin D derivatives with controlled PTH and elevated calcium × phosphate. *Clin J Am Soc Nephrol* 1:305–312.

Coyne D, Acharya M, Qiu P, *et al.* (2006) Paricalcitol capsule for the treatment of secondary hyperparathyroidism in stages 3 and 4 CKD. *Am J Kidney Dis* 47:263–276.

Cunningham J, Sprague SM, Cannata-Andia J, *et al.* (2004) Osteoporosis in chronic kidney disease. *Am J Kidney Dis* 43:566–571.

Delmez JA, Kaye M. (2001) Bone disease. In: Daugirdas JT, Blake PG, Ing TS (eds.), *Handbook of Dialysis*, 3rd ed., Lippincott Williams & Wilkins, Philadelphia, pp. 530–547.

Ersoy FF. (2007) Osteoporosis in the elderly with chronic kidney disease. *Int Urol Nephrol* 39:321–331.

Fischer D, Cline K, Plone MA, *et al.* (2006) Results of a randomized crossover study comparing once-daily and thrice-daily sevelamer dosing. *Am J Kidney Dis* 48:437–444.

Huart A, Kamar N, Lanau JM, *et al.* (2006) Sarcoidosis-related hypercalcemia in 3 chronic hemodialysis patients. *Clin Nephrol* 65:449–452.

Ishani A, Blackwell T, Jamal SA, *et al.* (2008) The effect of raloxifene treatment in postmenopausal women with CKD. *J Am Soc Nephrol* 19:1430–1438.

Kato A, Shinozaki S, Goga T, Hishida A. (2003) Isolated adrenocorticotropic hormone deficiency presenting with hypercalcemia in a patient on long-term hemodialysis. *Am J Kidney Dis* 42:E32–E36.

Miller PD. (2007) Is there a role for bisphosphonates in chronic kidney disease? *Semin Dial* 20:186–190.

Moe S, Drüeke T, Cunningham J, *et al.* (2006) Definition, evaluation, and classification of renal osteodystrophy: a position statement from Kidney Disease: Improving Global Outcomes (KDIGO). *Kidney Int* 69:1945–1953.

Moe SM, Drüeke T, Lameire N, Eknoyan G. (2007) Chronic kidney disease–mineral-bone disorder: a new paradigm. *Adv Chronic Kidney Dis* 14:3–12.

National Kidney Foundation. (2003) K/DOQI clinical practice guidelines for bone metabolism and disease in chronic kidney disease. *Am J Kidney Dis* 42:S1–S201.

Querfeld U, Salusky IB, Fine RN. (1988) Treatment of severe hypercalcemia with peritoneal dialysis in an infant with end-stage renal disease. *Pediatr Nephrol* 2:323–325.

Raggi P, Kleerekoper M. (2008) Contribution of bone and mineral abnormalities to cardiovascular disease in patients with chronic kidney disease. *Clin J Am Soc Nephrol* 3:836–843.

Ross EA, Tian J, Abboud H, *et al.* (2008) Oral paricalcitol for the treatment of secondary hyperparathyroidism in patients on hemodialysis or peritoneal dialysis. *Am J Nephrol* 28:97–106.

Saab G, Young DO, Gincherman Y, *et al.* (2007) Prevalence of vitamin D deficiency and the safety and effectiveness of monthly ergocalciferol in hemodialysis patients. *Nephron Clin Pract* 105:c132–c138.

Spasovski G, Vanholder R. (2007) Effect of lowering dialysate calcium on bone and mineral parameters related to adynamic bone disease. *Ther Apher Dial* 11:455–456.

Trimarchi H, Lombi F, Forrester M, *et al.* (2006) Disodium pamidronate for treating severe hypercalcemia in a hemodialysis patient. *Nat Clin Pract Nephrol* 2:459–463.

Wang IK, Shen TY, Lee KF, *et al.* (2004) Hypercalcemia and elevated serum 1, 25-dihydroxyvitamin D in an end-stage renal disease patient with pulmonary cryptococcosis. *Ren Fail* 26:333–338.

Wolf M, Shah A, Gutierrez O, *et al.* (2007) Vitamin D levels and early mortality among incident hemodialysis patients. *Kidney Int* 72:1004–1013.

19

Treatment of Renal Anemia

Bruce A. Pussell and Rowan G. Walker

The presence of anemia is almost universal in patients on dialysis or with moderate (glomerular filtration rate or GFR < 30mL/min) to severe (GFR < 15mL/min) chronic kidney disease (CKD). Anemia is primarily caused by a reduced erythropoietin production by the failing kidney. Symptoms of anemia can be present well before those of uremia, and can occur in some patients with only mild reduction in GFR (<60 mL/min). Correction of the anemia became possible 20 years ago with the introduction of human recombinant erythropoietin, or erythropoietic-stimulating agents (ESAs). Although there are no controlled trials comparing ESAs to transfusions, the potential benefits were immediately obvious and are listed in Table 19.1 (see also Eschbach *et al.* 1989).

19.1 Causes of Anemia in CKD

Decreased production of erythropoietin is not the only cause of anemia in CKD. Other causes are listed in Table 19.2. Similar findings are observed in patients who fail to respond to ESA therapy (Table 19.3).

19.2 ESA Prescription

19.2.1 *ESA Preparations and Dosing*

All marketed ESA preparations are effective in achieving target hemoglobin (Hb) concentrations. The choice between epoietin alpha, epoietin beta, and darbepoietin depends on individual patient needs, availability, and cost. ESAs have been shown to be effective when administered at intervals of 2–4 weeks, which may be useful when given subcutaneously in patients who are on peritoneal

Table 19.1   Potential benefits of correction of anemia in CKD.

Improved quality of life (including cognitive function, fatigue, weakness, and exercise tolerance)
Elimination of the need for regular blood transfusions
Decreased iron overload
Reduction in risk of transfusion-related viral transmission
Avoiding sensitization for subsequent transplantation
Reduction in left ventricular hypertrophy and heart failure
Reduction in overall mortality in dialysis patients
Possibly slowing the progression of CKD

Table 19.2   Causes of anemia in CKD.

Erythropoietin deficiency
Blood loss (hemodialysis puncture sites, gastrointestinal tract)
Iron deficiency
Vitamin deficiency (B_{12}, folate)
Hemolysis
Myelodysplasia
Malignancy

Table 19.3   Causes of iron deficiency in CKD.

Reduced dietary intake
Impaired intestinal absorption
Frequent blood loss from hemodialysis or blood tests
Use of ESAs
Chronic inflammation
Failure of adequate supplementation

---

dialysis or in those with CKD prior to commencement of dialysis. The original report by Eschbach *et al.* (1989) used a high starting dose of epoietin alpha of 150–300 U/kg reducing to 75 U/kg intravenously three times a week, which eliminated all transfusion requirements within 2 months. Lower starting doses increasing to achieve target Hb may be more cost-effective. Similarly, darbepoietin dosing ranges from 10 μg to 100 μg weekly. All ESAs should be titrated to the target Hb; however, there is wide variability depending on the starting Hb, mode of administration, target Hb level, and individual patient response.

19.2.2 Route of Administration

Although management of patients needs to be individualized, the subcutaneous route (SC) of administration may prove cost-effective in some patients by reducing the total weekly dose of ESAs. Kaufman *et al.* (1998), in a randomized crossover study, showed that the dose of epoietin needed to maintain target Hb was 30% lower in the SC group. However, there was a lot of variation, with some individuals needing more epoietin when switched from SC to intravenous (IV) administration. Patient convenience and comfort are often the factors determining the route of administration.

19.2.3 Precautions/Side-Effects

See Table 19.4.

19.3 Target Levels for Hemoglobin

In general, it is our practice to target a Hb level to that which is optimal for each individual patient depending on age, physical activity, and the presence of comorbidities (especially cardiovascular disease and diabetes). However, the current balance of evidence suggests that these targets should not exceed 13 g/dL for dialysis or CKD patients. Targets are necessary as starting points and are potentially useful in trying to maintain Hb levels without too much variability. The consensus based on the following guidelines and recently reported controlled trials suggests that a Hb range of 11–12 g/dL might be prudent in the majority of patients, bearing in mind the risk management.

Table 19.4   Precautions/Side-effects of ESAs.

Iron deficiency
Increased blood pressure
Convulsions
Myalgia
Hyperkalemia
Primary red cell aplasia (PRCA) (rare)

19.3.1 What the Guidelines Say

19.3.1.1 Australian Guidelines

The Australian guidelines (Caring for Australians with Renal Insufficiency or CARI) were first published in 2003 and updated in 2005 and 2008. A further update is pending. The only guideline based on level 1 evidence is that the Hb should not exceed 13 g/dL in patients with cardiovascular disease. Recommendations based on lesser evidence state a minimum Hb of 11 g/dL in dialysis patients.

19.3.1.2 Japanese Society for Dialysis Therapy

The Japanese guidelines, published in 2004, recommend a hemoglobin level of 10–11 g/dL, which is less than most other guidelines.

19.3.1.3 North American Guidelines

In dialysis and non-dialysis CKD patients receiving ESA therapy, the Kidney Disease Outcomes Quality Initiative (K/DOQI) gives a selected Hb target range of 11–12 g/dL.

19.3.1.4 United Kingdom Guidelines

Patients with CKD should achieve an outcome distribution of hemoglobin of 10.5–12.5 g/dL. Adjustments to ESA doses should be considered when Hb is <11 g/dL or >12 g/dL in order that the population distribution has the maximum proportion of patients in the range of 10.5–12.5 g/dL as is possible.

19.3.1.5 European Guidelines

The European guidelines recommend a hemoglobin level of >11 g/dL.

19.3.1.6 Canadian Guidelines

The Canadian guidelines recommend a hemoglobin level of 11–12 g/dL.

19.3.2 Recent and Relevant Trials

The use of ESAs to normalize hemoglobin may increase cardiovascular events, cause increased thrombosis of fistulas, and/or lead to poorly controlled hypertension. Figure 19.1 shows the results of some recent trials of high versus low hemoglobin targets, which has also been the subject of a meta-analysis by Phrommintikul et al. (2007).

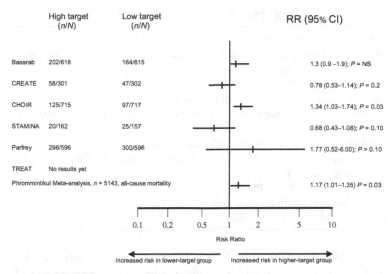

	High target (n/N)	Low target (n/N)	RR (95% CI)

Basarab 202/618 164/615 1.3 (0.9 –1.9); P = NS

CREATE 58/301 47/302 0.78 (0.53–1.14); P = 0.2

CHOIR 125/715 97/717 1.34 (1.03–1.74); P = 0.03

STAMINA 20/162 25/157 0.68 (0.43–1.08); P = 0.10

Parfrey 296/596 300/596 1.77 (0.52-6.00); P > 0.10

TREAT No results yet

Phrommintikul Meta-analysis, n = 5143, all-cause mortality 1.17 (1.01–1.35) P = 0.03

Risk Ratio 0.1 0.2 0.5 1 2 5 10

◄ Increased risk in lower-target group   Increased risk in higher-target group ►

Patient characteristics
Besarab *et al.*: 1233 patients on hemodialysis with cardiac disease.
Drueke *et al.* (2007) (CREATE): 603 patients with CKD, not on dialysis, with cardiac disease in 93%.
Singh *et al.* (2007) (CHOIR): 1432 patients with CKD, not on dialysis, with cardiac disease in 35%.
Ghali *et al.* (STAMINA): placebo vs. darbepoietin in 319 patients with cardiac disease but without CKD.
Parfrey *et al.*: 596 patients recently started on hemodialysis without symptomatic cardiac disease randomized to high (13.5–14.5 g/L) or low (9.5–11.5 g/L) hemoglobin.
Phrommintikul *et al.* (2007) : meta-analysis of 5143 patients in randomized controlled trials targeting different hemoglobin concentrations.
TREAT (see Mix *et al*, 2005). The trial is a 4000-patient randomised, double-blind, placebo-controlled trial in patients with CKD, Type 2 Diabetes and Anemia.

Fig. 19.1 Relative risk of high or low hemoglobin target on cardiovascular outcomes.

19.4 Failure to Respond to ESAs

Iron deficiency is the commonest cause of non-response to erythro-poietin (EPO) (Table 19.3). Other conditions that may be associated with poor response to ESAs are shown in Table 19.5.

19.4.1 *Iron Use in Anemia of CKD*

Iron metabolism in patients with CKD is characterized by reduced intake and poor absorption from the gastrointestinal tract. Effective use of ESAs requires increased iron levels to obtain an effective response.

Table 19.5   Failure to respond to ESAs.

Failure of iron absorption
Blood loss from gastrointestinal tract, dialyser cannulation site bleeding, frequent blood tests
Functional iron deficiency
Inflammation (inhibition of erythropoiesis)
Malnutrition (particularly carnitine, vitamin C, vitamin B_{12}, and folate)
Dialysis inadequacy
Angiotensin-converting enzyme inhibitors (ACEIs)
Bone marrow failure due to hyperparathyroidism, aluminum toxicity, or malignant infiltration
Primary red cell aplasia (PRCA)
Poor compliance with ESA therapy
Albumin and sensitivity to ESAs

Guidelines published by K/DOQI, Europe, and Australia all suggest that iron status should be regularly assessed by measurements of serum ferritin, transferrin saturation (TSAT), and/or percentage of hypochromic red blood cells (HRCs) and reticulocyte hemoglobin content (CHr). Target iron levels before commencing ESA therapy are: TSAT, >20%; ferritin, >100 µg/L; and HRCs, >6%. During ESA therapy, one should maintain adequate response with a TSAT > 20% and ferritin > 200 µg/L. Although there is little evidence to support an upper level, it is recommended to avoid intravenous iron if the ferritin is >500 µg/L.

Iron may be given orally or intravenously. Oral iron absorption is usually impaired in CKD, probably due to the chronic inflammatory state (see Horl 2007), but is used in patients on peritoneal dialysis or following transplantation. Following transplantation, oral iron administration may interfere with the absorption of other drugs and caution is warranted. Intravenous iron is usually preferred because of its efficacy and ease of use in patients on hemodialysis, where most protocols suggest 100 mg of iron sucrose infused near the end of hemodialysis weekly for five doses followed by repeat measurements of iron status; further dosing is then determined based on the response and follow-up levels. Intravenous iron is usually given as iron polymaltose or iron sucrose. Vitamin C supplements may need to be added during administration of iron.

As with patients with iron overload, there is a risk of bacterial infection during iron supplementation. Therefore, iron use should be suspended when infection is suspected.

19.5 Hemoglobin Variability

Hemoglobin cycling (or variability) was first described in 2005 by Fishbane and Berns, who observed the pattern of changes of hemoglobin concentration in individual patients over time. The features are summarized in Table 19.6. Variance is a statistical measure of the amount of variability, or spread, around the mean of the measurements. The frequency with which CKD patients maintain stable target Hb levels is very low, with only 6.5% of patients in one study maintaining stable Hb within the target range over a 6-month period (Ebben *et al.* 2006). The factors associated with Hb variability are summarized in Table 19.7.

Hemoglobin variability is not observed in a normal healthy population and may have an influence on outcomes, as it has been shown that a low Hb with high variability is possibly associated with clinical

Table 19.6   Hemoglobin variance.

Quantifies the amount of variability, or spread, around the mean of the measurements.
When considering target Hb levels, measurement of variance may indicate that the Hb level is well controlled.
Evidence is growing that Hb levels which are too high or too low may have clinically important implications.
Hb is associated with improved survival: 15% for every 1 g/dL.
No or less frequent ESAs are associated with a significantly higher risk of cardiac events and death compared to those receiving ESAs more frequently.
Decreasing Hb is an independent risk factor for death in patients with ischemic heart disease.

Table 19.7   Factors associated with hemoglobin variability.

Erythropoietin dose
Changes in or initiation of intravenous iron
Recent hospitalization
Chronic infection/inflammation
Hyperparathyroidism
Abrupt changes caused by bleeding or transfusion
Narrow target range
Variable target level and management protocols
Variation in individual patient response

complications such as ischemic heart disease, infections, and increased hospitalizations.

Suggested Reading

Besarab A, Reyes CM, Hornberger J. (2002) Meta-analysis of subcutaneous versus intravenous epoetin in maintenance treatment of anemia in hemodialysis patients. *Am J Kidney Dis* 40:439–446.

Drueke TB, Locatelli F, Clyne N, *et al.* (2007) Normalization of hemoglobin level in patients with chronic kidney disease and anemia. *N Engl J Med* 355:2071–2084.

Ebben JP, Gilbertson DT, Foley RN, Collins AJ. (2006) Hemoglobin level variability: associations with comorbidity, intercurrent events and hospitalizations. *Clin J Am Soc Nephrol* 1:1205–1210.

Eschbach JW, Abdulhadi MH, Browne JK, *et al.* (1989) Recombinant human erythropoietin in anemic patients with end-stage renal disease. Results of a phase III multicenter trial. *Ann Intern Med* 111:992–1000.

Fishbane S, Berns JS. (2005) Hemoglobin cycling in hemodialysis patients treated with recombinant human erythropoietin. *Kidney Int* 68:1337–1343.

Ghali JK, Anand IS, Abraham WT, *et al.* (2008) Study of anemia in heart failure trial (STAMINA-HeFT). *Circulation* 117:526–535.

Gilbertson DT, Ebben JP, Foley RN, *et al.* (2008) Hemoglobin level variability: associations with mortality. *Clin J Am Soc Nephrol* 3:133–138.

Horl WH. (2007) Clinical aspects of iron use in the anemia of kidney disease. *J Am Soc Nephrol* 18:383–393.

Kaufman JS, Reda DJ, Fye CL, *et al.* (1998) Subcutaneous compared with intravenous epoetin in patients receiving hemodialysis. Department of Veterans Affairs Cooperative Study Group on Erythropoietin in Hemodialysis Patients. *N Engl J Med* 339:578–583.

Mix T-C H, Brenner RM, Cooper ME, *et al.* (2005) Rationale — Trial to Reduce Cardiovascular Events with Aranesp Therapy (TREAT): Evolving the management of cardiovascular risk in patients with chronic kidney disease. *Am Heart J* 149:409–413.

Parfrey PS, Foley RN, Wittreich BH, *et al.* (2005) Double-blind comparison of full and partial anemia correction in incident hemodialysis patients without symptomatic heart disease. *J Am Soc Nephrol* 16:2180–2189.

Phrommintikul A, Haas SJ, Elsik M, Krum H. (2007) Mortality and target haemoglobin concentration in anaemic patients with kidney disease treated with erythropoietin: a meta-analysis. *Lancet* 369:381–388.

Remuzzi G, Ingelfinger JR. (2007) Correction of anemia — payoffs and problems. *N Engl J Med* 355:20–21.

Rossert J, Levin A, Roger SD, *et al.* (2006) Effect of early correction of anemia on the progression of CKD. *Am J Kidney Dis* 47:738–750.

Singh Ak, Szczech L, Tang KL, *et al.* (2007) Correction of anemia with epoetin alfa in chronic kidney disease. *N Engl J Med* 355:2085–2098.

Wolfe RA, Hulbert-Shearon TE, Ashby VB, *et al.* (2005) Improvements in dialysis patient mortality are associated with improvements in urea reduction ratio and hematocrit, 1999 to 2002. *Am J Kidney Dis* 45:127–135.

20

Bleeding Tendency and Hepatitis B Vaccination

Bo-Ying Choy and Kar Neng Lai

20.1 Management of Bleeding Tendency in Dialysis/Uremic Patients

Bleeding tendency has long been recognized in uremic patients. The etiology is multi-factorial, with abnormal platelet function and platelet–endothelium interaction being the major determinants of uremic bleeding.

20.1.1 *Factors Contributing to Bleeding Tendency*

These include the following:

- Defective platelet adhesion and aggregation

  (a) Abnormal expression of platelet surface receptors glycoprotein (GP) Ib (receptor for von Willebrand factor) and glycoprotein (GP) IIb/IIIa (receptor for fibrinogen)
  (b) Reduced platelet granule adenosine diphosphate and serotonin levels, and defective thromboxane A2 production

- Abnormalities of von Willebrand factor
- Increased platelet and endothelial production of nitric oxide, which inhibits platelet aggregation
- Anemia

  A normal hematocrit facilitates the flow of red blood cells in the midstream while displacing platelets closer to the endothelium. The proximity of the platelets and endothelium allow the platelets to react quickly to any injury of the vascular wall. Reduced red cell mass or increased vessel luminal diameter by nitric oxide will decrease the peripheral dispersion of platelets and their contact with the endothelial surface of the vessel wall.

- Uremic toxins

  High level of uremic toxin such as guanidinosuccinic acid impairs platelet function, probably through stimulation of production of nitric oxide.

20.1.2 Clinical Manifestations

- Easy bruising, mucosal bleeding, epistaxis, gingival bleeding, hematuria
- Gastrointestinal bleeding
- Bleeding in response to injury or invasive procedure

20.1.3 Prevention and Treatment

20.1.3.1 Prevention

Adequate dialysis

Dialysis can remove some of the uremic toxins. Activation of the GPIIb/GPIIIa receptors is also partially restored by dialysis. Peritoneal dialysis is preferred over hemodialysis, as this avoids the use of anti-coagulant and platelet–dialyser interaction.

Correction of anemia

Raising the hematocrit to 30% or above by recombinant human erythropoietin or blood transfusion enhances platelet adhesion and aggregation.

20.1.3.2 Treatment

Desmopressin (DDAVP)

DDAVP is used in patients with acute bleeding or in patients planned for invasive procedures such as percutaneous renal biopsy. DDAVP acts by increasing the release of factor VIII–von Willebrand factor multimers from endothelial storage sites. The dosing regime is summarized in Table 20.1. Tachyphylaxis develops with repeated dosing, probably because of the depletion of von Willebrand factor from the endothelial stores.

Table 20.1   Treatment of bleeding tendency in dialysis/uremic patients.

	Dose	Route	Onset of action	Duration of effect
Desmopressin (DDAVP)	0.3 μg/kg in 50 mL saline over 30 min	Intravenous[a]	1 h	4–8 h
	0.3 μg/kg	Subcutaneous	2 h	
	3 μg/kg	Intranasal	2 h	
Cryoprecipitate	10 unit over 30 min	Intravenous	1 h	24 h
Conjugated estrogen	0.6 mg/kg/day for 5 days	Intravenous[a]	6 h	14 days
	25–50 mg/day maximum for 7 days	Per oral	3–5 days	
	50–100 μg patch 2 times per week	Transdermal	1–2 days	

[a] Preferred route of administration.

Cryoprecipitate

Cryoprecipitate is rich in factor VIII, von Willebrand factor, and fibrinogen. Because of the risk of blood-borne infections and fluid overload, cryoprecipitate should be reserved for life-threatening bleedings that are resistant to treatment with DDAVP. The usual dose is 10 units intravenously over 30 min with onset of action within 1 hour. The maximum effect occurs in 4 h and lasts for 24 h.

Conjugated estrogen

Estrogen decreases nitric oxide production and increases the production of adenosine diphosphate and thromboxane A2. Administration of conjugated estrogen is useful for patients needing a more prolonged control of bleeding, as in patients undergoing planned surgery or patients with chronic gastrointestinal bleeding from telangiectasia. The effect is dose-dependent and limited by the side-effects of estrogen. The normal dosing regime is 0.6 mg/kg/day for 5 days with intravenous as the preferred route. The alternative is 25–50 mg per day orally for a maximum of 7 days or 50–100 µg transdermal estradiol twice weekly.

For intravenous treatment, the onset of action is 6 h. Maximum effect reaches in 5–7 days with total duration of action around 14 days.

20.2 Hepatitis B Vaccination

Hepatitis B virus (HBV) is a 42-nm double-stranded DNA hepadnavirus with an outer surface coat and inner nucleocapsid core. HBV infection is transmitted through percutaneous or mucosal exposure to infective blood or body fluid. Chronic hepatitis B infection, with its sequelae of liver cirrhosis, hepatocellular carcinoma, and liver failure, is associated with significant morbidity and mortality.

Patients with chronic renal failure (CRF) are more susceptible to HBV infection. Up to 60% of patients with CRF become chronic carriers after primary infection. The uremic state confers a reduced expression of the costimulating molecule B7 on antigen-presenting cells; this defect leads to a depressed T-cell activation response against the HBV viral particle, which explains the failure of viral clearance after primary infection. Cellular immunodeficiency also reduces the response of CRF patients to hepatitis B vaccination. The response rate of CRF patients after the standard three doses of intramuscular HBV vaccination is only 50%–60% as compared to 95% of normal individuals. Other contributing factors for the poor response include old age, malnutrition, inadequate dialysis, use of bioincompatible dialysers, anemia, iron overload, hyperparathyroidism, and human leukocytic antigens (including HLA-B8, SC01, and DR3). Patients who have initially mounted a good response to HBV vaccine also have a more rapid fall in their antibody titers with time.

The currently recommended hepatitis B vaccine is derived from hepatitis B surface antigen (HBsAg), produced through the recombinant DNA technique from yeast. It contains nonglycosylated HBV small S protein as the envelope antigen. A protective antibody response is defined as an antibody titer against HBsAg (anti-HBs) of ≥10 mIU/mL (IU/L). For immunocompromised patients and dialysis patients, it has been advocated to maintain an anti-HBs antibody titer > 100 mIU/mL (IU/L) to achieve adequate seroprotection.

Strategies to enhance the response of patients with CRF to HBV vaccination are summarized in Table 20.2. These include:

Table 20.2 Suggested sequential program for hepatitis B vaccination in patients with chronic renal failure.

Vaccination at early stage of chronic kidney disease (stage 3 or earlier).
Adequate dialysis as measured by Kt/V_{urea} in patients already on dialysis.
 Correction of anemia, malnutrition, and hyperparathyroidism, as well as use of biocompatible dialyzers.

Double-dose-enhanced vaccination schedule with yeast-derived recombinant HBV vaccine 40 μg intramuscularly at 0,1,6 months (3-dose regime) or 0,1,2,6 months (4-dose regime). Give one additional booster dose or an extra course of intramuscular vaccination if the response remains suboptimal after checking the anti-HBs antibody 4–6 weeks after the last dose of vaccine.

For patients not mounting any response to the intramuscular regime, intradermal vaccination with HBV vaccine 5 μg every two weeks for 8 doses or until seroconversion.

Consider trying recombinant vaccine with more immunogenic pre-S1/pre-S2 antigens, or the new adjuvant HBV-AS04 vaccine, with the same schedule as an intramuscular regime for patients who failed both standard intramuscular and intradermal vaccination.

Early vaccination

Vaccination of patients at an early stage of chronic kidney disease (stage 3 or earlier) is associated with better response, as compared to patients with advanced renal failure or patients already on dialysis.

Adequate and efficient dialysis

Adequately dialysed patients with a higher Kt/V_{urea} value are more likely to mount a better response to HBV vaccination than patients who are underdialysed. A positive correlation between the Kt/V_{urea} value and the anti-HBs antibody titer has been demonstrated. Correction of anemia, malnutrition, and hyperparathyroidism should be achieved before vaccination.

Augmented dosing

A higher dose of HBV vaccine in each inoculation and a higher total number of doses are associated with a higher response rate in patients with CRF. Double-dose-enhanced vaccination schedule with 40 µg/dose HBV vaccine intramuscularly at 0,1,6 months (three-dose regime) or 0,1,2,6 months (four-dose regime), with one additional booster dose or an extra course of intramuscular vaccination if the anti-HBs antibody titer checked 6 weeks after the last dose of vaccine remains suboptimal.

Intradermal vaccination

Meta-analysis of intradermal versus intramuscular vaccination against HBV in uremic patients shows that the former achieves a higher seroconversion rate. This finding occurs despite the fact that a lower dose of vaccine is used for intradermal inoculation. Intradermal vaccination has also elicited seroconversion in some patients who failed to response to the intramuscular regime.

Langerhans cells, which are important antigen-presenting cells, are present in the epidermis but not in subcutaneous tissues or muscle. Vaccines that are introduced via repeated intradermal injection will be retained for an extended period in the dermal region. Antigen persistence and appropriate antigen presentation via Langerhans cells stimulate the immune system more effectively to produce an adequate antibody response. HBV vaccine 5 µg intradermally every 2 weeks for eight doses or until seroconversion is recommended.

Recombinant vaccine with immunogenic pre-S1/pre-S2 antigens

The widely used yeast-derived recombinant HBV vaccine contains only the S antigen. The third-generation mammalian cell-derived recombinant vaccine contains, in addition, the highly immunogenic pre-S1/pre-S2 antigens which improve the efficacy of the vaccine. Patients with CRF who fail to respond to conventional HBV vaccine may consider trying the recombinant vaccine with pre-S1/pre-S2 antigens.

Co-administration of immunogenic/immunostimulant agents

Attempts to enhance the immune response to HBV vaccine via co-administration with zinc, levamisole, interferon-γ, interleukin-2, and granulocyte colony stimulatory factor have all been tried. A recently developed adjuvant system, HBV-AS04, composed of aluminum salt and MPL (3-O-desacyl-4'-monophosphoryl lipid A) has shown promising results. The new adjuvant system increases the antigen-presenting capacity via upregulation of the CD86 molecules and via an increased production of cytokines. Twenty-microgram HBV-AS04 given intramuscularly elicits earlier antibody response and higher antibody titers as compared to conventional intramuscular double-dose HBV vaccine, although the incidence of side-effects is also higher. HBV-AS04 is commercially available and can be considered for patients with renal insufficiency as the primary vaccination or as a booster after standard HBV vaccine priming.

In conclusion, patients with renal insufficiency are susceptible to hepatitis B infection. HBV vaccination should be considered early when a patient's immune system is still intact. Implementation of a HBV vaccination strategy in the early stages of chronic kidney disease increases the success rate of HBV vaccination, and is still the most cost-effective way of preventing HBV infection among patients on a dialysis program.

Suggested Reading

Bertino JS Jr, Tirrell P, Greenberg RN, *et al.* (1997) A comparative trial of standard or high-dose S subunit recombinant hepatitis B vaccine versus a vaccine containing S subunit, pre-S1, and pre-S2 particles for revaccination of healthy adult nonresponders. *J Infect Dis* 175:678–681.

Fabrizi F, Dixit V, Magnimi M, *et al.* (2006) Meta-analysis: intrademal vs. intramuscular vaccination against hepatitis B virus in patients with chronic kidney disease. *Aliment Pharmacol Ther* 24:497–506.

Girndt M, Köhler H, Schiedhelm-Weick E, *et al.* (1993) T cell activation defect in hemodialysis patients: evidence for a role of the B7/CD28 pathway. *Kidney Int* 44:359–365.

Hedges SJ, Dehoney SB, Hooper JS, *et al.* (2007) Evidence-based treatment recommendations for uremic bleeding. *Nat Clin Pract Nephrol* 3:138–153.

Kaw D, Malhotra D. (2006) Platelet dysfunction and end-stage renal disease. *Semin Dial* 19:317–322.

Kong NCT, Beran J, Kee SA, *et al.* (2008) A new adjuvant improves the immune response to hepatitis B vaccine in hemodialysis patients. *Kidney Int* 73: 856–862.

Mast EE, Weinbaum CM, Fiore AE, *et al.*; ACIP Centers for Disease Control and Prevention (CDC). (2006) A comprehensive immunization strategy to eliminate transmission of hepatitis B virus infection in the United States. Recommendations of the ACIP part II: immunization of adults. *MMWR Recomm Rep* 55(RR16):1–33.

Remuzzi G, Perico N, Zoja C, *et al.* (1990) Role of endothelium-derived nitric oxide in bleeding tendency of uremia. *J Clin Invest* 86:1768–1771.

Tang S, Lai KN. (2005) Chronic viral hepatitis in hemodialysis patients. *Hemodial Int* 9:169–179.

Zeigler ZR, Megaludis A, Fraley DS. (1992) Desmopressin (d-DAVP) effects on platelet rheology and von Willebrand factor activities in uremia. *Am J Hematol* 39:90–95.

21

Routine Investigations for Dialysis Patients

Sydney C. W. Tang

21.1 Predialysis Workup

The optimal timing for initiation of dialysis is still under debate, but it is generally accepted that preparation for dialysis should begin when stage 4 chronic kidney disease (CKD) is reached. Attention should be paid to the control of blood pressure, anemia, electrolyte disturbance, malnutrition, and psychosocial impact.

21.1.1 *Patient Selection*

With the escalating burden of CKD globally and the rising cost of renal replacement therapy, it may not be feasible to dialyze every patient who reaches end-stage renal disease (ESRD). Patients who may not benefit medically from renal replacement therapy may include those with the following conditions:

- Non-uremic dementia
- Severe psychiatric illness resulting in self-neglect, violence, or incompliance to medical instructions
- Irreversible neurological conditions, e.g. major stroke or severe neurodegenerative disease
- Advanced malignancy with limited life expectancy
- Severe debility without family support

21.1.2 *Patient Education*

This encompasses the psychological preparation to commence renal replacement therapy and the introduction of the various options of replacement therapy, including the different modes of peritoneal dialysis (PD) and hemodialysis (HD) together with surgical procedures for associated dialysis access. As such, this requires multidisciplinary predialysis management involving the nephrologist, nurse specialist, nutritionist, surgeon, and other relevant allied health professionals. In addition, patient-initiated self-help groups may sometimes play a counseling role.

The choice of dialysis, while theoretically should be patient-driven, is in practice often resource-driven. The first-line mode of therapy varies with different socioeconomic systems. For instance, HD is the predominant form of dialysis in the USA, while PD is most prevalent in Hong Kong. The conditions that contraindicate PD include colostomy, ileostomy, intra-abdominal fibrosis, poor person hygiene, and morbid obesity. Those that contraindicate HD include thrombosed central veins, severe heart failure, and major coronary artery disease.

21.1.3 Investigations

These include hematological, biochemical, and virologic (hepatitis B and C, and HIV status) examinations. For patients with transplant potential, cytomegalovirus (CMV), Epstein–Barr virus (EBV), and varicella zoster antibodies, as well as G6PD status, should be checked. For PD, attention should be paid to any previous lower abdominal surgery that may have caused peritoneal fibrosis. For HD, venous mapping may be required for some patients.

21.2 Routine Investigations During Maintenance Dialysis

The investigations differ according to the practice of different centers and the patient population. Some of the pertinent investigations for PD and HD patients are shown in Table 21.1.

21.3 Assessment of Suitability for Kidney Transplantation

Kidney transplantation provides the best potential for full rehabilitation or return to normal life, and maximizes survival for ESRD patients. However, not all patients with ESRD are suitable for transplantation, and the following salient considerations should be contemplated.

Table 21.1 Pertinent routine investigation protocol for maintenance dialysis.

Every 1–2 months	Every 3–4 months	Every 6 months	Every 12 months
Complete blood count	Fasting glucose and HbA1C (for DM subjects)	Lipid profile	PTH
Renal function	α-feto protein (for HBV/HCV carriers)	Fasting glucose	Aluminum
Ca/PO$_4$/ALP		Iron status	HBsAg/HBsAb
Liver function		PTH (for patients with known hyperparathyroidism)	Anti-HCV
		Anti-DNA, C3, C4 (for SLE patients)	Skeletal survey
		ANCAs (for patients with vasculitis)	CXR
		CRP	ECG
		Anti-HLA Ab (for patients on transplant waiting list)	Echocardiogram
			Peritoneal equilibration test (for PD patients)
			Kt/V assessment

Abbreviation: ALP, alkaline phosphatase; DM, diabetes mellitus; HBV, hepatitis B virus; HCV, hepatitis C virus; PTH, parathyroid hormone; SLE, systemic lupus erythematosus; ANCAs, antinuclear cytoplasmic antibodies; CRP, C-reactive protein; CXR, chest X-ray; ECG, electrocardiogram; Kt/V, marker of dialysis adequacy.

21.3.1 *Cause of Renal Failure*

This has an important bearing on the suitability and timing of transplantation. Patients with pathogenetic antibodies causing renal failure, such as anti-glomerular basement membrane (anti-GBM) disease, ANCA-associated rapidly progressive glomerulonephritis, and active lupus nephritis, should allow time (typically 6–12 months after initiating dialysis) for the disease to enter quiescence before being considered for transplantation workup. It is recommended that these pathogenetic antibodies should be undetectable for approximately 2 years before a renal transplantation is performed. Some diseases have high risk of recurrence, such as primary oxalosis, focal glomerulosclerosis, and IgA nephropathy, but they do not constitute an absolute contraindication to kidney transplantation.

21.3.2 *Comorbidities*

Comorbidities heavily impact on transplant suitability and outcome, and these considerations are summarized in Table 21.2.

21.3.3 *Laboratory Investigations*

These are summarized in Table 21.3.

Table 21.2 Comorbidities that affect suitability for kidney transplantation.

Condition	Considerations
Malignancy	Patients with malignant neoplasms within five years, except basal or cutaneous squamous cell carcinoma, should not be considered.
Infections	Patients with active infections, such as severe peritonitis or tuberculosis, should be temporarily withdrawn from the transplant waiting list until the infection is completed treated.
	Patients who are carriers of HBV or HCV without active hepatitis or cirrhosis can be considered, and post-transplant monitoring +/− antiviral therapy should be implemented.
	Whether HIV-infected subjects should be considered is debatable.

(Continued)

Table 21.2   (*Continued*)

Condition	Considerations
Vasculopathic states	Patients with extensive peripheral vascular disease are at risk of graft thrombosis after transplantation, and should undergo full angiographic workup, particularly of the iliac vessels. Patients with major coronary heart disease should undergo revascularization prior to transplantation.
Urogenital anomalies	Full urologic workup is needed before transplantation.
Poor neurological state	Patients with major psychosis, dementia, neurodegenerative disease, or stroke with severe residual neurological deficits should not be considered.
Other major organ failure	Patients with advanced cardiac or respiratory failure should not be considered. Patients with cirrhosis or liver failure can be individually considered for combined liver and kidney transplants.
High panel-reactive antibodies (PRAs)	Patients with history of blood transfusion, previous kidney transplants, and pregnancies are at risk of presensitization, and a high PRA level may contraindicate further transplantation, except in highly specialized centers that deal with such recipients.

Table 21.3   Laboratory investigations prior to kidney transplantation.

Hematology	Full blood count
	Clotting profile
	G6PD status
Biochemistry	Renal and liver function tests
	Fasting glucose and lipid profile
	Bone profile
	Iron status
Viral serology	HBsAg, anti-HBs, anti-HCV, anti-HIV
	HBV DNA (as indicated)
	CMV, EBV, varicella zoster
Cardiopulmonary function	CXR
	ECG
Immunology	Anti-nuclear factor, anti-dsDNA, C3, C4, CRP, ANCAs (if indicated)
	Direct microcytotoxicity test

Part III
Renal Transplantation

22

Pretransplantation Donor and Recipient Workup

Laurence K. Chan and Siu-Kim Chan

22.1 Recipient Selection and Pretransplant Evaluation

Treatment options for patients with end-stage renal disease (ESRD), or chronic kidney disease (CKD) stage 5, fall into three broad categories: hemodialysis, peritoneal dialysis, and transplantation. In most developed countries, there is a choice for each patient as to the modality of treatment that best suits the individual. Early referral of patients during the course of CKD permits better preparation for dialysis and transplantation. With improved transplant outcomes and the widespread expectation that renal transplantation will be available, the growth in the number of patients wanting or waiting for a transplant has outpaced the supply of available organs. It is therefore important that patients are referred early and that potential kidney transplant recipients are carefully evaluated in order to detect and treat coexisting illnesses which may affect survival after transplantation.

22.1.1 *General Considerations*

Most patients are transplanted after having been established on maintenance hemodiaysis or peritoneal dialysis. More recently, however, many patients are being transplanted before they require dialysis. Indeed, if the supply of kidneys were to increase, this shortcut would become an increasingly common practice. Transplantation before the commencement of dialysis (pre-emptive transplantation) has been convincingly shown to improve posttransplant patient and graft survival. Because of the varied course of advanced CKD, it is difficult to provide a precise point when referral for transplant should be made. However, patients with a glomerular filtration rate (GFR) in the 20's and patients whose course suggests they will be dialysis-dependent in 1 to 2 years should be referred.

The decision to place a patient on the waiting list for a transplant should be made jointly by the nephrologist and the transplant surgeon. All patients with ESRD should be considered for kidney transplantation, provided no absolute contraindications exist. Criteria for acceptance were more stringent in the past. Criteria for eligibility should be transparent and made available to patients and the public; eligibility should not be based on social status, gender, race, or personal or public appeal. Today, there are few absolute contraindications to a kidney transplantation and many of these contraindications are relative (Table 22.1). Conditions excluding a patient from renal transplantation would probably be:

- the presence of severe ischemic heart disease (although this might be approached by coronary artery bypass surgery, where appropriate, before transplantation)
- old age (over 75 years), although attitudes are still changing
- the presence of persistent infection or cancer — when a patient has had previous curative therapy for cancer, it is generally thought appropriate to wait for 2–5 years, with proven freedom from recurrence, before going ahead with transplantation (Table 22.2)
- patients with chronic illness with a life expectancy of less than 1 year
- poorly controlled psychosis and patients with active substance abuse.

Table 22.1 Contraindications to transplantation.

Absolute	Relative
Active infection	Renal disease with high recurrence rate
Disseminated malignancy	Refractory noncompliance
Extensive vascular disease	Urologic abnormalities
High risk for perioperative mortality	Active systemic illness
Persistent coagulation abnormality	Ongoing substance abuse
Informed patient refusal	Uncontrolled psychosis

Table 22.2 Recommendations for minimum tumor-free waiting periods.

Tumor type	Minimal waiting time
Bladder	
In situ	None
Invasive	2 years
Breast	
In situ	2 years
Regional lymph node/Bilateral disease	5 years
Colorectal	2–5 years
Lymphoma	2–5 years
Prostate	2 years
Renal cell carcinoma	None (incidental small tumor)
	2 years (<5 cm)
	5 years (>5 cm)
Skin (local)	
Basal cell	None
Squamous cell	Surveillance
Melanoma	5 years
Uterus	
Cervix (*in situ*)	None
Cervical (invasive)	2–5 years
Uterine body	2 years

Reference website: www.ipittr.uc.edu/.

Relative contraindications, which require careful evaluation and possible prior therapy as described below, include:

- active infection
- coronary heart disease
- cerebrovascular disease
- proven habitual medical noncompliance
- active HIV infection.

22.1.2 *Patient Education and General Evaluations*

The evaluation process is an opportunity to counsel patients about their treatment options and to advocate for their welfare (Table 22.3).

Table 22.3   Pretransplantation recipient medical evaluation.

History and physical examination
Social and psychiatric evaluation
Determination of primary kidney disease activity and residual kidney function
Dental evaluation
Laboratory studies:
  Complete blood cell count and blood chemistry
  HBsAg
  HCV
  HIV
  Cytomegalovirus and Epstein–Barr virus
  HLA typing and antibody screening
  Urine analysis and urine culture
Chest X-ray
Electrocardiogram
Special procedures for selected patients:
  Abdominal ultrasound of gallbladder
  Upper gastrointestinal study or endoscopy
  Barium enema or colonoscopy
  PPD skin test
  Treadmill/exercise electrocardiogram
  Thallium scan
  Angiogram: coronary
  Cystoureterography
Consults (optional):
  Psychiatric
  Gynecologic evaluation and mammography (for female >40 years)
  Urologic assessment (voiding cystoureterography, cystoscopy, or
    urodynamic studies in patients with vesicoureteric reflux, neurogenic
    bladder, bladder neck obstruction, or strictures)

A detailed medical history at the time of initial evaluation should be obtained. This assessment should include not only a complete medical evaluation and determination (where possible) of the underlying disease causing renal failure, but also a careful surveillance for problems that might arise. It is important to have social and psychiatric evaluation with a view to give support to these patients. A careful physical examination should be performed to identify coexisting cardiovascular, gastrointestinal (GI), or genitourinary (GU) disease. Additional examinations should assess pulmonary reserve, define potential sources of infection including dental caries, and assess the gynecologic risks for females. The laboratory evaluation should include routine hematologic tests to detect leukopenia or thrombocy-topenia, liver function tests including complete hepatitis and HIV profiles, viral titers, and urine cultures. Blood group should be tested with human leukocyte antigen (HLA) typing and a panel-reactive antibody assay to detect for previous sensitization. Certain radiologic procedures, in addition to chest X-ray, are routinely performed; these include ultrasonography (of the abdomen and pelvis to include the kidneys, ureters, and possibly a postvoid bladder image), echocardiography, thallium scintigraphy, and/or dobutamine stress echocardiography.

22.1.3 *Risk Factors*

Major risk factors that have an impact on the recipient include age, the presence of diabetes mellitus, arteriosclerotic heart disease, chronic pulmonary disorders, and malignancy. Patient compliance has also been identified as an important cause of late graft failure (Table 22.4).

22.1.3.1 *Age*

The very young patient (<5 years) and the elderly recipient do have a poorer patient and graft survival than patients of ages between these two extremes. A reluctance to accept transplantation in older patients was previously due to the belief that the perioperative and postoperative complication rates outweighed the advantages. However, with the improvements in perioperative management and immunosuppressive strategies, advanced age itself is no longer a contraindication to renal transplantation. Based on a retrospective analysis, it appears that older patients may have better immunologic survival despite the higher mortality from cardiovascular disease. One explanation may

Table 22.4 Factors influencing the outcome of cadaveric renal transplantation.

Immunologic	Nonimmunologic
Immunosuppressive protocol	Delayed graft function/ischemic time
Matching for HLA	Compliance
Sensitization	Cardiovascular disease
Rejection	Recipient age
	Center effect/clinical care
	Nephron dose/Donor and recipient sex

be an age-related change in immunologic function that confers less alloreactivity with aging. For this reason, many centers advocate the use of lower immunosuppression in elderly patients.

Transplantation can now be safely and successfully performed in the elderly patient, and will become much more widely practiced in this group of patients with ESRD. Recipient age alone should no longer be considered a contraindication to transplantation, since the age limit for being a transplant recipient has steadily increased. Indeed, many patients over the age of 65 years have been transplanted safely and with an acceptable rate of long-term graft function. Such patients are also candidates for extended-criteria donor kidneys.

22.1.3.2 *Obesity*

Obesity alone is rarely an absolute contraindication to transplantation, yet it is a well-defined risk factor. Lower graft survival rates as well as higher postoperative mortalities and complications have been demonstrated in patients with a body mass index (BMI) greater than 30 kg/m². The large body size is also a risk factor for progression and subsequent premature failure, due to the physiologic changes that have been linked to nephron hyperfiltration. Hence, weight reduction is important for an obese dialysis patient before proceeding to transplantation.

22.1.3.3 *Prior Kidney Transplantation*

Renal allograft failure is now one of the most common causes of ESRD, accounting for about 30% of patients awaiting renal transplantation. Graft survival of a second and/or third kidney transplant has been reported to be inferior to that of the first. Evaluation of a potential recipient for a second or third allograft requires careful attention to the reason for the graft failure. Factors to be assessed include (a) noncompliance with immunosuppressive medications, (b) loss of the graft in association with recurrent renal disease, and (c) high alloreactivity with high panel-reactive antibody (PRA) titers (PRA). These patients may also manifest complications of prior immunosuppressive therapy, and as such should be screened for complications associated with these medications (e.g. infection and malignancy).

No controlled prospective studies have been performed to determine the best method for tapering or withdrawal of immuno-suppression following renal allograft failure. Most centers have adopted a policy of immediate withdrawal of immunosuppression combined with pre-emptive nephrectomy for patients with early allograft failure; however, this practice is less common for patients with late graft failure. A longer tapering of immunosuppression may permit the maintenance of some residual renal function while on dialysis. Several small studies have noted that patients who have undergone transplant nephrectomy have higher PRAs than those undergoing dialysis with the allograft still in place. Further studies are needed to determine whether a slower tapering of calcineurin inhibitors or other immunosuppression can reduce the incidence of nephrectomy without untoward side-effects in these patients while on dialysis.

22.1.4 Specific Evaluations of Recipients

22.1.4.1 Immunologic Evaluation

In addition to determining HLA antigens at the A, B, C, and DR loci, the potential recipient's serum should be screened regularly for HLA antibodies. Prophylactic measures are most important in the management of presensitization leading to hyperacute and accelerated rejection. The avoidance of both ABO incompatibility and positive T-cell cross-matches has eliminated the major cause of hyperacute rejection seen in the early days of transplantation. The presence of lymphocyte cytotoxic antibodies in the patient's serum is due to sensitization to HLA antigens. It can occur after pregnancy, blood transfusion, and renal transplantation. Autoantibodies, on the other hand, often occur spontaneously and are not related to any obvious antigenic challenge.

One method of defining highly sensitized patients is to include subjects who at any time have developed lymphocytotoxic antibodies which react with ≥90% of random panel cells. One approach to this is by removing the anti-HLA antibodies prior to transplantation (e.g. via plasmaphoresis or using anti-CD20 monoclonal antibody), in addition to treatment with intravenous immunoglobulin (IVIG).

22.1.4.2 Cardiovascular Evaluation

Cardiovascular disease is a major cause of morbidity and mortality for the patient in ESRD, whether the patient remains on dialysis or chooses to have a kidney transplantation. It is therefore important to carefully screen the patient for any cardiovascular problem, especially in diabetic patients. Initial assessment of the severity of cardiovascular disease consists of careful clinical examination, an electrocardiogram (ECG), and X-ray of the chest and peripheral vessels for calcification. Evidence of moderate or severe myocardial ischemia is an indication for further investigation with thallium stress test, coronary angiography, and/or cardiac magnetic resonance imaging (MRI). Coronary artery bypass grafting should be considered prior to transplantation in the presence of severe angina or double- or triple-vessel disease. Any patient who has had a recent myocardial infarction should only be reassessed for a transplant 6 months after the incident.

Approximately 20% to 30% of diabetic transplant candidates have significant coronary artery disease, which may be asymptomatic. Since active intervention may improve patient outcome, noninvasive testing and, if indicated, cardiac catheterization should be performed prior to renal transplantation. For the nondiabetic, asymptomatic patient, extensive cardiac evaluation appears unnecessary, unless risk factors (such as smoking, hypertension, hyperlipidemia, and family history of heart disease) are present.

22.1.4.3 *Gastrointestinal Evaluation*

Although the incidence of peptic ulcer after renal transplantation is decreasing, complications of peptic ulcer such as perforation or hemorrhage are associated with high mortality in the transplant patient. For this reason, many centers actively screen patients for evidence of peptic ulceration before accepting them for transplantation, and in the past have been quite aggressive about the management of these patients before transplantation. Similarly, in patients with symptomatic cholelithiasis or asymptomatic gallstones demonstrated by ultrasonography, cholecystectomy should be performed to eliminate the risk of cholelithiasis and possible sepsis after transplantation. Patients with colonic disease, especially those with diverticulitis, should be evaluated with barium enema and colonoscopy and, if appropriate, should be treated with surgical resection prior to transplantation.

22.1.4.4 *Genitourinary Evaluation*

Accurate evaluation of the lower urinary tract function prior to transplantation is important to minimize postoperative urologic complications. The original renal disease must be clearly defined.

Any history of repeated urinary infections and current reports of urine cultures should be obtained. In the past, a voiding cystourethrogram was performed on all patients to evaluate the urinary tract for evidence of outflow obstruction or vesicoureteral reflux; it is now considered necessary only if there is clinical evidence of a bladder or ureteric abnormality. Cystoscopy and urodynamic studies should be performed in patients with evidence of bladder dysfunction. Urologic operations are necessary either to correct or improve obstructive lesions, or sometimes to provide a conduit in the presence of a neurogenic bladder or a previous cystectomy.

22.1.4.5 Hepatitis B Surface Antigen (HBsAg) Screening

Successful renal transplant in patients with positive HBsAg has been reported. However, when HBsAg-positive transplant patients are retrospectively compared with an age-matched group of hemodialysis patients known to be HBsAg-positive, the transplant patients have a higher frequency of chronic hepatitis and mortality due to hepatitis. The adverse effects are not apparent during the first 2 years after transplantation, but become evident over the long term. Hemodialysis patients have a high rate of HBsAg persistence but rarely develop chronic hepatitis, and the rate of seroconversion to surface antigen negativity is 15%–20% per year. Because of this, some centers do not recommend renal transplantation in chronic HBsAg carriers. This decision, however, should be individualized. The better quality of life of the transplant patient should be weighed against the low but definite risk of development of chronic liver failure.

In a study from the Necker Hospital, France (Fornairon *et al.* 1996), patient and graft survival rates were similar between HBsAg-positive and HBsAg-negative kidney recipients. These data suggest that renal transplantation may be appropriate for patients with chronic hepatitis irrespective of their hepatitis virus status. However, no patient should undergo transplantation when he or she has evidence of active hepatitis. Before transplantation, potential recipients should have stable liver enzymes, preferably less than two or three times normal for several months.

22.1.4.6 Hepatitis C Virus (HCV) Screening

Transplant recipients are potentially at risk of developing hepatitis C virus infection due to reactivation of pretransplantation HCV infection or to infection acquired from blood products or from HCV-infected organ donors. In potential recipients with serologic evidence of HCV, a liver biopsy should be performed to assess the histologic severity of the disease.

22.1.4.7 *HIV Screening*

The HIV antibody status of all potential donors and recipients should be determined before transplantation. Potential recipients who are highly sensitized may have false-positive enzyme-linked immunosorbent assay (ELISA) results because of a higher incidence of antibodies in their serum that react with HLA antigens on the target cell used in the serologic assay. The Western blot technique, which detects viral envelope protein, may be more accurate in these situations. Polymerase chain reaction (PCR) analysis to detect small amounts of HIV viral DNA in serum may further improve accuracy.

22.1.5 *Underlying Renal Diseases*

It is most important to assess the cause of the potential recipient's renal failure. The primary pathologies leading to renal failure are expected to influence the outcome, depending on the etiologic mechanisms, propensity for recurrence, and status of the immune system. The type of original kidney disease is not a contraindication to transplantation. However, the transplant team should inform their recipients that many diseases can recur in the allograft and, in some cases, lead to graft failure (Table 22.5). Examples include focal glomerulosclerosis, membranoproliferative glomerulonephritis, and primary hyperoxaluria, which may require a special approach and precautions.

22.1.5.1 *Oxalosis*

The early transplant experience was disappointing because of early graft failure due to recurrent urolithiasis, nephrocalcinosis, renal failure, and systemic oxalate deposition. The earlier recommendation to consider primary oxalosis as a contraindication to transplantation is now being challenged by recent reports of successfully prolonged graft function despite persistent hyperoxalosis. Those grafts with good long-term function have usually passed urine promptly after the operation and have had little rejection. To reduce the chances of

Table 22.5   Recurrent diseases in renal allografts.

Disease	Approximate recurrence rate (%)	Graft loss due to recurrence
Primary glomerulonephritis		
FSG	30–60	Common
HUS	20–50	Uncommon
Type I MPGN	20–30	Common
Type II MPGN	50–100	Uncommon
HSP	15–50	Uncommon
IgA nephropathy	40–50	Uncommon
Anti-GBM	25–50	Uncommon
Membranous GN	10–30	Uncommon
Systemic disease		
Oxalosis	80–100	Common
Cystinosis	50–100	Uncommon
Fabry's disease	<5	Common
Sickle cell disease	Rare	Common
Diabetes type I	100	Uncommon
SLE	3–10	Uncommon

Abbreviations: FSG, focal segmental glomerulosclerosis; HUS, hemolytic-uremic syndrome; MPGN, membranoproliferative glomerulonephritis; HSP, Henoch–Schönlein purpura; GBM, glomerular basement membrane; GN, glomerulonephritis; SLE, systemic lupus erythematosus.

oxalate accumulation, dialysis treatment or kidney transplantation should be considered when the GFR approaches 20 mL/min. Aggressive dialysis schedules should be implemented before transplantation to deplete the oxalate metabolic pool. Medical therapy with pyridoxine, neutral phosphate, and magnesium should be given after transplantation to reduce oxalate deposition and recurrence. Combined renal and hepatic transplantation has also been recommended as a more definitive approach, and early results have been encouraging.

Unlike primary oxalosis, which is a congenital condition with enzymatic defects in oxalate metabolism, secondary oxalosis is due to excessive intake or absorption of oxalates from the diet. Secondary oxalosis is seen primarily in fat malabsorption, short bowel syndrome after gastrointestinal surgery, and high-oxalate diets. For these patients, consideration should be given to reanastomosis of gastric bypass, hydration, and dietary restriction of oxalates. Good allograft function can be achieved when attention is paid to reduce the oxalate excretion load.

22.1.5.2 Amyloidosis

Recurrent nephrotic syndrome and graft failure can occur in primary and secondary amyloidosis, but there is some indication that patients with amyloid-induced renal disease do better after renal transplantation than with dialysis as replacement therapy. The graft survival of patients with amyloid-induced ESRD who receive transplantation now appears to be equal to the survival of non-amyloid-induced ESRD patients who receive transplants. Familial Mediterranean fever (FMF), rheumatoid arthritis, and osteomyelitis are the most common causes of secondary amyloidosis.

FMF is an autosomal recessive disorder that occurs in Sephardic Jews, Armenians, Turks, and Levant Arabs. In Israel, amyloidosis constitutes 6% of all patients on dialysis, compared to 0.6% in Europe. Although there has been a higher early mortality rate among transplanted patients in the past, the incidence of rejection episodes is now lower than in patients without amyloidosis. Reduced immunosuppression has reduced postoperative mortality and morbidity. Colchicine at 1–2 mg/day dramatically relieves the symptoms and reduces the incidence of FMF attacks.

22.1.5.3 Alport syndrome

Dialysis and transplantation pose no particular problems for patients with Alport syndrome. Recurrent disease has not been well documented. Improvement or stabilization of deafness after renal transplantation has occasionally been reported. There is a remote risk of developing de novo anti-glomerular basement membrane (anti-GBM) nephritis after transplantation.

22.1.5.4 Focal Segmental Glomerulosclerosis (FSG)

Recurrent focal sclerosis may be seen early after transplantation, presenting with nephrotic-range proteinuria and a rapid decline in renal function. Histologically, the features on light microscopy that permit categorization are focal and segmental sclerosis affecting a small number of glomeruli, often those in the deep juxtamedullary cortex. The development of foot process fusion can be immediately after transplantation and precede glomerular segmental sclerosis by weeks to months. The frequency of recurrence is about 20% in adults and may be as high as 40% in children. It is likely that some of these patients had secondary FSG due to nephron loss in reflux nephropathy, which would not be expected to recur in the transplant. Thus, the recurrence rate of primary FSG may be substantially higher than the reported values. Patients who presented with rapid progression of renal disease from the time of diagnosis of nephrotic syndrome to ESRD have a higher risk of recurrence. If a transplant patient lost his or her graft because of recurrent FSG, there is a 50% risk of subsequent allograft failure within 5 years of a second transplantation.

Treatment for recurrent FSG remains disappointing. Heavy proteinuria and nephrotic syndrome are usually resistant to steroids. Cyclosporine (CsA) has not proved effective in preventing recurrence. Because of the high risk of recurrence and rapid progression to ESRD, living donors generally are not used for the first allograft. Use of a cadaver kidney, however, is not precluded, since the disease will not recur in all cases and not all patients with recurrence will lose the graft. Some centers have also suggested that, if a first graft is lost to recurrent disease, a second transplant should be delayed for 1–2 years.

The rapidity of recurrence strongly suggests the presence of a circulating factor in primary FSG that is toxic to the capillary wall. It has been shown that serum from some patients with FSG increases the permeability of isolated glomeruli to albumin. Testing of pretransplant sera with this approach can be used to predict recurrence after transplantation. Use of a regenerating protein adsorption column or plasma exchange can reduce protein excretion in patients with recurrent FSG in the transplant. More prolonged remissions have been achieved using plasma exchange that is initiated promptly after onset of proteinuria or the combination of plasma exchange and cyclophosphamide. These prolonged beneficial results have also been reported in children treated with plasma exchange and cyclophosphamide.

22.1.5.5 *Anti-Glomerular Basement Membrane (Anti-GBM) Disease*

Based on histology and fluorescence study, anti-GBM disease is associated with a recurrence rate of over 50% in the allograft. However, only 25% of patients with biopsy-proven IgG staining along the capillary wall have evidence of clinical disease activity. Furthermore, graft failure due to disease recurrence is less common. Although engraftment during the presence of anti-GBM antibodies has been reported to be successful, many transplant centers still prefer serologic quiescence of anti-GBM antibody production for 6–12 months before proceeding with transplantation to reduce the risk for recurrent anti-GBM disease. Despite delaying transplantation to allow anti-GBM antibodies to fall, recurrence has been reported.

22.1.5.6 *Hemolytic-Uremic Syndrome (HUS)*

HUS has a recurrence rate of 20%–50%. It has pathologic features common to the small-vessel findings in acute vascular rejection, CsA toxicity, and malignant hypertension. The recurrence rate is higher in recipients of living-related transplants. Live kidney donation should proceed with caution in view of the possibility of a familial tendency to an abnormality of prostacyclin synthesis. A meta-analysis of 159 grafts in 126 patients by Ducloux *et al.* found that recurrent HUS was significantly associated with the older age onset of HUS, short duration between disease onset and ESRD or transplantation, use of living-related donors, and, to a lesser degree, administration of calcineurin inhibitors (CsA or tacrolimus). In high-risk patients with a history of HUS, prevention by the administration of low-dose aspirin and dipyridamole should be used. Calcineurin inhibitors and antilymphocyte serum should be used with caution in these patients.

22.1.5.7 *Type I Membranoproliferative Glomerulonephritis (MPGN)*

The frequency of recurrence of type I MPGN is estimated to be 20%–30%. Approximately 30%–40% of patients with recurrent type I MPGN will lose their allograft. Graft rejection is often a confounding factor. Reduced C3 levels before transplantation usually return to the normal range after transplantation and do not correlate with disease activity.

22.1.5.8 *Type II MPGN (Dense Deposit Disease)*

The recurrence rate of type II MPGN is reported to be 50%–100%, with graft failure in 20%–50%. Proteinuria with or without hematuria is the usual clinical presentation. Decrement in serum C3 levels and appearance of C3 nephritic factor may be present in some cases. Recurrence is usually evident within the first year after engraftment. The unique ultrastructural appearance of extensive deposit within the basement membrane allows this diagnosis to be made with certainty both before and after transplantation.

22.1.5.9 IgA Nephropathy (IgAN)

Recurrence of mesangial IgA deposits in the renal allografts occurs with a recurrence rate ranging from 13% to 60% of patients with IgAN. The longer the duration of follow-up of the patients after transplantation, the more likely the affected patients become symptomatic and the higher the reported incidence of recurrent disease. The recurrence is due to the deposition of IgA with an abnormal glycosylation profile unique to patients suffering from IgAN. Recurrent disease exhibits considerable clinical similarities with primary IgAN. An estimated 10-year incidence of graft loss due to recurrent IgAN of 9.7% was reported by the Australia and New Zealand Dialysis and Transplant Registry (ANZDATA), which contains 532 allograft recipients with primary IgAN.

Observations from Choy *et al.* (2003) suggest that the impact of other factors, including recurrent disease, on graft survival becomes more apparent on long-term follow-up (>12 years). Recurrent IgA nephropathy runs an indolent course similar to primary IgAN with a favorable outcome in the initial 10 years posttransplant, and thereafter its contribution to graft loss becomes more significant.

22.1.5.10 Diabetes Mellitus

Although the diabetic patient is a high-risk candidate for transplantation, it is now generally accepted that transplantation is the treatment of choice for many of these patients. Recurrence of diabetic nephropathy in type I diabetic recipients is a late and slowly developing complication. The frequency and natural history of recurrence in type II diabetic recipients remain to be elucidated.

There is an increasing use of combined kidney and pancreas transplantation in selected patients with ESRD due to diabetes. Pancreas transplantation is performed mostly with a simultaneous kidney from the same donor. Benefits of pancreas transplantation include better glycemic control and improvement in some of the secondary complications of diabetes. As of 2003, more than 21 000 pancreas transplants were reported to the International Pancreas Transplant Registry. Patient survival and pancreas graft survival rates continue to improve, with data from US centers demonstrating 95% and 86% 1-year patient and graft survival rates, and 85% and 70% 5-year patient and graft survival rates, respectively.

With the increase in utilization of living donors for kidney transplantation, solitary pancreas transplant after kidney transplant (PAK) has grown in popularity, comprising over 25% of pancreas surgery cases. However, debate has arisen regarding the benefit derived from this strategy, as one study suggests an increase in mortality in patients who undergo PAK when compared to patients who remain on the waiting list for pancreas transplantation.

22.2 Live Donor Evaluation

22.2.1 *Background*

The shortage of kidneys, improvements in techniques and care, and the use of new treatments have made live kidney donation a viable option. An increase in the number of living donors (including living unrelated donors) may ameliorate this trend. The number of living donors is currently greater than the number of deceased donors. Living kidney donor transplantation is expected to grow, especially in light of the fact that a high graft survival rate has been found associated with these donors. Most of the living kidney transplants are from directed donors. Possible donors include family members (i.e. sibling, parent) or genetically unrelated individuals (i.e. spouse, friend, acquaintance, or another person who has an emotional bond or rapport with the recipient). In rare instances, a directed donor may know of a particular recipient in need of a donated organ and only develop a relationship with that recipient for the purpose of the transplant (e.g. church members, individuals who respond to public or media notice).

The ethics committee of the Transplantation Society had developed a guideline on live kidney donors' care in a forum held in 2004. It stressed that both directed and nondirected live kidney donation should receive complete medical and psychological evaluations to protect donor safety and autonomy. This guideline was further clarified in 2008 by the Declaration of Istanbul, sponsored by The Transplantation Society, World Health Organization, and International Society of Nephrology. Donors are accepted if they are medically and psychosocially suitable. After ABO compatibility and a negative cross-match are assured, the donor evaluation process can begin.

22.2.2 *Aim of Live Donor Evaluation*

- To determine if an individual is a suitable donor by psychological and medical evaluation.
- Psychological assessment should exclude psychological problems complicating the donation.
- Medical assessment should exclude medical conditions prohibiting donation, and assess the risk of the potential donor.

22.2.3 *Process of Live Donor Evaluation*

22.2.3.1 *Evaluation of Donor Risk*

- Risk associated with general anesthesia.
- Assessment of cardiovascular, pulmonary, and thromboembolic risks should be individualized.
- Surgical risks and benefits of open nephrectomy versus laparoscopic nephrectomy.
- General risk of kidney donation on mortality and morbidity.
- Risk of development of ESRD after kidney donation.
- Risk during donor evaluation.
- Benefits and risks associated with the discovery of certain medical conditions such as malignancy and infections like HIV (including treatment risk and psychological impact, change of insurance status after the discovery of certain diseases, risk associated with contrast imaging).

22.2.3.2 *Medical Assessment of Donors*

- To exclude conditions prohibiting donation (Table 22.6).
- To determine donor anatomy.

History

- Family history

  ○ Kidney-specific disease, including polycystic kidney disease and reflux disease.
  ○ General history including hypertension, diabetes, autoimmune disease.

Table 22.6 Exclusion criteria for live kidney donation.

Age under 18 years
Diabetes
Hypertension — well-controlled hypertensive donors using not more than
  1 antihypertensive medication can be considered
Chronic lung disease
Major and intermediate predictors of cardiovascular risk for noncardiac
  surgery as proposed by the American College of Cardiology; donors with
  minor predictors require individualized consideration
Metastatic malignancy or recent malignancy
Bilateral nephrolithiasis, single stones with high probability of recurrence
Proteinuria >300 mg/day
Hematuria — usually requires renal biopsy to exclude kidney disease
Infective disease (including hepatitis B, hepatitis C, HIV, syphilis,
  tuberculosis (especially urinary tuberculosis))
Creatinine clearance less than 80 mL/min/1.73 m^2
Urological abnormalities (preclude successful organ harvesting)
Morbid obesity with BMI >35

- Personal history
  - Kidney-specific personal history, including proteinuria, hematuria, recurrent urinary tract infection, hypertension, diabetes, nephrolithiasis, gouty arthritis, autoimmune disease.
  - General personal history, including ischemic heart disease, chronic lung disease, infection like tuberculosis, hepatitis status, malignancy, coagulopathy.
- Smoking and alcohol abuse.
- Allergic history.
- Active and past medications (especially analgesic use).
- Psychiatric history (including history of psychiatric illness, depression).
- Social history.
  - Enquiry about employment status, financial status, family relationship.

Physical examination

Calculate BMI by measuring body height and body weight. Blood pressure monitoring is important; it is preferably measured by ambulatory blood pressure monitoring (ABPM). Physical examination should focus on cardiovascular examination, especially signs of peripheral vascular disease.

Urinalysis

Dipstick urinalysis is a quick and convenient way to assess possible signs of current kidney disease, like proteinuria and hematuria. Asymptomatic pyuria should warrant further investigation to exclude urinary tuberculosis, which is a contraindication for kidney donation.

A 24-h urine sampling is routinely done to quantify proteinuria and to measure creatinine clearance as a surrogate of glomerular filtration rate.

General blood test

- Complete blood count, liver and kidney function test, bone profile, uric acid level, coagulation profile (including prothrombin time and activated partial thromboplastin time)
- Diabetic screening by measuring fasting blood glucose. Those of impaired fasting glucose should have the test repeated.
- Measurement of fasting lipid profile should be performed to help assess the cardiovascular risk.

Malignancy screening

Age- and sex-specific malignancy screening should be performed. Family history of malignancy should be enquired as reference. Specifically, breast, cervical, prostate and colorectal cancer screening can be performed according to prevailing guidelines.

Screening of transmissible infections

The aim of infectious disease screening is twofold. It serves to screen for transmissible infections that preclude organ donation. It also provides specific information about the risk of developing infection in recipients after transplant. Donor treatment is indicated in certain infections.

Screening for possible increased risk of infection after transplant in recipients:

- Cytomegalovirus (CMV)
- Epstein–Barr virus (EBV)

Other infection screening:

- Hepatitis B virus (HBV) surface antigen and anti-HBc antibody
- Anti-HCV antibody
- HIV-I, HIV-II
- Syphilis (VDRL test)

- Other infective disease screening as indicated (e.g. strongyloidosis, brucellosis, toxoplasmosis, malaria)
- Tuberculosis — Donors with treated tuberculosis should receive extensive investigation to exclude urinary tuberculosis. Focus should be put on the evidence of sterile pyuria and anatomical abnormality of the urinary tract.

Anatomical assessment

Kidney ultrasound is a good imaging modality to assess the possibility of cystic disease for donors with a family history of polycystic kidney disease. It can also serve as rapid screening for structural abnormality and stone disease, if they are suspected due to pre-existing donor factors.

Various imaging techniques can be employed to assess the anatomy of the kidneys specific for transplant, notably the number of renal arteries. Computed tomography (CT) angiogram or magnetic resonance (MR) angiogram are good alternatives for conventional angiography to minimize patient morbidity. They can also show the size of the kidneys and the presence of renal stone or other anatomical abnormalities. The decision of which kidney to harvest depends on the expertise of the transplant surgeon, but usually the one with the least abnormalities is left for the donor.

Immunological assessment

- Blood grouping
- HLA typing
- Cross-matching

Other investigations

Routine chest X-ray is performed to assess the chronic pulmonary condition and rule out active lung disease. Pulmonary function test may be required if chronic disease is suspected and in old-age donors. Reference values of FVE_1 (forced expiratory volume in 1 second) and FVC (forced vital capacity) are similar to other upper abdominal operations.

ECG should be performed in all donors. Further cardiovascular risk stratification can be made by performing stress test if risk factors are present for cardiovascular diseases.

Psychological assessment

Donors should be evaluated by a psychologist, a psychiatrist, or an experienced social worker. Appropriate referral should be made if psychological or psychiatric problems are identified in the donors. The assessment involves two processes: the evaluation and the explanation of psychosocial consequences.

Psychosocial evaluation:

- To assess the donor's ability to consent and ability to understand the process and risks of donation.
- To evaluate the psychological issues complicating donation.
- To evaluate the financial situation of the donor and identify possible financial complications after donation.
- To exclude the possibility of coercion.
- To identify and refer any psychiatric illnesses.

Explanation of psychosocial consequences:

- To inform the donor that the change of health status after donation may affect the future health insurance.
- To inform the donor that the health information obtained during medical and psychosocial evaluation will be treated as an ordinary medical record, and additional protection of personal health information will not be provided.

22.2.4 *Informed Consent*

22.2.4.1 *Principles of Informed Consent in Live Kidney Donation*

This is to educate potential donors on the process of medical and psychosocial evaluations leading to kidney donation. They were given a detailed explanation on the risks of donation and the benefits for recipients after transplant. In addition, donors should be reassured that they have the right to withdraw at any stage of donor evaluation and that the reason for doing so will be kept secret if they wish; a general explanation like medical unsuitability will be given to the recipient.

22.2.4.2 *Process of Informed Consent*

- Fully explain the process of donor evaluation and the risks associated with the evaluation.
- Psychosocial assessment will be performed by specialized personnel, who can be a nurse specialist, an experienced social worker, or a clinical psychologist or psychiatrist.

- A written document in the donor's native language should be provided to explain in detail the process and risks of live kidney donation, including medical, psychological, and financial risks.
- Alternative forms of treatment other than kidney transplantation should be mentioned. The benefits and risks of kidney transplant in recipients should be fully explained.
- The success rate and survival benefit of kidney transplant should be given; these should be adjusted to the recipient's specific condition, if appropriate. The donor should understand that details of the recipient's medical conditions should be kept secret and cannot be given during the explanation process.
- Donors will be given an appropriate period of time to reflect on their concerns before making the decision whether or not to donate.
- Donors should be reassured that their donations are free from coercion and originated from altruistic acts.
- Donor follow-up will be provided. Financial implications on follow-up should also be addressed. The donor's health details and outcome data will be collected for future analysis.

22.2.5 *Donor Nephrectomy*

The surgical procedures and risks regarding donor nephrectomy should be explained clearly to potential donors.

22.2.5.1 *Standard Open Nephrectomy*

The standard method for removing a kidney from a living donor is through a flank incision by open nephrectomy. The approach to the kidney — usually the left kidney, since it has a longer renal vein — may be either below or through the bed of the twelfth rib using a retroperitoneal approach or rarely via an anterior transperitoneal approach using a midline incision. Care must be given to retraction of the kidney during its removal so as to avoid traction injury of the renal artery; and dissection in the hilum of the kidney, particularly between the ureter and the renal artery, should be avoided to prevent damage to the ureteric blood supply. Furthermore, in removing the ureter down to the brim of the pelvis, care should be taken to leave an adequate amount of periureteric tissue.

22.2.5.2 *Laparoscopic Nephrectomy*

Living donor nephrectomy for transplantation can also be performed by the laparoscopic approach. The techniques of endoscopically assisted nephrectomy are now well established. Over the last few years, there has been an increased rate of donation with laparoscopic donor nephrectomy. This approach results in less postoperative surgical pain, a shorter hospital stay, and a quicker recovery than the standard open donor nephrectomy.

22.2.6 *Expansion of Living Donor Pool*

There have been multiple efforts to expand the living related as well as unrelated donor pool. One method is the establishment of a paired kidney exchange program. In this system, kidney donors who are ABO-incompatible with their intended recipients participate in a Paired exchange program, resulting in an expanded availability of organs. This type of program has been successfully initiated in certain geographic areas. Another strategy is to consider a nondirected live kidney donor. These individuals or altruistic kidney donors offer to donate a kidney, but do not identify the specific recipient. In the 2005 Scientific Registry of Transplant Recipients Report, there were 88 nondirected donations (among a total of 2343 living unrelated donors).

22.3 Deceased (Cadaver) Donor Evaluation

22.3.1 *Background*

Deceased or cadaver donors should be the major source of kidneys for transplantation. However, there is a far greater demand for than supply of deceased organs. Therefore, several approaches have been taken to increase the number of organs for transplantation. These include the use of marginal donors by expanding the criteria that define a suitable organ donor and increasing donor consent through public education efforts. Medical evaluation of potential deceased donors is summarized in Table 22.7. Table 22.8 depicts the essential laboratory tests for potential deceased donors.

Table 22.7   Medical evaluation of potential deceased donors.

Diagnosis of brain death
  Preconditions
    Comatose patient on ventilator
    Positive diagnosis of cause of coma (irremediable structural brain damage)
  Exclusions
    Primary hypothermia (<33°C)
    Drugs
    Severe metabolic or endocrine disturbances
  Tests
    Absent brainstem reflexes
    Apnea (strictly define)
No pre-existing renal disease
No active infection (HIV, HTLV-1, HTLV-2, active HSV encephalitis)

Table 22.8   Essential laboratory tests in potential deceased donors.

Basic tests	Complete blood count, liver and renal function test, clotting profile
Autoimmune markers	ANA, C3/C4, Ig pattern
Serology	HBsAg, anti-HBs, anti-HBc, anti-HCV, anti-HIV-I/II, serologies for CMV/EBV/VZV
	Other tests for potential infections
Sepsis screening	Urine microscopy and culture, blood culture
Tissue typing	ABO blood group, HLA typing, cross-matching

22.3.2 *Aim of Cadaveric Kidney Donor Evaluation*

- To identify conditions that preclude kidney donation
- To categorize donors into different donor groups
- To provide information on organ matching and organ allocation
- To identify risk factors that could affect the outcome of transplant in the future.

22.3.3 *Brain-Dead Donors versus Donation After Cardiac Death*

Deceased donors can be divided in two groups: brain-dead (BD) donors, and donation-after-cardiac-death (DCD) donors or non-heart-beating donors. Although brain-dead (or "heart-beating") donors are considered dead, the donor's heart continues to pump and maintain blood circulation. This makes it possible for surgeons to start operating while the organs are still perfused. The criteria for the diagnosis of brain death have been well defined in most Western countries, although the requirements vary little from country to country. The general acceptance of brain death and improved preservation in recent years has led to the supply of better-quality kidneys and the establishment of organ-sharing programs to match donor and recipient on the basis of ABO blood group compatibility and HLA matching.

22.3.3.1 *Definition of Brain Death*

Brain death is defined as the irreversible loss of brain stem reflexes, irreversible coma, and loss of respiratory center function, or as the loss of intracranial blood flow. The medical practitioner certifying brain death should not be the officer authorizing removal of tissue, proposing to remove the tissue, or attending to a recipient of the tissue to be removed. The process of brain death certification should be well documented and established by experienced clinicians, with the help of confirmatory investigations if necessary.

22.3.3.2 *Diagnostic Procedure*

Determination of cause of coma

- The cause of coma should be established before the process of brain death test. It may be obvious if it is the result of brain trauma, intracranial hemorrhage, or complication following neurosurgery. However, the cause may be more difficult to establish if coma follows cardiac arrest or severe circulatory insufficiency with an undetermined period of cerebral anoxia.
- The comatose patient is apneic and ventilated. The effect of muscle relaxants or other drugs with similar effect should be excluded.
- Potentially reversible causes of coma should be excluded, especially the effect of sedatives or muscle relaxants. Toxicology screening may be helpful to exclude drug effect. An appropriate antidote for opioids or benzodiazepines should be given if their effect is suspected. There should be no profound abnormality of the serum acid base, electrolytes, or glucose level. Hypothermia should be excluded and no brain death should be considered if the core temperature falls below 35°C.

Clinical examination of brain stem function

- Both pupils are fixed in diameter and do not respond to changes in the intensity of light.
- Corneal reflex is absent in both eyes.
- The vestibulo-ocular reflex is absent. Ocular movements should be absent in response to head turning or instillation of ice-cold water to the external auditory meatus. This test may not be appropriate in patients with cervical spine trauma.
- No motor responses within the cranial nerve distribution can be elicited by adequately painful stimulation of any somatic area.
- There is no gag reflex.
- There is no cough reflex on suctioning.
- Apnea test should be performed after the brain stem function tests mentioned above. Absence of respiratory effort should be demonstrated when the patient is disconnected from the mechanical ventilator for long enough to ensure that the arterial $PaCO_2$ rises above 8.0 kPa and the pH falls below 7.3.

Confirmatory tests

These should be done if the cause of coma is unclear and the clinical condition precludes full assessment of brain stem function. This could be due to possible drug and metabolic effects, cervical cord trauma, or severe hypoxemia and hemodynamic instability precluding apnea test. These tests primarily demonstrate the absence of intracranial blood flow:

- Radiocontrast cerebral angiography by injection of contrast under high pressure or digital subtraction technology
- Cerebral scintigraphy, e.g. technetium ^{99m}Tc-HMPAO scintigraphy

22.3.4 *Organ Harvesting and Preservation Before Transplant*

22.3.4.1 *Donor Preservation*

Following brain death, diabetes insipidus develops due to brain injury with increase in urinary sodium and volume output. Structural damage ensues, together with inflammatory changes. Donor preservation should be optimized by providing hemodynamic, metabolic, and respiratory support. Use of desmopressin in excessive urine output greater than 250 mL/h is warranted. Mean arterial pressure should be maintained above 60 mmHg, while judicial use of vasopressors and fluid resuscitation are indicated in most of the cases. Replacement of hormones like thyroxine and corticosteroid may be indicated in selected donors.

Most kidneys will be removed as part of a multiple-organ harvesting procedure in which not only the kidneys, but also the liver and heart (and occasionally the lungs and pancreas) are removed. This necessitates coordination and careful cooperation between the interested parties. The technique of *in situ* perfusion and *en bloc* dissection has evolved as the standard. With experience and care, a donor may provide all of the above organs, all of which can be satisfactorily transplanted.

22.3.4.2 *Renal Preservation*

There are two methods of preservation: simple cold storage in ice after flushing with a hypothermic solution to give a renal core temperature of 0°C, and a more complicated approach of continuous perfusion of the kidney with an oxygenated colloid solution. The simple cold-storage approach is more commonly used because it provides adequate preservation for at least 24 h. The kidneys are initially flushed free of blood with a cold solution via the aorta and renal artery while the kidney is *in situ*. Preservation solution serves to prolong the cold ischemic time when the kidney is bathed below 4°C. The aim of this procedure is to reduce the chances of posttransplant acute tubular necrosis (ATN), which could affect the long-term graft function and survival. The most commonly used preservation solutions currently include the University of Wisconsin (UW) solution and the histidin-tryptophan-ketoglutarate (HTK) solution. Bath solutions are shown to have similar outcome in kidney preservation. Newer agents have been studied extensively to help prevent ATN. Purine nucleotide precursors have been tried with variable results. Calcium channel blockers may be added to preservation solution, as it has been shown that intracellular calcium accumulation is associated with organ dysfunction following ischemic injury.

In the absence of any warm ischemia, which is generally the case with a brain-dead donor on a ventilator, immediate function can be obtained in most kidneys with up to 24 h of preservation and even after 48 h of preservation in some patients. However, from 24 h onward, most kidneys will have a significant period of delayed function, ranging from a week to several weeks, and there will be a significant incidence of permanent nonfunction.

Unlike simple cold storage, machine preservation is more complex and expensive with limited benefits. With this system, a cold perfusate — either plasma protein fraction (PPF) or albumin — is used to perfuse the kidney at low pressures using either pulsatile or continuous perfusion, with the perfusate being oxygenated within the circuit. Both the temperature and the pressure of the perfusate are monitored, and the flow is generally kept at 1–3 mL/g of kidney per min. Progressively rising resistance with a fall in flow rates and a rise in pressure indicates inadequate preservation.

22.3.5 *Deceased Kidney Donor Classification*

Organs recovered from brain-dead donors constitute the largest number of transplants, and they are called standard criteria donors (SCDs). Marginal donors include those having certain characteristics which could affect the graft outcome in the future, or organs from donors that were declared cardiac death; they are now categorized into expanded criteria donors (ECDs) and donation-after-cardiac-death (DCD) donors, respectively. With the ongoing organ shortage, such marginal donors are being utilized to help shorten the waiting list and are allocated to the recipients affected least with such "marginal kidneys".

While DCD donors are easily identified, the differences between SCDs and ECDs are controversial. The classification protocol adopted by the USA defines ECDs as those kidneys donated with risk of graft failure >1.7. Risk factors of graft failure identified include age, history of hypertension, cerebrovascular accident as cause of death, and creatinine level >1.5 mg/dL. Donors of age 60 years or above and those aged 50–59 years with any two of the remaining three risk factors are classified as ECDs.

The use of ECD kidneys remains a challenge in the transplant community. Key issues such as how to allocate these kidneys and the ways to achieve the best outcome are yet to be resolved. Studies have shown that ECD kidneys provide survival benefit in those patients waiting for longer than 1350 days, or those with a waiting time shorter than 1350 days but older than 40 years. It has to be emphasized that the successful use of ECD kidneys relies on an efficient allocation system. The utilization of kidneys from marginal donors due to other risk factors is subjected to individual consideration. Information about the use of ECDs should be given to the recipient, and informed consent should be obtained. Kidneys from the ECDs should be allocated to those who have consented to have such a category of kidney only.

22.3.6 *Procedure of Cadaveric Donor Evaluation*

22.3.6.1 *History and Physical examination*

Social history is important to exclude high-risk factors. Medical history is important for donor evaluation. History of hypertension, diabetes, hepatitis status, autoimmune disease, and malignancy may preclude donation. Cause of death is important to classify donors into different categories, if not prohibit from donation. The clinical course before donation should be carefully sought, including use and dose of inotropes, blood pressure trend, urine output, and signs of infection. Body weight should be measured during physical examination, which is an important factor in determining donor–recipient size mismatch.

22.3.6.2 *Post-retrieval Biopsy*

In order to more accurately predict the prognosis of the harvested kidney, post-retrieval biopsy may be performed before the kidney is transplanted into the recipient. Criteria for discarding the kidney include the degree of glomerulosclerosis, fibrosis, thrombosis, and necrosis. More than 20% of glomerulosclerosis is regarded as a relative contraindication for the use of the harvested kidney. However, the biopsy should only be performed if it affects the decision of transplant.

22.3.6.3 *Contraindications to Deceased Kidney Donation*

These include active communicable infections and HIV infection. Donation from donors of high-risk social background may be relatively contraindicated, as HIV antibody may not appear in early infection. Donors with chronic hepatitis B and C are usually not accepted. Urinary tract infection should be treated before organ donation. Metastatic cancers are also contraindicated, except certain histologic types of brain tumors.

22.3.7 *Key Issues in Deceased Kidney Allocation*

Allocation of the deceased or cadaveric kidney in general follows a point system, except in a few circumstances. This point system follows a number of principles, including waiting time, HLA matching status, and recipient age. Incremental life-years from transplantation (LYFT) vary from patient to patient. Prioritization is being considered for those with the greatest medical urgency and for those with the best expected posttransplantation survival.

The following are key issues in constructing such a point system:

- Waiting time and recipient age — Priority is usually given to those with the longest waiting time under the rule of fairness. Younger patients are also given priority, as they should have better outcome with transplant and the kidneys are best utilized.
- Matching of ABO blood group — In order to be fair to the blood group O recipients, kidneys from blood group O donors are reserved to them.
- Priority of zero-mismatch recipients — In general, zero-mismatch recipients are given priority in receiving the kidneys. This principle aims at providing kidneys to those having the best outcome.
- Priority of recipients with medical emergency — Subject to the physician's opinion, those patients who have failed dialysis due to various reasons and are medically suitable for kidney transplant should be given priority to receive the kidneys.
- Allocation to recipients with high panel-reactive antibody (PRA) level — A suggestion has been made to give priority to those with the highest PRA level among the recipient pool. This is because if they are not given kidneys early on, their chances of successful transplant will be much lowered due to the high immunogenicity developed.
- Allocation of ECD and DCD kidneys — These kidneys should be allocated to recipients with prior consent for accepting such organs. Target recipients are those believed to benefit most, including older patients and those with a long waiting time.

Suggested Reading

Bunnapradist S, Danovitch GM. (2007) Evaluation of adult kidney transplant candidates. *Am J Kidney Dis* 50:890–898.

Chan L, Wiseman A, Wang W, *et al.* (2007) Outcomes and complications of renal transplantation. In: Schrier RW (eds.), *Diseases of the Kidney and Urinary Tract,* 8th ed., Lippincott Williams & Wilkins, Baltimore, pp. 2553–2611.

Choy BY, Chan TM, Lo SK, *et al.* (2003) Renal transplantation in patients with primary immunoglobulin A nephropathy. *Nephrol Dial Transplant* 18:2399–2404.

Delmonico F; Council of the Transplantation Society. (2005) A report of the Amsterdam Forum on the Care of the Live Kidney Donor: data and medical guidelines. *Transplantation* 79(6 Suppl):S53–S66.

Ducloux D, Rebibou JM, Semhoun-Ducloux S, *et al.* (1998) Recurrence of hemolytic-uremic syndrome in renal transplant recipients: a meta-analysis. *Transplantation* 65:1405–1407.

Fornairon S, Pol S, Legendre C, *et al.* (1996) The long-term virologic and pathologic impact of renal transplantation on chronic hepatitis B virus infection. *Transplantation* 62:297–299.

Guidelines on certification of brain death. Hong Kong Society of Critical Care Medicine. http://www.fmshk.com.hk/hksccm/inside5.htm/.

Kasiske BL, Cangro CB, Hariharan S, *et al.* American Society of Transplantation. (2001) The evaluation of renal transplant candidates: clinical practice guidelines. *Am J Transplant* 1(Suppl 2):3–95.

Kasiske BL, Ramos EL, Gaston RS, *et al.* (1995) The evaluation of renal transplant candidates: clinical practice guidelines. *J Am Soc Nephrol* 6:1–34.

Ojo AO. (2005) Expanded criteria donors: process and outcomes. *Semin Dial* 18:463–468.

Organ Procurement and Transplantation Network (OPTN). (2007) Resource document for informed consent of living donors. http://www.unos.org/ContentDocuments/Informed_Consent_Living_Donors.pdf/.

Organ Procurement and Transplantation Network (OPTN). (2008) Guidance for the development of program-specific living kidney donor medical evaluation protocols. http://www.unos.org/SharedContentDocuments/Program_Specific_Living_Kidney_Donor_Med_Eval_Protocols.pdf/.

Pascual J, Zamora J, Pirsch JD. (2008) A systematic review of kidney transplantation from expanded criteria donors. *Am J Kidney Dis* 52:553–586.

Steinman TI, Becker BN, Frost AE, *et al.* (2001) Guidelines for the referral and management of patients eligible for solid organ transplantation. *Transplantation* 71:1189–1204.

United Networks for Organ Sharing. Policy 3.5. (2008) Organ distribution: allocation of deceased kidneys. http://www.unos.org/PoliciesandBylaws2/policies/pdfs/.

23

Management Guidelines Peritransplantation

Jeremy R. Chapman

This chapter describes the sequence of events after the call that "there is a patient coming in for transplantation". This scenario occurs between 60000 and 100000 times a year in hospitals all over the world. With some minor exceptions, based upon geographical risks of certain infectious diseases, what happens over the next 24 hours is almost always the same, no matter who is being transplanted or where it is occurring. This chapter is designed to bring a sense of calm and order to replace the immediate sense of panic in such situations.

There are standard practices that protect the patient and maximize the chances of a successful transplant. The chapter does not include the operation, but does include the assumption that there is a team of people responsible for these crucial hours. That team includes the surgeon; physician; nurses; organ donor coordinators; physiotherapists; and those who work in imaging, pharmacy, and pathology departments. Only the surgeon can do the transplant operation; but without the rest of the team, grafts will be lost unnecessarily over the next 24 hours (Fig. 23.1).

23.1 The Recipient Before Transplantation

The previous chapter has detailed the recipient workup confirming a prior evaluation for suitability for transplantation. The immediate pretransplant assessment is thus designed to reassure the surgeon and anesthetist that the patient remains suitable to transplant. The essential starting point is as follows.

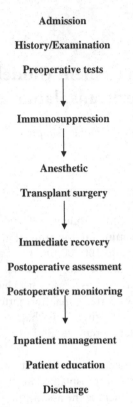

Admission

History/Examination

Preoperative tests

Immunosuppression

Anesthetic

Transplant surgery

Immediate recovery

Postoperative assessment

Postoperative monitoring

Inpatient management

Patient education

Discharge

Fig. 23.1   Perioperative care of the renal transplant recipient.

23.1.1 *Previous Medical History*

- Cause of end-stage kidney failure
- History of assessment and placement on the transplant waiting list/decision to proceed to transplantation, including tests performed (electrocardiogram (ECG), chest X-ray (CXR), coronary angiogram, etc.) and medical and surgical assessments
- Previous transplantation history
- Comorbid diseases

    o Cardiac disease
    o Chronic infectious disease (e.g. tuberculosis, regional chronic infectious disease such as Chagas disease in South America and schisomiasis in Middle East)
    o Acute infectious disease (e.g. urinary tract infection, respiratory infection, dialysis access sepsis, dental abscess, peritonitis)

- o Cancer (exclusion criterion if recent, unless non-melanoma skin cancer)
- o Respiratory disease
- o Diabetes mellitus
- o Gastrointestinal disease
- o Liver disease (e.g. hepatitis, cirrhosis, cholecystitis)
- o Cerebrovascular and neurological disease
- Dialysis history
- Anesthetic history
- Blood transfusion history (especially note recent transfusions and ensure that the sample used for the cross-match has been taken at least 2 (preferably, 4) weeks after the last transfusion)
- Smoking, alcohol consumption
- Pregnancies
- Allergies
- Medication (concentrate on potential drugs that may interact with immunosuppressives; see Table 23.1)

The focus of the history must include recent events that have occurred since the patient was last assessed for the transplant waiting list. The intent of the medical history is to uncover those events that may threaten the safety of the patient during surgery and in the immediate postoperative period. The knowledge and understanding of the transplant procedure by the patient and their family must also be considered, to ensure that they are properly informed of the risks that they are undertaking. A social history will provide a guide to the postoperative family support that the patient will receive, and will ensure that problems which arise with work and domestic responsibilities are resolved or are at least resolvable.

Most transplant programs will have a standard *pro forma* used for acceptance for transplantation that will contain much of this information. This will be helpful, since admission for deceased donor transplantation is always a hurried affair. The anesthetist, surgeon, and nurse will be urging speed and may overturn the normal order of events — instead of moving smoothly from history through examination and investigation and then to therapy — investigation and medication may well precede history and examination, which in themselves may be concurrent and occur almost as the patient is wheeled out of the ward on the way to the operating theater. It is vital that each link is put into place, since mistakes occur when routine issues are overlooked, with potentially dreadful consequences to the patient.

Table 23.1 Examples of drug interactions with cyclosporine or tacrolimus.

Precautionary note: A detailed reference listing of drug interactions should be sourced whenever the prescription of a drug with potential interaction is being considered. All drugs which interact with the ABC transporter system or with the metabolism of drugs by the liver cytochrome P450 system must be checked before prescribing them to a patient using immunosuppressants.

Examples of drugs which increase cyclosporine and/or tacrolimus blood levels:
Antiretroviral agents
Azithromycin
Chloroquine
Clarithromycin
Clotrimazole
Dapsone
Diltiazem
Erythromycin
Fluconazole
Grapefruit juice
Itraconazole
Ketoconazole
Miconazole
Midazolam
Nicardipine
Nifedipine
Omeprazole

Examples of drugs which decrease cyclosporine and tacrolimus blood levels:
Antacids
Anticonvulsants (e.g. phenytoin, carbamazapine, phenobarbitone)
Dexamethasone
Rifampicin
St. John's wort

Examples of other significant drug interactions with cyclosporine and tacrolimus:
Aminoglycosides — enhance nephrotoxicity
Cisplatin — enhances nephrotoxicity
Sirolimus — alters absorption if co-administered, alters intracellular calcineurin inhibitor (CNI) concentrations

23.1.2 *Physical Examination*

- Cardiovascular system examination
- Respiratory system examination
- Abdominal examination

- Neurological examination (central/peripheral)
- Dialysis access examination (peritoneal or vascular, concentrating on infection risk).

The patient will be under considerable stress, especially if the transplant is from a deceased donor and is thus being performed in an atmosphere of urgency. The patient may have been on the waiting list for some years, and may thus lie about their current history to minimize and explain away their symptoms rather than miss the chance of the transplant. For example, "It was only a little bit of chest pain, I think I strained myself lifting something or I slept badly" may in fact be a classic description of unstable angina in the patient being assessed for a transplant! It is important to be aware of this problem and protect the patient from themselves and their anxiety to be suitable for transplantation, through proper examination and investigation.

23.1.3 *Pretransplant Investigation*

A variety of tests will have been performed in the transplant list workup and it is important to view these and have them available for the anesthetist and surgeon, such as an abdominal computed tomography (CT) scan, urodynamic studies, previous stress cardiac tests, or coronary angiography. The most important pretransplant investigations that must be undertaken immediately before surgery are those that are designed either to provide the basis for proceeding to a safe anesthetic or to serve as baselines for postoperative investigations.

23.1.3.1 *Tests Required for a Safe Anesthetic*

- Chest radiograph
- Respiratory function tests if appropriate (e.g. peak flow if asthmatic)
- ECG
- Electrolyte tests (especially potassium)
- Hematology tests (hemoglobin, white cell count, platelets)
- Coagulation tests if potentially anticoagulated.

23.1.3.2 *Tests Required for a Safe Transplant*

- ABO blood group test
- Human leukocyte antigen (HLA) typing (HLA-A, HLA-B, HLA-DR)

- Pretransplant antibody screening (e.g. panel-reactive antibody (PRA) and/or luminex antibody screening and specificity)
- Cross-match test against the donor lymphocytes (e.g. cytotoxicity cross-match, flow cytometry cross-match)

23.1.3.3 *Tests Required as Baselines for Postoperative Monitoring*

- Biochemistry tests (renal and liver function, calcium, phosphate)
- Infectious disease serology tests (HIV, hepatitis B and C, CMV, EBV, herpes varicella zoster, syphilis, plus tests for local/regional infectious risks)
- Pretransplant serum for storage (e.g. for confirmation of cross-match tests)
- Midstream urine test (if the patient still passes urine)
- Nasal and rectal swabs (to detect colonization with resistant organisms)

23.1.4 *Informed Consent*

A decision will be made in most transplant units about the general plan for immunosuppression, and it must be communicated to the recipient before their consent to the operation is signed (see Tables 23.2 and 23.3 for approaches to immunosuppression). Consent to undertake a surgical procedure has its own rules and rationales in all countries of the world, but only a limited number of operations carry lifelong risks from medication as a direct consequence of the procedure (e.g. cardiac valve replacement may carry an analogous risk with the need for lifelong anticoagulation). Informed consent for renal transplantation requires not only understanding of the planned immunosuppression, but also relevant information about donor factors that are known to impact on short- and long-term outcomes.

There is a strong and widely held view that it is inappropriate to address complex consent issues, such as the decision to proceed with an extended-criteria donor or one with a possible higher risk of disease transmission, at the time of a deceased donor transplantation. It is deemed to be more appropriate to have resolved those decisions at the time of wait listing, and thus the preoperative consent is merely a confirmation of previous decisions.

Table 23.2   Classification of patients based upon immunological risk.

Low risk	First transplant
	Nulliparous female
	Living related donor, and 3/6 HLA mismatch or better
	Low panel-reactive cytotoxic antibodies (<20%)
	Negative cross-match (T and B cells)
Medium risk	HLA mismatch
	Multiple transfusions
	Multiparous
	Poor HLA match
	Panel-reactive cytotoxic antibodies (between 20% and 80%)
High risk	High panel-reactive cytotoxic antibodies (>80%)
	Previous failed transplant (especially if rejected acutely)
	HLA mismatch (specific to known antibody or prior antigen mismatch)
	Positive cross-match

Notes: The presence of any one factor is sufficient to increase the patient to a higher risk level. HLA matching is usually defined at a broad allele level for HLA-A, HLA-B, and HLA-DR. Since each individual has two antigens at each locus, the total is scored out of 6. Since the relevant biological reaction is the recipient response to mismatched antigens carried on the graft, the HLA match result is expressed as the mismatch of donor antigens to recipient antigens (e.g. 3/6 HLA mismatch means that the graft carries 3 antigens that the recipient does not express).

23.1.5 *Is It Safe to Send the Patient to the Theater?*

If all is well with the preoperative assessment and informed consent, then there is no more to do as the patient now proceeds to the operating theater and this chapter will await their safe return. However, the patient may require action before it is safe to proceed. Dialysis or reversal of anticoagulation may be required, and decisions may need to be made about infection risks and the potential requirement for preoperative culture and antibiotics. The cardiac status may have changed since the waiting list evaluation and decision taken on suitability. In a well-managed unit, it is only very rarely that the transplant is called off at this point, but patients can change their minds and new events may intervene. The route to the operating theater must not be a foregone conclusion.

23.2 Investigations After Renal Transplantation

"The transplant patient is on their way back from the theater."

Transplant units around the world vary with respect to the location of immediate anesthetic recovery. An operating suite recovery room, an intensive care unit, a high dependency ward, and a well-staffed and well-equipped transplant isolation room in a transplant or renal ward are all appropriate, provided that there is sufficient equipment and that well-trained staff are instantly available. Those staff need to attend not only to the airways and oxygen saturation, but also to the blood pressure, venous filling pressure, pain control, fluid and electrolyte replacement, and immunosuppression. The most-needed tests are those that are directed towards assessment of the kidney and maintenance of its perfusion. The least important test is the standard assessment of recovery of wakefulness: "Hello Mrs X, can you hear me?" For this reason, most transplant units either send renal staff to the recovery room or train the intensive care or recovery room staff in transplant management. No matter where the patient is cared for, the prescription of fluid and replacement of electrolytes is an urgent priority.

23.2.1 *Immediate Assessment and Management*

23.2.1.1 *History of the Operation*

- Donor organ perfusion
- Number of renal arteries and veins anastomosed
- Post-revascularization perfusion of the kidney
- Urine production on the operating table
- Blood loss and fluid replacement volumes in the operating theater
- Duration of total cold and warm ischemia times
- Untoward surgical problems
- Anesthetic issues, including medications administered, peroperative blood pressures and central venous pressures, ventilation and oxygenation.

23.2.1.2 *Physical Examination*

- Vital signs (respiration, oxygen saturation, blood pressure, central venous pressure, pulse rate, temperature — all measured at least hourly)

- Hydration status (skin turgor, jugular venous pressure and filling, mucous membranes)
- Abdomen (distension, bowel sounds, wound bleeding, graft palpation, graft bruit, drains and drain fluid)
- Bladder catheter, urine volume measured hourly, urine color (blood staining or frank blood), urine biochemistry (Na^+, K^+ if volumes greater than 1 L/h)
- Chest and cardiovascular examination
- Neurological state, including pain control
- Skin pressure point protection.

23.2.1.3 *Investigations*

- Chest radiograph
- Blood biochemistry and hematology (monitor regularly)
- Duplex ultrasound of the renal blood flow (some units perform an ultrasound examination routinely early after return from the operating room; and others, only if there are problems)

There are three important rules in the immediate assessment of the patient:

The kidney will probably be as well perfused as the feet

So if the patient has cold and poorly perfused feet, then the kidney is likely to be similarly underperfused and the patient needs more intravascular volume using plasma substitutes or normal saline replacement.

If the patient has a fever, it will be due to rejection

Only when rejection is ruled out should one resort to the explanation that the fever is due to infection or an allergic response. Especially in the early postoperative period, fever due to infection is not common; however, when there is accelerated or hyperacute allograft response manifest in these first hours, it is often accompanied by fever and it is a bad diagnosis to miss.

Act now

Immediate action should be taken, especially if there is a lack of urine flow unless due to acute tubular necrosis (ATN), which is almost inevitable as a result of donor factors or recipient operative problems.

The greatest risk of graft loss is in the first few hours; more importantly, the majority of causes of graft loss at this time are reversible if diagnosed and treated early. The best diagnostic test is duplex ultrasound to examine blood flow and urinary obstruction, but if the renal vasculature is kinked or thrombosed there are only a few minutes available in which to rescue the graft. There is no substitute for immediately returning the patient to the operating theater if vascular compromise is suspected.

23.2.2 Problems Faced Immediately After Surgery

It is important to combine information from examination of the patient with regular measurement of standard parameters. Each transplant unit will have a protocol for measurement, based upon the availability of equipment and the nursing and medical resources available. Careful and regular assessment will identify problems quickly, permit diagnosis, and facilitate intervention.

23.2.2.1 No Urine Flow[a]

- Underperfused kidney due to low blood pressure, reduced intravascular blood volume, or cardiac failure
- Blocked catheter
- Blocked ureter
- Kinked/Thrombosed renal artery or renal vein
- Acute tubular necrosis
- Hyperacute rejection

23.2.2.2 Hypoxic/Low Blood Oxygen Saturation

- Airway obstruction
- Incomplete reversal of muscle paralysis
- Narcotization
- Hypoglycemic coma
- Monitor or probe dysfunction
- Fluid overload
- Aspiration pneumonia
- Pulmonary embolus
- Cardiac failure

---

[a] Think prerenal, renal, and postrenal.

23.2.2.3 *Hypotension*

- Reduced intravascular volume (bleeding)
- Postoperative vasodilation in an underfilled patient
- Gastrointestinal volume pooling associated with ileus
- Septic shock
- Myocardial ischemia/Myocardial infarction
- Pulmonary embolus
- Hyperacute rejection
- Anaphylactic reaction to medication

23.2.2.4 *Failure of Plasma Creatinine to Fall in the First 24 h Despite Urine Output*

- Acute tubular necrosis
- Hyperacute/Accelerated rejection
- Urinary leak and reabsorption of urine
- Partial ureteric obstruction
- Drug nephrotoxicity

23.2.2.5 *Electrolyte Disorders*

- Hyponatremia/Hypernatremia
- Hypokalemia/Hyperkalemia
- Hypocalcemia
- Hypoalbuminuria
- Hypoglycemia/Hyperglycemia

23.3 Prophylactic Immunosuppression

It is essential that every transplant program has a standard immuno-suppressive protocol. In the early 1990s, there was little in the way of viable alternative immunosuppression, but during the past 5 years it has become clear that there are many alternatives which deliver effective immunosuppression. It is possible to identify patients preoperatively who fall into one of three broad categories: low, standard, and high immunological risk (Table 23.2). Donor organs can be classified into two categories for the likelihood of immediate graft function: standard risk and high risk/marginal criteria/extended criteria. Using these two classifications, it is possible to draw up a protocol for selecting immunosuppression (Fig. 23.2).

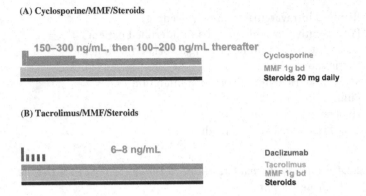

(A) Cyclosporine/MMF/Steroids

150–300 ng/mL, then 100–200 ng/mL thereafter

Cyclosporine
MMF 1g bd
Steroids 20 mg daily

(B) Tacrolimus/MMF/Steroids

6–8 ng/mL

Daclizumab
Tacrolimus
MMF 1g bd
Steroids

Fig. 23.2   Standard "low dose" target doses and levels, adapted from the Symphony study protocol.

The common combinations of drugs used for standard-risk patients are more variable now than 10 years ago, though a recent trial has demonstrated the superiority of low-dose tacrolimus, mycophenolate mofetil, and low-dose corticosteroids with an anti-IL2 receptor blocker induction agent providing the lowest rate of acute rejection and the least adverse events. Some regulatory authorities do not recognize this clinical reality, and cling to the view that cyclosporine should be substituted for tacrolimus in this standard triple therapy regimen. The cost of drugs is a very relevant factor in many parts of the world and financial pressures may lead individuals to make different decisions, since the drugs are relatively expensive in all parts of the world. The use of biological induction agents also varies from unit to unit and country to country. In the USA, for example, induction with antithymocyte globulin is almost standard practice; while it is reserved for high-immunological-risk patients in most other countries. The concept of triple therapy with or without an induction agent is, nevertheless, imbedded in most transplant programs. The use of three drugs allows synergy to be gained for immunosuppressive effect, while keeping the doses and thus adverse events of each agent to a minimum. The biology of graft rejection also determines that the highest-intensity immunosuppression is employed in the first weeks after transplantation, and that long-term maintenance doses can be much reduced.

Table 23.3 provides a guide to the selection of immunosuppression. The next sections describe each class of agent, with major

Table 23.3 General principles in the combination of immunosuppressive agents for renal transplantation.

Agent	Low risk	Standard risk	High risk	Initial non-function
Anti-IL2R antibody Antithymocyte antibody	+/−	+	+	+/−
Corticosteroids	+/−	+	+	
Cyclosporine Tacrolimus	+ or +	+ or +	+	+/− or +/−[b]
Azathioprine Mycophenolates	+ or +	+ or +	+	+
Sirolimus Everolimus	In place of CNI[a]	In place of CNI	−	−

Notes: One agent needs to be selected from each cell these treatments need to put into cells (five in total) to make sense of this comment.

+/− implies that the agent is not always used in that risk group.

[a] Most common therapies involve a calcineurin inhibitor (CNI), with cyclosporine being the lower-cost alternative to tacrolimus. Recent approaches to avoiding CNI therapy have involved the use of sirolimus or everolimus.

[b] CNI is often delayed until graft function is evident, using antithymocyte globulin (ATG) to provide early immunosuppression.

advantages and disadvantages of each serving as a quick reference guide. One must be familiar with the package insert information in each immunosuppressive agent, since the following descriptions are not a substitute for the carefully created detailed information contained with each drug.

23.3.1 *Anti-interleukin 2 (IL2) Receptor Antibodies*

"Induction" implies the use of an agent in the early posttransplant period to augment immunosuppressive potency at that time. The biological agents that can be used in this manner are either directed at whole human thymocytes (e.g. antithymocyte globulin, ATG) or at specific targets on the surface of functional T lymphocytes (e.g. CD3 T cells in the case of OKT3, or the IL2 receptor). There are two anti-IL2 receptor antibodies available on the market, with slightly different biological properties based upon differences in their molecular structure.

Basilixumab is a chimeric antibody produced from the combination of the variable region of a mouse monoclonal antibody and a human IgG constant region. Daclizumab, on the other hand, is a human antibody onto which have been grafted just the complementarity-determining region of a mouse monoclonal antibody directed at the IL2 receptor. This difference leads to a longer biological half-life for daclizumab, but both agents last for at least 1 month after the last dose.

Clinical research strategies for the two agents were also slightly different, with basilixumab used in two fixed doses at day 0 and day 4 posttransplant, while daclizumab was developed using a strategy of five two-weekly injections starting on day 0 and finishing at 8 weeks. The former strategy affords protection from rejection for up to 60 days; and the latter, for about 120 days.

There have been many trials of these agents and two meta-analyses, which clearly demonstrate their effectiveness in reducing acute rejection, graft loss, and patient loss. They are also distinguishable for being amongst the limited number of drugs that seem to have few, if any, adverse reactions. Since they are effective and have no adverse reactions associated with their use, the only reason not to use one of these agents is cost. The reality is that about 9 patients need to be treated to avoid one acute rejection episode and 45 to avoid one patient death, so 45 multiplied by the cost of treating one patient equals the value of a life!

23.3.2 Standard Triple Therapy

The standard combination of three drugs grew out of the late 1980s, when transplant programs were working out how to use cyclosporine. The first studies were done with cyclosporine as an additive to standard therapy, but this proved to be too immunosuppressive. It was then used alone or with steroids, and was effective but nephrotoxic, so a strategy was developed to combine the three agents available at that time — cyclosporine, azathioprine, and corticosteroids — but at lower doses. No formal clinical trials of this strategy were developed to prove the superiority of this approach, but through the 1990s this was universally adopted as standard practice. The development of tacrolimus as an alternative to cyclosporine, and the two mycophenolate agents (Mycophenolate mofetil and mycophenolate sodium) as alternatives to azathioprine, gave scope for improvement in results.

Each drug has adverse events associated with it, and the majority of adverse events are dose- and/or blood-level-related. The flexibility of the triple therapy regimens is that each drug can be dosed depending upon each individual's responses. It would be much easier to manage if there was a reliable measure of the level of immunosuppression, but this does not exist and in fact is in itself a delusion. The agents each impact on different parts of the immune cascade and are not really additive in any biological sense, since control of the T-cell response cannot be exercised without attention to control of B cells.

23.3.2.1 Corticosteroids

The majority of protocols include corticosteroids at doses of around 20 mg of prednisolone. Steroid-free regimens are being utilized for low-risk patients, but always in conjunction with high levels of induction antibody (such as ATG or alemtuzumab) in combination with tacrolimus and a mycophenolate. Some units use a high-dose (500–1000 mg) intravenous dose of methylprednisolone at the operation, and others do not. Steroid reduction to a baseline of 10 mg or 5 mg starts at a variable time after transplantation, depending upon the early course of the patient.

The side-effect profile of corticosteroids is too well known to detail here, but the characteristic Cushingoid facies and central obesity that were a universal feature of transplant recipients a decade ago have almost vanished due to lower dosing and steroid-avoidance strategies.

23.3.2.2 Calcineurin Inhibitors

The most effective advancement in renal transplantation was made in the mid-1980s with the introduction of cyclosporine (ciclosporin). Rejection rates dropped dramatically and graft survival rates immediately improved by 20% or more with its use. Further gradual improvements took the next 5 to 10 years, as units learned to manage the agent. It is very effective in controlling rejection and provides good levels of immunosuppression in a narrow therapeutic window. The mechanism of action is well known and involves reversible inhibition of the calcineurin pathway of T-cell activation.

The problem with both cyclosporine and tacrolimus is that they exhibit on-target and off-target toxicity. That is, overimmunosuppression is too easy to achieve and drug–drug interactions can lead to considerable changes in blood levels without dose changes. The second problem is toxicity, especially to the kidney (see Chapter 32), and allied problems with gout and hypertension (cyclosporine) or posttransplant diabetes (tacrolimus). Blood level measurement is essential for the safe prescription of both drugs, which cannot be used in fixed doses because of the high degree of individual variability and multiple drug interactions with both absorption and metabolism through the ATP-binding cassette (ABC) transporter system and cytochrome P450 metabolic pathway.

Both calcineurin inhibitors (CNIs) are used from the first day of transplantation in most patients. The starting doses vary, depending upon the transplant program and the use of concomitant medications. Intravenous preparations are available but little used because of their toxicity profiles. Drug interactions, such as that between diltiazem or ketoconazole and cyclosporine, may be used deliberately to reduce the costs of therapy by cutting the dose of cyclosporine substantially. The standard approach is to select a dose and measure trough levels each morning after transplantation, and thereafter adjusting the dose to achieve target levels. An example of standard-risk protocol target levels is shown in Fig. 23.2. The side effects of CNIs are outlined in Table 23.4. Those that are more prominent with cyclosporine include hypertension, gum hypertrophy, hypercholesterolemia, and gout; while the most prominent issues with tacrolimus are neurotoxicity in the short term and posttransplant diabetes in the

Table 23.4   Adverse event profiles of cyclosporine and tacrolimus.

Cyclosporine	Adverse event	Tacrolimus
+++	Nephrotoxicity	++
−	Neurotoxicity	++
−	Hallucination	++
+/−	Tremors	++
++	Gum hypertrophy	+/−
++	Hypertension	+
++	Hyperkalemia	+
+	Hyperuricemia/Gout	−
+	Posttransplant diabetes	++
+	Hyperlipidemia	+/−
−	Hair loss	+
++	Hypertrichosis	−
+/−	Arthralgia	−

long term. A list of the commonest drug interactions is provided in Table 23.1. It is important to consider carefully the introduction of any of these agents and to measure blood levels regularly in order to allow for dose adjustment.

23.3.2.3 Antiproliferatives

Azathioprine was first used in the early 1960s and only superceded in the late 1990s by mycophenolate mofetil and mycophenolate sodium. They both act to reduce proliferation through the inhibition of nucleotide synthesis. Azathioprine is much less expensive and thus still widely used globally, with well-known adverse impacts upon bone marrow synthesis requiring careful monitoring of white blood cell and platelet counts. There is one important drug interaction with allopurinol that interferes with the metabolism of the active compound 6-mercaptopurine, leading to dangerous overimmunosuppression.

Two mycophenolate molecules are available on the market, both being converted to the active agent mycophenolic acid. There are few differences between mycophenolate mofetil and mycophenolate sodium, though there is the suggestion that the latter has fewer gastrointestinal side effects. Both lead to increased cytomegalovirus (CMV) infection and there is a suspicion that, in conjunction with tacrolimus, they are responsible for the epidemic of BK virus nephropathy which has occurred in the last 10 years.

Blood level measurement is not routinely employed for either azathioprine or mycophenolates, despite suggestions that this would improve outcomes. Measurement of 6-mercaptopurine has proved technically difficult and the kinetics of the mycophenolates require at least an AUC (area under the curve) analysis, with multiple blood samples taken over 3 or 4 h.

23.3.3 Sirolimus/Everolimus

Sirolimus and everolimus represent a new class of agents, targeting the downstream pathway of the IL2 receptor and other growth factors through inhibition of the target of rapamycin (TOR). TOR inhibitors, sometimes also called proliferation signal inhibitors (TORis/PSIs), have profoundly different effects on CNIs and the antiproliferative agents (azathioprine and the two mycophenolates). Immunosuppressive potential is less than the CNIs when combined with myeophenolate mofetil, but they have been used to replace CNIs when graft function declines late after transplantation. The best place for these drugs is still to be defined, largely because of the adverse event profile. TOR inhibition affects many growth factors in addition to IL2, and early in the clinical trials was observed to impair wound healing through reduction in fibrogenesis. While this attribute would be desirable in long-term allografts where chronic fibrosis is a defining cause of progressive deterioration in graft function, it is a problem in the first weeks since it impairs wound healing. There are also complex and less-well-understood effects on glomerular podocytes as well as a number of tedious side effects such as mouth ulcers, acneiform rashes, and peripheral edema. There is also a synergistic impact on CNI nephrotoxicity when sirolimus and cyclosporine are combined, probably mediated through intracellular accumulation of cyclosporine in the presence of sirolimus. When either is combined with mycophenolates, there is a combined influence on the bone marrow that makes anemia a more common event. Blood levels are easily measured for both agents, with recommended levels of 4–8 ng/mL when used in combination with other immunosuppressants.

There are some major beneficial effects of these agents, such as the reduction in cancer risk and frank regression of Kaposi's sarcoma, when patients are converted to sirolimus or everolimus. Controlled trials have demonstrated that patients who tolerate the drugs in the long term do extremely well, with improving renal function.

The current conclusion is that these agents have a defined place in patients with cancer or higher-than-average skin cancer risk, and they are the standard care in patients with Kaposi's sarcoma. They can be used *de novo*, provided that the surgeon does not use absorbable sutures and keeps the skin clips in for at least 3 weeks. Lymphoceles are also more common, unless the surgeon pays particular attention to the ligation of cut lymphatics. Most use occurs later after transplantation with conversion from standard triple therapy at 3, 6, or 12 months, to avoid long-term CNIs. Indeed, conversion will probably be the long-term strategy that will provide the dominant use of these two drugs.

23.4 Highly Sensitized Recipients

Assessment of allosensitization has undergone a revolution in the past few years with the introduction of solid-phase assays of antibody specificity. Exposure of an individual to foreign HLAs leads to an immune response which may yield memory T cells and antibodies specific for the HLAs that they were exposed to. The main causes of sensitization are pregnancy, blood transfusion, and organ or cell transplantation, all of which share the feature that the patient is exposed intravenously to cells bearing foreign HLA molecules. Multiple exposures, and the environment in which the exposure occurs, determine the degree of alloimmune response. The majority of highly sensitized patients have received multiple blood transfusions without the protection of a white cell filter and/or have lost a previous renal transplant from acute rejection, although both of these factors are becoming uncommon and the number of highly sensitized patients is dropping on most transplant waiting lists. Patients who have suffered such exposure develop antibodies to many different HLA epitopes or to broad foreign HLAs or antigen groups, so they react to cells from many different potential donors. The panel-reactive antibody (PRA) level is a measure of the percentage of potential donors on a panel of different individuals to which they react in a standard complement-dependent cytotoxicity test. A highly sensitized patient is usually defined as one who reacts to >80% of the panel. It is very hard to find suitable donors for these patients — hence, the focus on allocating kidneys to such highly sensitized patients when there is a negative cross-match between the donor and recipient.

The situation has been made more confusing by the development of very sensitive solid-phase assays in which a single allele of a HLA molecule is attached to a bead, rather than relying upon donated lymphocytes which express at least two HLA-A, HLA-B, and HLA-DR molecules. This has yielded much new information, including a growing understanding of the role of donor-specific antibodies posttransplantation. The technique has, however, identified patients with low levels of antibodies to the HLAs of a potential donor, not apparent in the standard complement-dependent cytotoxicity test or even in the more sensitive flow cytometry test. Are these relevant and do they preclude transplantation? The answer is not clear, especially in the presence of today's powerful immunosuppression.

It is clear that transplantation of a patient who has become highly sensitized is a more challenging experience than if the patient is unsensitized. Assessment and determination of the therapeutic approach requires individualized approaches.

23.4.1 Assessment of the Sensitized Patient

- Sensitization history (blood transfusions, pregnancies, prior transplants)
- PRA levels in current and past serum samples
- Antibody specificity to HLAs
- Solid-phase assay of antibody (class I and class II screening assays)
- Solid-phase assay of antibody (class I and class II specificity)
- Cross-match between donor and recipient (peak sensitized and current serum samples)
- Complement-dependent cytotoxicity (T and B lymphocytes)
- Flow cytometry cross-match (T and B lymphocytes)
- Autologous cross-match to identify autoreactive antibodies.

23.4.2 Approaches to Transplantation of the Sensitized Patient

- Avoid HLAs to which the patient is sensitized.
- Avoid current serum-positive cross-match donors.
- Desensitize patients with an anti-CD20 monoclonal antibody, rituximab (50–375 g/m^2 in a single dose), and plasmaphoresis.
- Desensitize patients with intravenous pooled immunoglobulin.
- Use ATG induction therapy.
- Conduct posttransplant monitoring of donor-specific antibodies and plasmaphoresis.

23.5 Other Prophylactic Measures

Part of the success of transplantation has in fact come not from the increased safety of the immunosuppressants, but from the additional measures that are now routinely implemented to protect the recipient from the consequences of immunosuppression. Diseases that caused early mortality of transplant recipients in the 1970s and 1980s would continue to devastate the results were it not for prophylaxis against infection. It is thus routine for patients to leave the hospital taking at least eight different drugs in complicated schedules that alter on a daily basis. Education and systems such as individualized weekly dosette boxes, which contain a full week's medications laid out for each time point, are essential if patients are to take these critical medications reliably.

23.5.1 Prophylaxis for Pneumocystis Pneumonia

Pneumocystis pneumonia (PCP) used to cause severe disease about 3 months after transplantation in a significant proportion of immunosuppressed patients. Now called *Pneumocystis jirovecii,* the agent causes a characteristic syndrome including nonproductive cough, dyspnea, significant oxygen desaturation, and a "white-out" on chest X-ray. It is rarely seen now because of the effectiveness of co-trimoxazole prophylaxis. A single daily dose (480 mg) is sufficient to prevent disease and most units continue therapy to 6 or 12 months after transplantation. Daily dapsone (50–100 mg/day) and/or trimethoprim (25–50 mg twice weekly) is an alternative for the patient allergic to sulphonamides. An additional benefit of co-trimoxazole is that it also halves the rate of urinary tract infection.

23.5.2 *Prophylaxis for Cytomegalovirus*

Cytomegalovirus (CMV) is a common pathogen that most people encounter before the age of 20 years. The majority of recipients are thus immunized against CMV and the majority of donors carry the virus. Transplants can be divided into four groups based upon the donor and recipient CMV status: D+R+, D–R+, D–,R–, and D+R–. Of these, the first is the commonest situation, while the last provides the most serious risk for disease transmission. CMV can also be transmitted through blood transfusion, and so consideration should be given to using CMV-negative blood donations for patients who are D–R–.

Prophylaxis against infection is standard practice in most units for the first 3 to 6 months in all patients except D–R–, using valganciclovir, ganciclovir, or valacyclovir in appropriate doses for renal function. An alternative strategy is to monitor the development of CMV infection and treat it pre-emptively when CMV appears in the blood, but the cost is about the same as blanket prophylaxis. Patients at the greatest risk of serious disease are those treated with ATG or OKT3.

23.5.3 *Prophylaxis for Mycobacterium Tuberculosis*

Tuberculosis is a common problem in patients who have lived in endemic areas before transplantation. The approach to treatment/prophylaxis varies, depending upon the geographic area and drug availability. In developed countries, the tendency is to use isoniazid (300 mg/day) for 6 to 12 months with liver enzymes monitored regularly; while units in endemic areas often use a full treatment course of triple therapy, despite the problems that arise from drug interactions with cyclosporine and tacrolimus.

23.5.4 *Prophylaxis for Gastrointestinal Disease*

Patients at risk of transmission of hepatitis B should have been vaccinated prior to transplantation (see Chapter 20). For hepatitis B carriers, the use of lamivudine should be continued for at least 12 months. Peptic ulceration was a considerable problem in the early days of transplantation because of high steroid doses and lack of good medical therapy; it is now uncommon with most patients being given proton pump inhibitors while on corticosteroids. Oral and esophageal candidiasis can be prevented by the use of regular oral nystatin (500 000 units qid) or amphotericin lozenges during the early period of maximal immunosuppression.

23.5.5 *Prophylaxis for Cardiovascular Disease*

The biggest problem in the medium-to-long term for almost all transplant recipients is excessive weight gain as a result of corticosteroid use, unrestricted diet, and poor exercise regimen. It is important to commence education as early as possible, even though many are malnourished at the time of transplantation. Many dialysis patients will have been able to manage blood pressure through fluid balance management, but after transplantation 80% will become hypertensive and require therapy. The choice of primary agent varies, with many units avoiding angiotensin-converting enzyme (ACE) inhibitors and angiotensin II receptor blockers in the early weeks, but using them preferentially in the medium and long term. Beta blockers and calcium channel antagonists are often the agents of choice in the early days. Finally, there are relatively few patients who avoid hyperlipidemia, especially with the use of agents that increase cholesterol levels (cyclosporine and TOR inhibitors); thus, the use of statins has become routine.

23.6 Checklist When Discharging the Patient from the Ward

- Completed posttransplant education, especially about medication
- All medication provided:
  - o Immunosuppression
  - o Prophylaxis for infection
  - o Prophylaxis for gastrointestinal disease
  - o Prophylaxis for cardiovascular disease

- Summary of transplant surgery and early posttransplant course

- Follow-up plans clearly communicated
- Reminder that patients can write anonymously to the family of deceased donors to convey their gratitude for the new life that they have ahead of them.

Suggested Reading

Allison AC, Eugui EM. (2000) Mycophenolate mofetil and its mechanisms of action. *Immunopharmacology* 47:85–118.

Ekberg H, Tedesco-Silva H, Demirbas A, *et al.*; ELITE-Symphony Study. (2007) Reduced exposure to calcineurin inhibitors in renal transplantation. *N Engl J Med* 357:2562–2575.

Gallagher MP, Hall B, Craig J, *et al.*; Australian Multicenter Trial of Cyclosporine Withdrawal Study Group and the ANZ Dialysis and Transplantation Registry. (2004) A randomized controlled trial of cyclosporine withdrawal in renal-transplant recipients: 15-year results. *Transplantation* 78:1653–1660.

Kasiske B, Cosio FG, Beto J, *et al.* (2004) Clinical practice guidelines for managing dyslipidemias in kidney transplant patients: a report from the Managing Dyslipidemias in Chronic Kidney Disease Work Group of the National Kidney Foundation Kidney Disease Outcomes Quality Initiative. *Am J Transplant* 4(Suppl 7):13–53.

Kasiske BL, Vazquez MA, Harmon WE, *et al.* (2000) Recommendations for the outpatient surveillance of renal transplant recipients. American Society of Transplantation. *J Am Soc Nephrol* 11(Suppl 15):S1–S86.

Mathew TH. (1998) A blinded, long-term, randomized multicenter study of mycophenolate mofetil in cadaveric renal transplantation: results at three years. Tricontinental Mycophenolate Mofetil Renal Transplantation Study Group. *Transplantation* 65:1450–1454.

Mota A, Arias M, Taskinen EI, *et al.*; Rapamune Maintenance Regimen Trial. (2004) Sirolimus-based therapy following early cyclosporine withdrawal provides significantly improved renal histology and function at 3 years. *Am J Transplant* 4:953–961.

Nankivell BJ, Borrows RJ, Fung CL, *et al.* (2003) The natural history of chronic allograft nephropathy. *N Engl J Med* 349:2326–2333.

Vitko S, Margreiter R, Weimar W, *et al.* (2005) Three-year efficacy and safety results from a study of everolimus versus mycophenolate mofetil in *de novo* renal transplant patients. *Am J Transplant* 5:2521–2530.

24

Prophylaxis, Monitoring, and Preemptive Therapy for Potential Complications After Renal Transplantation

Sing-Leung Lui

24.1 Prophylaxis Against Peptic Ulceration

Peptic ulcer disease used to be a common and potentially fatal complication after renal transplantation. Risk factors for posttransplant peptic ulcer disease include:

- past history of peptic ulcer disease
- use of high doses of corticosteroids
- cigarette smoking
- concomitant use of ulcerogenic agents such as aspirin or non-steroidal anti-inflammatory drugs (NSAIDs).

In recent years, because of the widespread use of H_2-receptor antagonists and proton pump inhibitors, the incidence of peptic ulcer disease and peptic ulcer-related complications (such as gastrointestinal bleeding and gastric perforation) has declined substantially. It is now a common practice in most renal transplant centers to prescribe prophylactic H_2-receptor antagonists or proton pump inhibitors to all renal transplant recipients for the first 6 months after transplantation.

24.2 Prophylaxis and Treatment of Tuberculosis

Posttransplant tuberculosis (TB) is an important infective complication of renal transplantation, and is associated with significant mortality and morbidity. The prevalence of TB among renal transplant recipients varies from less than 1% in Western countries to 5% in the Middle East to nearly 15% in the Indian subcontinent. The majority of posttransplant TB cases are due to reactivation of latent foci of *Mycobacterium tuberculosis*. Extrapulmonary and disseminated TB is more common among renal transplant patients than in the general population. The initial presentation of posttransplant TB is usually nonspecific, and atypical presentations are not uncommon. A high index of suspicion is therefore needed to ensure early diagnosis and prompt the initiation of anti-TB treatment.

Prophylactic anti-TB treatment is indicated in renal transplant patients who have:

- past history of tuberculosis
- radiological evidence of old pulmonary tuberculosis
- close contact history with infectious patients
- positive tuberculin skin test (in nonendemic areas).

The usual prophylactic regimen is isoniazid 300 mg daily for 9–12 months.

The European Best Practice Guidelines recommend treating renal transplant recipients with active TB in the same way as in the general population — i.e. quadruple therapy with isoniazid, rifampicin, pyrazinamide, and ethambutol for the first 2 months, followed by isoniazid and rifampicin double therapy for 4 months. The usual dosages of the commonly used anti-TB drugs are listed in Table 24.1. Ethambutol can be omitted if the resistance rate to isoniazid in the community is low (<4%). Other authorities, however, advocate extending the total duration of anti-TB treatment in renal transplant recipients to 9–12 months.

Anti-TB treatment in renal transplant patients is associated with two special issues. This first issue is potential drug interactions between anti-TB drugs and concurrent immunosuppressive medications. Rifampicin is a potent inducer of the cytochrome P450 3A enzymes, which are involved in the metabolism of calcineurin inhibitors (cyclosporine and tacrolimus) and rapamycin. Co-administration of rifampicin with these immunosuppressive drugs will increase their clearance and lead to a significant reduction in their serum levels, which in turn may predispose the patient to the occurrence of acute allograft rejection. Appropriate dosage adjustment of the immunosuppressive drugs and close therapeutic drug monitoring, especially during the initiation and immediately after the cessation of anti-TB treatment, are warranted.

Table 24.1   Usual dosage of anti-TB drugs.

Drug	Dosage
Isoniazid	300 mg daily
Rifampicin	450 mg daily (BW < 50 kg)
	600 mg daily (BW ≥ 50 kg)
Pyrazinamide	1.5 g daily (BW < 50 kg)
	2.0 g daily (BW ≥ 50 kg)
Ethambutol	15 mg/kg daily

BW: Body weight.

The second issue relates to the increased risk of drug-induced hepatotoxicity (usually due to isoniazid) during anti-TB treatment in renal transplant patients. Transient and mild elevation of alanine aminotransferase (ALT) or aspartate aminotransferase (AST) is commonly observed during anti-TB treatment in renal transplant patients. However, if the serum levels of ALT or AST rise to more than three times the upper limits of normal, discontinuation of isoniazid needs to be considered. The risk of isoniazid hepatotoxicity is enhanced by chronic alcohol consumption, hepatitis B carrier status, and concomitant use of rifampicin.

24.3 Prophylaxis and Treatment of Candidiasis

Candida species are the most common pathogens causing fungal infection after renal transplantation. The clinical manifestations of *Candida* infection range from mucocutaneous candidiasis and urinary tract infection to disseminated candidiasis. Risk factors for the development of *Candida* infections in renal transplant recipients include:

- increasing age
- prolonged use of antibiotics
- diabetes mellitus
- heavy immunosuppression
- long duration of dialysis before the transplantation.

Oral and esophageal candidiasis can be prevented by regular use of oral nystatin solution (500 000 units) every 6 h for the first 3 months posttransplantation. Unlike patients with liver or lung transplants, routine use of prophylactic antifungal drugs in renal transplant recipients is not justified.

Amphotericin B is the mainstay treatment for patients with invasive candidiasis. The usual dosage regimen is 0.5–1 mg/kg body weight by slow intravenous infusion once daily for 14 to 21 days. Appropriate reduction in the level of immunosuppression is an important adjunct to the amphotericin B therapy. Nephrotoxicity is the main adverse effect of amphotericin B in renal transplant patients, particularly among those taking calcineurin inhibitors. For those patients who are unable to tolerate the conventional amphotericin B or who have developed significant nephrotoxicities, the liposomal formulation of amphotericin B can serve as a useful alternative. Infections caused by *Candida albicans* can also be treated with oral fluconazole (400 mg on the first day, followed by 200 mg daily). *Candida* species other than *Candida albicans* are usually fluconazole-resistant and have to be treated with amphotericin B. The use of newer antifungal agents such as caspofungin and voriconazole in the treatment of posttransplant *Candida* infection remains to be established.

24.4 Prophylaxis and Treatment of Pneumocystis Pneumonia

Pneumocystis pneumonia (PCP) is a serious opportunistic infection after renal transplantation and can cause fatality within a short time after disease onset. The risk of developing PCP is highest within the first 3–6 months after transplantation and after intensification of immunosuppression, as in the case of pulse steroid therapy for acute rejection.

Because of the serious nature of PCP, all renal transplant recipients should receive prophylaxis against *Pneumocystis jirovecii* (formerly known as *Pneumocystis carinii*). The usual prophylactic regimen consists of low-dose oral co-trimoxazole (trimethoprim-sulfamethoxazole), 480 mg daily for the first 6 months after renal transplantation. Patients who have been treated with pulse methylprednisolone or lymphocyte-depleting antibodies should be given co-trimoxazole prophylaxis for 3 months. Patients who are allergic to co-trimoxazole or G6PD-deficient can be treated with pentamidine inhalation (300 mg once every month) for 6 months instead.

The cardinal features of PCP in renal transplant recipients include:

- fever
- nonproductive cough

- shortness of breath
- profound hypoxemia with a relative lack of abnormal physical signs.

Chest X-ray typically shows a bilateral diffuse ground-glass appearance, although it can appear normal. The clinical condition of patients with PCP can deteriorate rapidly. The diagnosis can be established by demonstrating the presence of *Pneumocystis jirovecii* in the bronchoalveolar lavage using fluorescein-labeled monoclonal antibody staining. Early diagnosis and prompt initiation of treatment are crucial to the successful eradication of the infection. Treatment of PCP entails the use of high-dose co-trimoxazole (trimethoprim-sulfamethoxazole), 120 mg/kg body weight daily to be given in 2–4 divided doses for 14 days. Co-trimoxazole should be given intravenously in patients who have severe disease with marked hypoxemia; milder disease can be treated with oral co-trimoxazole. The major side effects of co-trimoxazole therapy are nephrotoxicity and myelosuppression.

24.5 Monitoring and Preemptive Therapy for Cytomegalovirus Disease

Cytomegalovirus (CMV) infection is the most common infective complication after renal transplantation. The risk of developing CMV infection is highest during the first 4–6 months posttransplantation if anti-CMV prophylaxis has not been administered. Renal transplant recipients who are CMV-seronegative are particularly at risk of developing CMV infection if they receive allografts from CMV-seropositive donors. They are also more prone to develop tissue-invasive CMV disease, recurrent CMV disease, and ganciclovir-resistant CMV infection. The CMV serostatus of both the donor and the recipient should therefore be determined before or at the time of transplantation to identify susceptible patients who might benefit from preventive measures. Patients who have been treated with increased immunosuppression, especially lymphocyte-depleting antibodies, are also at increased risk of CMV infection.

Active CMV infection (as evidenced by elevated CMV pp65 antigen levels) can be asymptomatic. Alternatively, patients with active CMV infection might present with fever, malaise, leucopenia, and thrombocytopenia. Tissue-invasive CMV disease, on the other hand, can manifest as pneumonitis, colitis, enteritis, hepatitis, or retinitis.

Table 24.2 Dosage adjustment for ganciclovir in patients with renal impairment.

CrCl	Dosage
≥70 mL/min	5.0 mg/kg every 12 h
50–69 mL/min	2.5 mg/kg every 12 h
25–49 mL/min	2.5 mg/kg every 24 h
10–24 mL/min	1.25 mg/kg every 24 h
<10 mL/min	1.25 mg/kg 3 times/week after hemodialysis

CrCl: creatinine clearance.

CMV disease might also cause direct allograft dysfunction and increase the risk of acute rejection.

Patients with active CMV disease should be treated with ganciclovir, given as an intravenous infusion over 1 hour at a dosage of 5 mg/kg body weight every 12 h. The dosage of ganciclovir should be adjusted in patients with impaired renal function (Table 24.2). Reduction of immunosuppression should be considered, especially in patients with severe disease manifestations. The duration of ganciclovir treatment should be at least 14–21 days or longer until the CMV viremia disappears. Development of ganciclovir-resistant CMV disease should be suspected if the patients remain symptomatic or have persistent viremia after 2 weeks of ganciclovir therapy. Ganciclovir-resistant CMV disease can be treated with newer antiviral agents such as foscarnet or cidofovir; however, these two drugs should be used with caution in patients with renal insufficiency as both drugs are potentially nephrotoxic.

All CMV-seronegative recipients of kidney allografts from CMV-seropositive donors should receive prophylactic anti-CMV treatment starting at the time of the transplantation. They can be treated with either:

- oral ganciclovir (1 g three times daily);
- valganciclovir, a prodrug of ganciclovir (900 mg once daily); or
- intravenous infusion of ganciclovir (5 mg/kg body weight once daily for 2 weeks), followed by oral valganciclovir (900 mg daily).

The total duration of prophylaxis should be at least 12 weeks.

All other renal transplant recipients should be monitored closely for the development of CMV viremia during the first 4 months after the transplantation. The CMV pp65 antigenemia assay is commonly employed to detect CMV viremia. Other methods of CMV viremia detection include CMV polymerase chain reaction (PCR) and hybrid capture DNA. Typically, the CMV antigenemia assay is performed weekly for the first 8 weeks posttransplantation and then fortnightly for another 8 weeks. The CMV pp65 antigenemia assay should also be performed weekly for 8 weeks in patients who have received lymphocyte-depleting antibodies or pulse steroid therapy. Patients with an increasing number of CMV pp65 antigen-positive leukocytes should be treated with intravenous ganciclovir, 5 mg/kg body weight once daily, until the CMV pp65 antigenemia test turns negative (preemptive therapy).

An alternative to the preemptive approach to prevent CMV disease in renal transplant recipients is to give all transplant recipients prophylactic oral ganciclovir (1 g three times daily) or valganciclovir (900 mg daily) during the first 3 months posttransplantation — e.g. universal prophylaxis. The choice of preemptive therapy versus universal prophylaxis is a matter of institutional preference.

Suggested Reading

EBPG Expert Group on Renal Transplantation. (2002) European best practice guidelines for renal transplantation. Section IV: long-term management of the transplant recipient. IV.7. Late infections. *Nephrol Dial Transplant* 17(Suppl 4):36–43.

Fishman JA. (2007) Infection in renal transplant recipients. *Semin Nephrol* 27:445–461.

John GT, Shankar V. (2002) Mycobacterial infections in organ transplant recipients. *Semin Respir Infect* 17:274–283.

Kotton CN, Fishman JA. (2005) Viral infection in the renal transplant recipient. *J Am Soc Nephrol* 16:1758–1774.

Ponticelli C, Passerini P. (2005) Gastrointestinal complications in renal transplant recipients. *Transpl Int* 18:643–650.

Silveira FP, Husain S. (2007) Fungal infections in solid organ transplantation. *Med Mycol* 45:305–320.

Singh N. (2003) Fungal infections in the recipients of solid organ transplantation. *Infect Dis Clin North Am* 17:113–134.

Weikert BC, Blumberg EA. (2008) Viral infection after renal transplantation: surveillance and management. *Clin J Am Soc Nephrol* 3:S76–S86.

25

Medical Complications After Renal Transplantation

Daniel T. M. Chan

This chapter discusses the management of common medical complications after kidney transplantation. The importance of prevention and early detection cannot be overemphasized. In this regard, many of the complications are potentially preventable by judicious choice of optimal immunosuppressive regimens, taking into consideration the characteristics of patients and their risk profiles.

25.1 Acute Rejection

This usually presents with an increase in serum creatinine by 10% or more over 1–2 days. Graft tenderness, reduced urine output, and/or fever is only present in severe cases. Other causes of renal allograft dysfunction need to be excluded, such as obstructive uropathy, renal vascular complications, and nephrotoxicity due to calcineurin inhibitor (CNI) or other agents. The incidence of acute rejection in patients treated with triple immunosuppression comprising corticosteroid, tacrolimus, and mycophenolate mofetil is approximately 8%–15%. Diagnosis of rejection should be confirmed with graft biopsy, which should be reported in a standardized format according to the Banff classification. Histological features of acute rejection include tubulointerstitial lymphocyte infiltration, endarteritis, glomerulitis, fibrinoid necrosis of the arterial wall, and in severe cases hemorrhage. Hyperacute and accelerated acute rejection are due to preformed antibodies against donor antigens. Humoral rejection is characterized by positive C4d immunohistochemical staining in the allograft biopsy. Assay for donor-specific antibodies is indicated in C4d-positive rejections. Cell- and antibody-mediated alloimmune responses are not mutually exclusive, but often coexist in variable predominance.

Treatment for an acute rejection episode takes into consideration the histological findings on allograft biopsy, the time from transplantation, the prevailing immunosuppressive regimen, history of sensitization, and prior induction therapy, and includes the following options alone or in combination:

- Pulse methylprednisolone 0.5–1 g daily intravenously for 3 days
- Increase in maintenance immunosuppression with or without a change in immunosuppressive medications
- Anti-lymphocyte treatment — e.g. antithymocyte globulin for 10–14 days or monoclonal anti-CD3 antibody (OKT3) for 7–10 days. Premedication with methylprednisolone and antihistamine as well as close monitoring is required especially after the initial doses because of the cytokine release syndrome, which can present with fever, chills and rigor, hypotension, diarrhea, and dyspnea. Avoidance of fluid overload reduces the risk of pulmonary edema.
- Plasmapheresis and/or intravenous gamma globulin — for antibody-mediated rejection
- Anti-CD20 — as adjunctive therapy (single dose, 50–375 mg/m^2) for T-cell-poor C4d-positive antibody-mediated rejection or B-cell-rich C4d-negative cellular rejection

25.2 Infective Complications

25.2.1 *Cytomegalovirus (CMV) Disease*

Primary CMV infection occurs in CMV-seronegative subjects who receive kidneys from CMV-seropositive donors, and the incidence of CMV disease is over 80% under these circumstances. It is thus obligatory to determine the CMV antibody status of the potential kidney transplant recipient and donor prior to transplantation. CMV disease can also occur in kidney recipients who are CMV-seropositive prior to transplantation, consequent to reactivation of viral replication or superinfection by another viral strain. Clinical manifestations of CMV disease include fever, leukopenia, thrombocytopenia, elevated transaminase levels, and pneumonitis. CMV retinitis, typically found in patients with AIDS, is relatively uncommon in kidney transplant recipients. Most CMV disease occurs within 6 months after transplantation or high-dose immunosuppressive therapy. Biologic therapy targeting T lymphocytes and high-dose mycophenolate mofetil treatment increase the risk of CMV disease.

25.2.1.1 *Practical Points*

- A CMV-seronegative subject who receives a kidney from a CMV-seropositive or CMV non-typed donor should receive prophylactic treatment for at least 3 months.
- CMV-seropositive recipients who have received anti-T-cell antibody treatment can be considered to receive prophylactic treatment for 3 months.
- All patients should have surveillance for the early detection of CMV disease after transplantation. This includes monitoring the level of pp65 antigenemia for at least 3 months and when clinically indicated. In subjects who are CMV-seronegative at transplantation, serial serologic testing is indicated to detect seroconversion. The pp65 antigenemia assay can also be used to monitor the efficacy of antiviral treatment.
- Pre-emptive treatment should be considered in asymptomatic patients with CMV pp65 antigenemia and a recent history of pulse steroid or anti-T lymphocyte therapy.

25.2.1.2 *Prophylactic Treatment*

- Hyperimmune globulin, duration 6–16 weeks (dosing regimen varies according to preparation) — need to monitor for the development of anaphylaxis, and should be avoided in patients with IgA deficiency.
- Ganciclovir i.v. 5 mg/kg q12h
- Ganciclovir p.o. 1 g tid
- Valganciclovir p.o. 900 mg daily

Dose adjustment according to renal function is applicable to both ganciclovir and valganciclovir.

25.2.1.3 *Treatment Options*

- Ganciclovir i.v. 5 mg/kg q12h for at least 14 days
- Ganciclovir i.v. for at least 5 days, followed by p.o. 1 g tid for 2 weeks or longer

- Foscarnet i.v. 60 mg/kg q8h for 2–3 weeks to be considered in patients with ganciclovir-resistant CMV — dose adjustment required in patients with impaired renal function; hydration is essential to minimize nephrotoxicity; also need to watch out for complications such as hypocalcemia, hypomagnesemia, hypokalemia, anemia, marrow suppression, and penile ulceration.

25.2.2 *Pneumocystis jirovecii Pneumonia*

Pneumocystis pneumonia occurs mostly within the first 6 months of renal transplantation or after increase of immunosuppression (such as for the treatment of acute rejection). The incidence is over 10% in the absence of prophylaxis, and is associated with considerable mortality. Characteristic manifestations include hypoxia, dyspnea, and dry cough, with relatively minor auscultatory signs. Increase in circulating lactic dehydrogenase levels is nonspecific. Chest radiograph can show bilateral perihilar airspace abnormalities or scattered patchy interstitial ground-glass opacities, but radiographic abnormalities can be subtle. High-resolution computed tomograpy (CT) scan, which shows areas of ground-glass attenuation with a background of interlobular septal thickening in a patchy or nodular distribution, increases the sensitivity of diagnosis. Differential diagnoses include other causes of interstitial pneumonitis, such as CMV pneumonia or rapamycin-associated pneumonitis. The diagnostic yield with bronchoalveolar lavage is over 90%.

Prophylaxis is essential and highly effective. Patients with normal glucose-6-phosphate dehydrogenase (G6PD) status can be given trimethoprim-sulfamethoxazole (80 mg and 400 mg, respectively) daily for 6 months. Aerosolized pentamidine, 300 mg monthly, can be given to patients with G6PD deficiency or who are intolerant to trimethoprim-sulfamethoxazole. Treatment of pneumocystis pneumonia is with intravenous trimethoprim 15–20 mg/kg/day and sulfamethoxazole 75–100 mg/kg/day divided into three or four doses. Other potential treatment options include intravenous pentamidine, atovaquone, clindamycin, and dapsone with trimethoprim.

25.2.3 *Viral Hepatitis B and C*

25.2.3.1 *Points to Note in the Management of Viral Hepatitis B or C in Kidney Transplant Recipients*

- Matching of donor and recipient status for hepatitis B or C is essential to prevent transmission through the transplanted organ.

Potential kidney recipients who are seronegative for both HBsAg and anti-HBs should receive hepatitis B vaccination, the latter at double-dose when the renal failure is moderate to severe (also refer to Chapter 20).

- Pretransplant liver biopsy is advisable in patients with clinical suspicion of cirrhosis. Combined liver and kidney transplantation is an option for selected patients.
- Quantitative assays of serum HBV DNA or HCV RNA are helpful tools to detect impending flares of liver disease.
- Increase in viral replication usually precedes biochemical flares. Flares can occur very rapidly in immunosuppressed individuals.
- Manifestations of liver disease related to hepatitis B or C in kidney transplant recipients can take the form of fulminating hepatitis, fibrosing cholestatic hepatitis, chronic active hepatitis, or progressive cirrhosis.
- Treatment with conventional interferon has been associated with deterioration of allograft function and graft loss. Preliminary data suggest that pegylated interferon might be better tolerated, but this awaits confirmation with more extensive experience. The use of interferon preparations demands cautious consideration of its potential risk and benefit. Significant hemolytic anemia may result from the combined use with ribavirin.
- Surveillance for hepatocellular carcinoma with regular alpha fetal protein assay and liver ultrasonogram, as well as attention to complications of cirrhosis or portal hypertension, should be part of the long-term management of kidney allograft recipients infected with hepatitis B or C.

25.2.3.2 *Specific Points in the Management of Hepatitis B in Kidney Transplant Recipients*

- Although HBeAg seropositivity has been associated with unfavorable liver outcome in organ transplant recipients, HBeAg status is not a reliable predictor of the clinical course at the level of individuals.
- For HBsAg-positive kidney transplant recipients, management in the early posttransplant period entails the use of antiviral nucleoside/nucleotide analog treatment either prophylactically or pre-emptively. The latter is coupled with monitoring of the circulating HBV DNA level, with 1.0×10^5 copies/mL (0.4 pg/mL) usually taken as the threshold for treatment.

- Both lamivudine and telbivudine can be used as first-line antiviral treatment of hepatitis B in kidney transplant recipients, although lamivudine is not preferred in view of the associated high incidence of drug resistance, due to the selection of YMDD variants with prolonged treatment.
- Lamivudine resistance can be managed by add-on adefovir, substitution with entecavir, or substitution with tenofovir. More data are awaited on the relative efficacy of these approaches.
- The optimal duration of antiviral treatment for hepatitis B in kidney transplant recipients is controversial. The risk of selecting drug-resistant viral variants needs to be taken into consideration. Attempts to discontinue treatment probably should be deferred until the treatment has been given for at least 9 months, and when viral replication has been satisfactorily suppressed for at least 3 months. The serum HBV DNA level must be monitored frequently after stopping treatment, since rebound occurs in around half of these patients.

25.2.4 *Polyoma BK Virus Disease*

Polyoma BK virus is a DNA virus that is ubiquitous in the adult population. Primary infection is asymptomatic. Immunosuppression predisposes towards viral reactivation, and the incidence of reactivation and the risk of BK virus nephropathy vary according to the degree of immunosuppression. The incidence of significant BK virus infection has increased following the combined use of tacrolimus, mycophenolate mofetil, and corticosteroid — coupled with antibody induction — in kidney transplantation.

Clinical manifestations of BK virus infection include viruria, viremia, ureteric stenosis, hemorrhagic cystitis, and BK virus nephropathy which is associated with a high incidence of graft loss. Viral reactivation is evident from the detection of urinary decoy cells, which are uroepithelial cells with enlarged nuclei and basophilic ground-glass intranuclear inclusions, and viruria. Since BK viremia portends adverse clinical outcomes, quantitation of BK viremia is a useful diagnostic tool, and a level above 10 000 copies/mL has been proposed as presumptive of BK virus nephropathy. Definitive diagnosis depends on the demonstration of cytopathic changes in the renal tubular epithelium of the graft biopsy, often accompanied by focal tubular cell injury and necrosis. In patients subjected to potent immunosuppression, periodic screening for urinary decoy cells (e.g. every 3 months for the first 2 years, then less frequently) is advisable. Positive results should be followed by viremia quantitation and graft biopsy, if necessary.

Reduction of immunosuppression is central in the management of BK virus disease. Replacement of mycophenolate mofetil with leflunomide — 100 mg/day for 3–5 days followed by 20–60 mg daily to aim for trough levels of 50–100 µg/mL — has been associated with a favorable outcome. Treatment with cidofovir — 0.25–1 mg/kg given every 2 weeks for four or more doses — may also be considered, but attention to its nephrotoxic effect is warranted. Intravenous immunoglobulin — 0.5–2 g/kg for 5–7 days — may be considered in patients with concomitant acute rejection. Pre-emptive reduction of immunosuppression is advisable in patients with persistent viremia. Viremia load should be monitored every 2 weeks during treatment.

25.2.5 *Varicella Zoster Virus Infection, Tuberculosis, and Candidiasis*

Herpes zoster affects up to 10% of kidney transplant recipients, mostly within the first year after transplantation. Most patients present with dermatomal disease, but disseminated or visceral disease can occur. The majority of adults have prior exposure to the virus and the disease is due to reactivation of latent infection. Vaccination is recommended in nonimmune subjects prior to transplantation, since primary infection after transplantation has been associated with increased mortality. Acyclovir or valacyclovir provides effective treatment.

Prophylaxis with isoniazid 300 mg daily for 1 year appears effective and well tolerated in kidney transplant recipients who have a history or radiological features of previous tuberculosis. Many of the drugs used in the treatment of tuberculosis alter the metabolism of CNIs (see Chapter 33). It is thus important to monitor their blood levels, and adjust the doses in anticipation of the forthcoming changes.

Oral or esophageal candidiasis usually occurs within the first 3–4 months after kidney transplantation. Nystatin syrup 500 000 U q.i.d. can be given as prophylaxis for 3 months.

25.3 Chronic Renal Allograft Dysfunction

There is a strong relationship between acute rejection and long-term kidney allograft survival. However, while the incidence of acute rejection has decreased considerably with advancements in immunosuppressive regimens, a concomitant improvement in long-term kidney allograft survival is less remarkable. Clinically significant chronic allograft dysfunction affects up to one third of renal allograft recipients on long-term follow-up.

25.3.1 *Factors that Affect Long-Term Renal Allograft Function*

- Renal allograft status — potential impact of donor age, ethnicity, and body-size mismatch between donor and recipient
- Perioperative nephron injury — potential effects of brain death, cardiac arrest, and ischemia-reperfusion injury
- Acute or subacute rejection
- Drug nephrotoxicity
- Systemic abnormalities — effects of hypertension, diabetes mellitus, and hyperlipidemia
- Renovascular diseases
- Recurrent or *de novo* renal parenchymal disease
- Nephropathy due to BK polyoma virus infection
- Obstructive uropathy or reflux nephropathy, with or without pyelonephritis

The Banff 2005 classification recommended that the diagnostic label of "chronic allograft nephropathy" be replaced with "interstitial fibrosis and tubular atrophy, no evidence of any specific etiology"; while all potential etiological or mechanistic factors that could contribute to progressive allograft dysfunction should be actively sought and intervened. In addition, there is accumulating evidence of chronic antibody-mediated alloimmune rejection causing allograft dysfunction in some patients.

CNI nephrotoxicity is characterized histologically by arteriolar hyalinosis with peripheral hyaline nodules, and tubular cell injury with isometric vacuolization. Manifestations of nephrotoxicity can be acute or chronic, both presenting with an increase in the serum creatinine level. While the susceptibility differs between individuals, in general acute nephrotoxicity is unlikely when the 12-h trough cyclosporin level does not exceed 250 µg/L or the 12-h trough tacrolimus level does not exceed 8 ng/mL. Drug interactions with CNIs are discussed in Chapter 33. Renal allograft function has been reported to stabilize or improve in some patients following CNI minimization or withdrawal, although it is difficult to predict which patients may benefit from this approach.

Proteinuria is an independent risk factor for graft failure. Urine protein excretion should be regularly monitored in kidney transplant recipients. Proteinuria can result from chronic allograft injury, recurrent or *de novo* glomerulopathies, drug-related nephropathy, disease in native kidneys, renal vein thrombosis, and reflux nephropathy. Nonspecific measures to reduce proteinuria include optimal blood pressure control and blockade of the renin-angiotensin system.

25.4 Gastrointestinal Complications

Multiple factors contribute to an increased risk of peptic ulceration after kidney transplantation, including the use of high-dose corticosteroid, gastric irritation by immunosuppressive medications, and *Helicobacter pylori* colonization. Historically, peptic ulcer has been a significant cause of morbidity and mortality. Prophylaxis with an H_2-receptor antagonist or a proton pump inhibitor for approximately 6 months is associated with decreased incidence of peptic ulceration. Gastrointestinal upset may be precipitated by corticosteroids or other immunosuppressive agents. Enteric-coated mycophenolic sodium may be tried in patients who do not tolerate mycophenolate mofetil, although the benefit is probably marginal. Nystatin is often prescribed in the first few months to prevent oroesophageal candidiasis.

25.5 Graft Renal Artery Stenosis

Clinical manifestations of graft renal artery stenosis include abdominal bruit, hypertension, renal impairment, and less commonly thromboembolism resulting in patchy infarction. Doppler ultrasonogram offers high diagnostic sensitivity, but is operator-dependent. Carbon dioxide or conventional angiogram provides a definitive diagnosis prior to intervention by angioplasty with or without stenting or vascular reanastomosis.

25.6 Malignancies and Posttransplant Lymphoproliferative Disorder (PTLD)

The increase in risk varies between different malignancies. Those affecting the lung, gastrointestinal tract, prostate, and breast are severalfold more common in kidney transplant recipients compared to age- and gender-matched controls; while the risks of Kaposi's sarcoma, non-melanomatous skin cancers in Caucasians, and PTLD are increased by more than 100-fold.

Viral infection presents an additional risk or modulating factor, such as the increased risk of hepatocellular carcinoma in subjects with chronic hepatitis B or C infection, the role of Epstein–Barr virus (EBV) infection in PTLD, the role of polyoma virus in uroepithelial tumor, and the role of human herpes virus type 8 in Kaposi's sarcoma. In patients with a history of malignancy, the inclusion of an mTOR inhibitor in the immunosuppressive regimen is reasonable considering its potential antitumor effect.

Surveillance for tumor development should be applied to patients at risk, and these include regular skin examination once or twice every year, annual testing for prostate-specific antigen, fecal occult blood and age-appropriate colonoscopy, breast examination, mammogram, and cervical smear examination. Chronic hepatitis B or C carriers should have regular blood tests for alpha-fetal protein every 3 to 4 months and a yearly liver ultrasonogram. Ultrasonogram of the native kidneys should be performed annually in patients with acquired cystic disease.

PTLD can range from a relatively more benign form of polyclonal proliferation to more malignant varieties with clonal chromosomal abnormalities. It can be nodal or extranodal, localized or disseminated. An association with EBV is not universal. Reduction of immunosuppression remains a pivotal element in the management of PTLD, with a response rate of up to 50%. Other modalities of treatment include surgical resection and chemotherapy. The role of antiviral therapy is controversial, while the use of anti-CD20 antibodies has been associated with encouraging results.

25.7 Metabolic Complications

Common metabolic complications after kidney transplantation include hyperlipidemia, hyperglycemia, hyperuricemia, obesity, and metabolic syndrome. Immunosuppressive medications can contribute to these metabolic abnormalities. Corticosteroid leads to obesity, hypertension, glucose intolerance, and hyperlipidemia in a dose-dependant manner. Tacrolimus, when given together with high-dose corticosteroid, may induce hyperglycemia and posttransplant diabetes mellitus in susceptible individuals. CNIs can also lead to hypertension, hyperuricemia, and hyperlipidemia. The lipid profile should be determined at baseline, then after 3–6 months, and then at least on an annual basis. Hyperlipidemia should be treated to aim for targets of LDL cholesterol < 2.6 mmol/L, non-HDL cholesterol < 3.4 mmol/L, and triglyceride < 1.7 mmol/L. Muscle enzyme levels should be monitored in patients receiving lipid-lowering treatment with statins or fibrates.

25.8 Cardiovascular Complications and Hypertension

Cardiovascular disease is a major cause of death in long-term kidney transplant recipients. Risk factors for vascular complications that are potentially amenable to treatment include:

- smoking
- hypertension
- dyslipidemia
- diabetes mellitus
- obesity and physical inactivity
- impaired renal function
- proteinuria
- hyperparathyroidism

Although there is insufficient data to recommend routine screening for cardiovascular disease, a proactive approach for early diagnosis and intervention is reasonable in kidney transplant recipients with risk factors, especially considering the increasing availability of noninvasive diagnostic investigations.

Hypertension (blood pressure above 120/80 mmHg) affects approximately 80% of kidney transplant recipients. Potentially reversible causes of hypertension include graft renal artery stenosis and the effect of CNIs or corticosteroid. Calcium channel blockers might exacerbate CNI-induced gingival hyperplasia. Drug interactions, such as the inhibition of CNI metabolism by diltiazem, should be noted. Beneficial effects on proteinuria, preservation of renal function, and cardiac function have been observed with inhibition or blockade of the renin-angiotensin system; but caution should be exercised in case of undiagnosed graft renal artery stenosis, hyperkalemia, or anemia.

25.9 Erythrocytosis and Anemia

Erythrocytosis may develop after kidney transplantation and persist for months. Adequate hydration is important, and treatment with an angiotensin-converting enzyme inhibitor or angiotensin receptor blocker may be necessary, especially when the hematocrit is above 55% in males or 50% in females. Renal ultrasonogram should be arranged to look for acquired cystic disease in the native kidneys.

Anemia may be associated with mycophenolate mofetil or azathioprine treatment, deficiency states, parvovirus infection, or rarely hemolysis due to lymphocytes of donor origin.

25.10 Hyperparathyroidism, Renal Osteodystrophy, and Osteoporosis

The levels of serum calcium, phosphate, and when indicated parathyroid hormone should be monitored after kidney transplantation. Tertiary hyperparathyroidism can improve spontaneously over 6 to 12 months after transplantation. Favorable results have been reported with the use of calcimimetics. Surgical parathyroidectomy may be necessary in some patients, especially when there is calciphylaxis or persistent hypercalcemia.

Accelerated bone loss occurs within the first 6 months after kidney transplantation, due to the following reasons:

- Corticosteroid treatment
- Previous osteodystrophy
- Persistent hyperparathyroidism
- Metabolic acidosis
- Smoking
- Hypogonadism

Diagnosis of osteoporosis or osteopenia is by dual energy X-ray absorptiometry scan of the lumbar spine or hip. Treatments include hormonal replacement, calcium and vitamin D supplement, correction of metabolic acidosis, and bisphosphonates.

Suggested Reading

Chan TM, Fang GX, Tang CSO, *et al.* (2002) Pre-emptive lamivudine therapy based on HBV DNA level in HBsAg-positive kidney allograft recipients. *Hepatology* 36:1246–1252.

Chan TM, Tse KC, Tang CSO, *et al.* (2004) A prospective study on lamivudine-resistant hepatitis B in renal allograft recipients. *Am J Transplant* 4:1103–1109.

Solez K, Colvin RB, Racusen LC, *et al.* (2007) Banff '05 Meeting Report: differential diagnosis of chronic allograft injury and elimination of chronic allograft nephropathy. *Am J Transplant* 7:518–526.

Solez K, Colvin RB, Racusen LC, *et al.* (2008) Banff '07 classification of renal allograft pathology: updates and future directions. *Am J Transplant* 8:753–760.

Part IV
Special Renal Investigations

26

Diagnosis of Renal Tubular Acidosis

James C. M. Chan

26.1 Introduction

Renal tubular acidosis (RTA) is characterized by systemic metabolic acidosis due to acidification defects on different segments of the renal tubules, and is classified into various types according to the sites of the defects. Four types of RTA are well described:

- Classic, type 1 or distal RTA is characterized by an inability to excrete adequate amounts of hydrogen ions at the distal renal tubule, resulting in hyperchloremic metabolic acidosis, high urinary pH, hypercalciuria, and hypocitraturia, which increase the risk of nephrocalcinosis.
- Type 2 RTA, also known as proximal RTA, is due to a bicarbonate reabsorption defect at the proximal renal tubule. This renal bicarbonate wasting gives rise to systemic metabolic acidosis, which is associated with minimum hypercalciuria and an inconsequential risk of nephrocalcinosis.
- Type 3 RTA is a subtype of type 1 RTA, usually seen in premature infants with a mild distal acidification defect combined with small proximal bicarbonate wasting. Both defects resolve naturally as the kidneys mature.
- Type 4 RTA, due to aldosterone deficiency or resistance, is characterized by a *hyperkalemic* metabolic acidosis, in contrast to the *hypokalemia* of the other types of RTA. In children with any type of RTA, growth retardation is a significant consequence of chronic metabolic acidosis.

26.2 Classification of RTA

26.2.1 *Primary Type 1 RTA*

- This is due to a defect in maintaining the pH gradient and in hydrogen ion secretion in the distal renal tubule.
- Most cases are sporadic, but familial cases have been described and associated with gene mutations.
- Type 1 RTA with nerve deafness and autosomal dominant transmission has been linked to chromosome 17q21–q22.
- For those without hearing defect and autosomal recessive transmission, the gene defect has been linked to chromosome 7q22–q34.

26.2.2 *Primary Type 2 RTA*

- This is transient in neonates due to proximal tubular bicarbonate wasting, which may resolve spontaneously as the kidneys mature.
- The adult-onset type 2 RTA is persistent.
- Familial cases are linked to chromosome 5p15.3.
- For cases with carbonic anhydrase deficiency, type 2 RTA is transmitted by an autosomal recessive gene linked to chromosome 8q22 and is associated with osteopetrosis and cerebral calcification.

26.2.3 *Primary Type 4 RTA*

- This has been described in early childhood and is transient.

26.3 Clinical Picture

RTA can develop secondary to a host of conditions, ranging from adverse reactions to medications to endocrine disorders. Tables 26.1, 26.2, and 26.3 list the causes of secondary type 1, type 2, and type 4 RTA, respectively.

26.3.1 *Clinical Features of Type 1 and Type 2 RTA*

- Polyuria and polydipsia are common presenting complaints, and are consequences of the chronic hypokalemia and hypercalciuria of type 1 RTA and the severe bicarbonaturia of type 2 RTA, respectively.
- Constipation results from muscle weakness of hypokalemia, which is encountered in both type 1 and type 2 RTA.

Table 26.1   Causes of secondary type 1 (distal) RTA.

Tubulointerstitial and other renal disorders
  Obstructive uropathy
  Medullary sponge kidney
  Kidney transplantation
  Pyelonephritis
  Nephrocalcinosis induced by vitamin D intoxication, hyperparathyroidism,
    idiopathic hypercalciuria, Wilson disease, hyperthyroidism

Genetically transmitted systemic diseases
  Ehlers–Danlos syndrome
  Marfan syndrome
  Osteopetrosis with associated nerve deafness
  Sickle cell disease
  Elliptocytosis
  Carbonic anhydrase deficiency
  Hereditary fructose intolerance
  Fabry disease
  Dent disease
  Carnitine palmitoyl transferase deficiency

Autoimmune disease
  Sjögren syndrome
  Hypergammaglobulinemia
  Systemic lupus erythematosus
  Chronic active hepatitis
  Thyroiditis
  Primary biliary cirrhosis
  Fibrosing alveolitis
  Polyarteritis nodosa
  Rheumatoid arthritis

Toxin- or drug-induced
  Amphotericin B
  Lithium
  Analgesics
  Cyclamate
  Toluene
  Mercury

Hyponatremic states
  Nephrotic syndrome
  Hepatic cirrhosis

Miscellaneous conditions
  Leprosy
  Sodium depletion

Table 26.2   Causes of secondary type 2 (proximal) RTA.

Drug-induced
  Gentamicin
  Cadmium
  Streptozotocin
  Lead
  Mercury
  Maleic acid
  Coumadin
  6-mercaptopurine
  Ifostamide
  Sulfonamide
  Acetazolamide
  Outdated tetracycline
  Valproic acid
  Carbonic anhydrase inhibitor

Interstitial kidney diseases
  Medullary cystic disease
  Kidney transplantation
  Balkan nephropathy
  Chronic renal vein thrombosis
  Sjögren syndrome

Inborn errors of metabolism
  Cystinosis
  Hereditary fructose intolerance
  Lowe syndrome
  Tyrosinemia
  Galactosemia
  Wilson disease
  Pyruvate carboxylase deficiency
  Metachromatic leukodystrophy
  Glycogen storage disease

Dysproteinemic states
  Amyloidosis
  Multiple myeloma
  Light chain disease
  Monoclonal gammopathy

(Continued)

Table 26.2 (*Continued*)

Miscellaneous
  Vitamin D deficiency, dependence, or resistance
  Nephrotic syndrome
  Leigh syndrome
  Paroxysmal nocturnal hemoglobinuria
  Congenital heart disease
  Malignancy

Table 26.3   Causes of secondary type 4 RTA.

Aldosterone resistance
  Obstructive uropathy
  Pseudohypoaldosteronism
  Chronic tubulointerstitial nephritis with salt wasting
  Induced by drugs (e.g. prostaglandin inhibitors, captopril, cyclosporine, spironolactone, amiloride, triamterine, heparin)

Aldosterone deficiency
  Congenital adrenal hyperplasia (21-hydroxylase deficiency)
  Addison disease
  Bilateral adrenalectomy
  Isolated hypoaldosteronism
  Inherited corticosterone methyloxidase deficiency

Aldosterone deficiency with hyporeninemia
  Diabetes mellitus
  Pyelonephritis
  Interstitial nephritis
  Gout
  Nephrosclerosis

Miscellaneous
  Renal transplantation
  Lupus erythematosus
  Acute glomerulonephritis
  Kidney amyloidosis
  Renal vein thrombosis
  Type 4 RTA induced by drugs (e.g. heparin, methicillin, potassium-sparing diuretics, prostaglandin inhibitors, captopril, cyclosporine)
  Potassium supplementations may aggravate type 4 RTA

- Nephrocalcinosis, which characterizes undiagnosed and inadequately treated type 1 RTA, results from hypocitraturia coupled with hypercalciuria.
- The metabolic acidosis of type 1 RTA due to a lack of adequate hydrogen ion secretion requires skeletal buffering of the positive hydrogen ion balance, and gives rise to the often-significant hypercalciuria.
- Nephrocalcinosis is not common in type 2 RTA because the severe bicarbonate wasting gives rise to metabolic acidosis without positive hydrogen ion balance.
- Thus, without hydrogen ion accumulation to stimulate skeletal buffering, there is no hypercalciuria or hypocitraturia, so patients with type 2 RTA incur a minimal risk of nephrocalcinosis.

26.3.2 Differences in Clinical Features between Pediatric and Adult RTA

- Anorexia, vomiting, and failure to thrive develop as presenting features of infants with RTA.
- An infant with undiagnosed and untreated type 1 RTA may present with life-threatening acidosis. Long-standing acidosis causes growth retardation.
- Adults with type 1 RTA usually present with recurrent renal calculi, nephrocalcinosis, osteomalacia, rickets, myalgia, and arthralgia.

26.3.3 Clinical Features of Type 4 RTA

- Adults with type 4 RTA often present with evidence of hyporeninemia and hypoaldosteronism, especially associated with compromised renal function from the underlying prostatic hypertrophy, obstructive uropathy, diabetes mellitus, or drug-induced interstitial nephritis.
- Neonates or children with type 4 RTA due to aldosterone deficiency from 21-hydroxylase insufficiency or from aldosterone resistance from posterior urethral valve obstruction may present earlier only with symptoms and signs of volume depletion.

26.4 Laboratory Measurements in Diagnosing RTA

The serum anion gap is the difference between the sum of cations (sodium plus potassium) and the sum of anions (chloride plus total CO_2); the normal value is 12 mEq/L. The use of the serum anion gap in the differential diagnosis of metabolic acidosis is presented in the algorithm in Fig. 26.1.

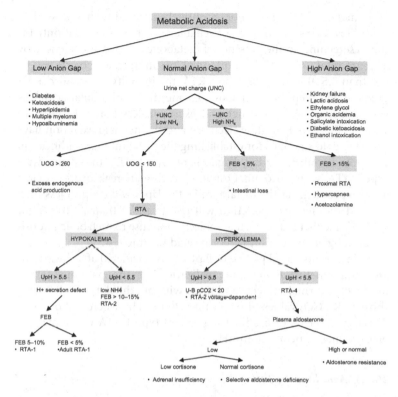

Fig. 26.1 Algorithm for diagnosis of different types of RTA. UNC: urine net charge, calculated as urine sodium plus potassium minus chloride; UOG: urine osmolality gap; FEB: fractional excretion of bicarbonate; RTA: renal tubular acidosis; UpH: urine pH; U-B pCO$_2$: urine minus blood partial pressure of CO$_2$.

The urinary net charge (UNC) is taken as a surrogate for the urinary ammonium content, and is calculated by urinary sodium plus potassium minus chloride. Positive UNC values indicate low ammonium concentrations, while negative UNC values indicate high ammonium concentrations.

Fractional excretion of bicarbonate (FEB) is calculated as [urinary bicarbonate × plasma creatinine] divided by [plasma bicarbonate × urine creatinine] multiplied by 100%. After sodium bicarbonate supplementation to achieve steady-state acid-base homeostasis, an FEB exceeding 10%–15% suggests proximal or type 2 RTA; while FEB values of less than 5% indicate that the proximal tubular reabsorption of bicarbonate is normal, which is compatible with distal, type 1 RTA.

Urinary pH (UpH) is more accurately assessed with a glass electrode. The urine dipstick is not reliable and should be used only for initial screening. In the presence of metabolic acidosis as evidenced by a serum total $CO_2 < 17.5$ mEq/L, the UpH in normal subjects will be less than 5.5. But in distal, type 1 RTA, the inability to establish a pH gradient will keep the UpH above 5.5 and the distal tubular acidification defect will keep the net acid excretion less than 70 μEq/min/ 1.73 m^2. The UpH by glass electrode and the net acid excretion have been the gold standard for establishing the distal tubular acidification defect and confirming the diagnosis of type 1 RTA. In patients with type 2 RTA, with a proximal tubular bicarbonate reabsorption defect and no problems at the distal tubule, the UpH will drop to less than 5.5 and the net acid excretion will rise to more than 70 μEq/min/ 1.73 m^2, like that in the normal subject's response to metabolic acidosis induced by an ammonium chloride acid loading test.

Urine minus blood pCO_2 (U-B pCO_2) is calculated after bicarbonate supplements achieve normalization of the patient's serum total CO_2. Normal subjects and those with proximal, type 2 RTA will show U-B pCO_2 values of better than 20 mmHg; whereas those with distal, type 1 RTA or gradient-dependent type 1 RTA will show U-B pCO_2 values of below 20 mmHg.

26.4.1 Acid loading Test

- This test confirms the diagnosis of RTA in patients with inconsistent metabolic acidosis or those with incomplete RTA.
- It can maximally test the acidifying capability of the kidneys.
- Ammonium chloride (75 mEq/m^2 or 0.1 g/kg) administered orally in gelatin-coated capsules induces a significant metabolic acidosis, as evidenced by a serum total $CO_2 < 17.5$ mEq/L, within 3 h and a compensatory renal UpH of less than 5.5 in normal subjects.
- In subjects with a distal tubular inability to acidify, the UpH will be in excess of 5.5 and the net acid excretion will be <70 μEq/min/ 1.73 m^2.
- The UpH of patients with proximal RTA will fall below 5.5 and the net acid excretion will be in excess of 70 μEq/min/1.75 m^2.

Spontaneous metabolic acidosis with serum total $CO_2 < 17.5$ mEq/L, avoids the need to use acidifying salts, and should be taken advantage of immediately by testing the UpH in a freshly collected urine sample. A layer of mineral oil over the urine sample to prevent loss of CO_2 is still advocated, but freezing for up to 1 week can prevent such loss if UpH and net acid excretion are performed immediately upon thawing as shown by Yang *et al.* (1981).

26.4.2 Furosemide Test

- After an overnight fast and previous normal sodium diet, if the UpH is less than 5.5, the renal tubular acidification is intact and the furosemide test is avoided.
- If the UpH is over 5.5, then an oral dose of furosemide 40 mg is given to a normal 70-kg patient.
- Urine is collected every 30 min for up to 5 h.
- RTA is diagnosed if the UpH persists above 5.5 at the end of the test (Penney and Oleesky 1999).
- A recent test combining furosemide (40 mg) plus fludrocortisone (1 mg) is as effective as the ammonium chloride acid loading test in establishing the diagnosis of distal, type 1 RTA (Walsh *et al.* 2007).

26.5 Diagnostic Approach

The earlier the diagnosis of RTA is made and treated, the less the consequential damage from hypercalciuria and nephrolithiasis. The nephrocalcinosis of distal, type 1 RTA will persist even with early treatment, but renal function will not deteriorate if the patients are compliant with treatment. Patients with type 2 or type 4 RTA have minimal risk of nephrocalcinosis because of the lack of hypercalciuria in the former and the high excretion of calcium-chelating citrate in the latter.

Neonates and infants with RTA present with tachypnea, i.e. respiratory compensation for the metabolic acidosis. Irritability, vomiting, polyuria, polydipsia, and failure to thrive are nonspecific signs and symptoms (Table 26.4). Growth retardation and rickets in the child and osteomalacia in the adult patient are the chief complaints; these may be accompanied by neuromuscular weakness from the chronic hypokalemia, presenting as constipation, fatigue, and myalgia, which may progress to muscular paralysis. Acute urinary calculi presenting as renal colic may pass and turn into dull abdominal pain. Nephrocalcinosis is without symptoms except for mild, intermittent hematuria and/or proteinuria, and is often picked up by ultrasound of the kidneys in connection with other examinations.

Table 26.4 Neonatal failure to thrive and normal anion gap metabolic acidosis.

Obstructive uropathy
Congenital hypothyroidism
Early chronic kidney failure
Distal renal tubular acidosis
Bicarbonate wasting: proximal renal tubular acidosis, diarrhea, intestinal
  fistula, ureterosigmoidostomy, drug-induced (calcium chloride,
  cholestyramine, magnesium sulfate)
Acid loading (ammonium chloride, arginine hydrochloride)

In contrast to the hypokalemic symptoms dominating type 1 and type 2 RTA, patients with type 4 RTA often present with features associated with hyperkalemia and hypovolemia secondary to hyporeninemia and hypoaldosteronism. Fever from those with severe volume depletion may be confused with infectious episodes.

A careful history taking may reveal similar symptoms in family members. Other family members may already be suffering from hearing loss, osteopetrosis, Fanconi syndrome, and other disorders as listed in Tables 26.1–26.3 for secondary RTA. They should all undergo physical examination, urinalysis, and blood chemistries.

Figure 26.1 offers a strategy for the diagnostic workup of RTA in its various spectra. Depending on the stage of diabetic ketoacidosis, the anion gap can be low or high; otherwise, the anion gap can differentiate the conditions with metabolic acidosis into three major categories. Most patients with RTA have a normal anion gap, with additional information gleaned from examination of the UNC. With high ammonium concentrations as suggested by a negative UNC, an FEB of over 15% confirms the diagnosis of proximal, type 2 RTA. If the FEB is less than 5%, there is no significant bicarbonate wasting from the proximal tubules and so other sites for bicarbonate wasting will need to be sought, including gastrointestinal losses.

Figure 26.1 also suggests that a positive UNC, namely a low urinary ammonium, should prompt an examination of the urine osmolality gap (UOG) in mmol/L, which is calculated as (urine osmolality) − [(urine sodium) × 2] − [(urine potassium) × 2] − (urine chloride) − (urine glucose):

- Low urinary ammonium coupled with high UOG > 260 mmol/L points to excessive endogenous hydrogen ion production as the cause of metabolic acidosis.

- High urinary ammonium coupled with low UOG < 150 mmol/L points to RTA as the cause of metabolic acidosis.

The next step is to determine how the acidosis is related to the status of serum potassium concentrations, i.e. whether it is hyperkalemia or hypokalemia.

26.5.1 *Hyperkalemic Metabolic Acidosis*

- Hyperkalemic metabolic acidosis with UpH less than 5.5 points to type 4 RTA, which requires the determination of plasma aldosterone. If this is high or normal, the likely diagnosis is type 4 RTA from aldosterone resistance (obstructive uropathy or other underlying conditions).
- Hyperkalemic metabolic acidosis with UpH less than 5.5 and low plasma aldosterone may suggest adrenal insufficiency, requiring a low plasma cortisone to confirm the diagnosis.
- In cases of hyperkalemic metabolic acidosis with UpH less than 5.5 and low plasma aldosterone, a normal cortisol suggests selective aldosterone deficiency.
- Hyperkalemic metabolic acidosis but with UpH over 5.5 points to voltage-dependent RTA, in which case the U-B pCO_2 will show values of less than 20 mmHg.

26.5.2 *Hypokalemic Metabolic Acidosis*

- Hypokalemic metabolic acidosis with UpH less than 5.5 associated with an FEB of over 10%–15% supports the diagnosis of proximal, type 2 RTA.
- Hypokalemic metabolic acidosis with UpH greater than 5.5 and FEB less than 5% supports the diagnosis of adult type 1 RTA.
- In infants, hypokalemic metabolic acidosis with UpH greater than 5.5 and FEB of 5%–10% supports the diagnosis of type 1 RTA.

Acknowledgments

This work was supported by National Institutes of Health grants DK50419 and DK07761.

Suggested Reading

Chan JCM, Santos F. (2007) Renal tubular acidosis in childhood. *World J Pediatr* 3:92–97.

Herrin JT. (2004) Renal tubular acidosis. In: Avner ED, Harmon WE, Niaudet P (eds.), *Pediatric Nephrology*, Lippincott Williams & Wilkins, Philadelphia, pp. 757–776.

Nicoletta JA, Schwartz GJ. (2004) Distal renal tubular acidosis. *Curr Opin Pediatr* 16:194–198.

Penney MD, Oleesky DA. (1999) Renal tubular acidosis: a review. *Ann Clin Biochem* 36:408–422.

Quigley R. (2006) Proximal renal tubular acidosis. *J Nephrol* 19:S41–S45.

Walsh SB, Shirley DG, Wrong OM, Unwin RJ. (2007) Urinary acidification assessed by simultaneous furosemide and fludrocortisone treatment: an alternative to ammonium chloride. *Kidney Int* 71:1310–1316.

Yang SC, Wellons MD, Chan JCM. (1981) The effects of long-term freezing preservation on urinary titratable acid and ammonium. *Clin Biochem* 4:45–46.

27

Treatment of Renal Tubular Acidosis

James C. M. Chan

27.1 Treatment of Type 1 and Type 2 Renal Tubular Acidosis (RTA)

27.1.1 *Bicarbonate Replacement*

In a patient with hypercapnea from severe metabolic acidosis, as evidenced by a serum total CO_2 of less than 12 mEq/L, intravenous sodium bicarbonate ($NaHCO_3$) is given to achieve rapid correction. The formula to calculate the amount of sodium bicarbonate is as follows:

[desired change in serum bicarbonate × body weight in kg × 0.6]

One milliliter of 8.4% $NaHCO_3$ contains 1 mEq of bicarbonate. The last figure in the equation above (i.e. 0.6) is the distribution space of bicarbonate in the body, which is 60% of the body weight. Half of the total dose of sodium bicarbonate is given in the first hour, and the rest over the next 24 hours. It is standard care during bicarbonate infusion to monitor the serum potassium and calcium concentrations.

In patients with a less severe degree of metabolic acidosis, as evidenced by a serum total CO_2 better than 12 mEq/L, oral supplementation of sodium bicarbonate or other alkaline medications — such as the more palatable Shohl's solution or Bicitra containing sodium citrate and citric acid — can be used. Bicitra solution has a slight fruity taste and provides base at a dose of 1 mEq/mL. Polycitra K solution contains potassium citrate, providing 2 mEq/mL of base as well as 2 mEq/mL of potassium to correct both the metabolic acidosis and the concurrent hypokalemia in many cases of type 1 RTA.

In order to maintain consistent correction of metabolic acidosis in type 1 RTA, sodium bicarbonate or sodium citrate solutions need to be given every 6–8 h round the clock. This schedule becomes a great problem in achieving patient compliance. The total dose of base needed to neutralize the endogenous production of net acid in the adult is 2 mEq/kg/day, given in divided doses. Because infants and young children with a more rapid growth rate incur a higher rate of endogenous net acid production, the alkaline dosages needed to maintain correction have been shown by Santos and Chan (1986) to be 3.5 mEq/kg/day for both infants and children.

Patients with type 2 RTA require a larger amount of base to keep up with the bicarbonate wasting by the proximal renal tubules. Thus, dosages of Bicitra or Polycitra solutions that provide base up to 14 mEq/kg/day in divided doses are often needed. It is uncertain how compliant patients are when such large doses are prescribed and administered as frequently as every 6 h. The involvement of school nurses and teachers, in addition to that of the patient and family, in order to achieve this rate of administration becomes a constant struggle, even with the best intentions of all concerned. It is now advocated that the total daily QID doses be rearranged to a TID schedule with doubling of the Bicitra dose at bedtime (based on the rationale that better correction of acidosis during sleep promotes growth hormone effectiveness). This TID schedule encourages better patient compliance compared to the QID schedule.

27.1.2 Potassium Replacement

The potassium supplements in treating hypokalemia are different between type 1 and type 2 RTA. With type 1 RTA, as the metabolic acidosis is corrected with base therapy, the doses of potassium become less. In contrast, with type 2 RTA, the potassium supplements required to maintain potassium homeostasis become larger as the acidosis is corrected. This is an important point, as mentioned by Sebastian et al. (1971), because the hypokalemia — unless recognized and treated — may be life-threatening, especially when compounded by intercurrent infections.

27.2 Treatment of Type 4 RTA

The hyperkalemia which characterizes type 4 RTA requires dietary restriction of potassium intake plus the use of loop diuretics to increase potassium excretion. Some patients may benefit from potassium binders to reduce the intestinal absorption of this ion.

Type 4 RTA due to congenital adrenal hyperplasia requires replacement with fludrocortisones 0.05–0.15 mg/m²/day. Concurrent blood pressure monitoring is mandatory.

To correct the metabolic acidosis, sodium bicarbonate or sodium citrate solutions are used as discussed for the other types of RTA.

Suggested Reading

Chan JCM, Scheinman JI, Roth KS. (2001) Renal tubular acidosis. *Pediatr Rev* 22:277–287.

Herrin JT. (2004) Renal tubular acidosis. In: Avner ED, Harmon WE, Niaudet P (eds.), *Pediatric Nephrology*, Lippincott Williams & Wilkins, Philadelphia, pp. 757–776.

Hui J. (2005) Renal tubular disorders. In: Chiu MC, Yap HK (eds.), *Practical Paediatric Nephrology. An Update of Current Practices*, Medcom Ltd, Hong Kong, pp. 196–208.

Santos F, Chan JCM. (1986) Renal tubular acidosis in children: diagnosis, treatment and prognosis. *Am J Nephrol* 6:289–295.

Scheinman SJ, Guay-Woodford LM, Thakker RV, *et al.* (1999) Genetic disorders of renal electrolyte transport. *N Engl J Med* 340:1177–1187.

Sebastian A, McSherry E, Morris RC Jr. (1971) Renal potassium wasting in renal tubular acidosis (RTA): its occurrence in types 1 and 2 RTA despite sustained correction of systemic acidosis. *J Clin Invest* 50:667–678.

Part V

Radiology in Renal Patients

28

Imaging and Interventional Treatment of Nephrological Problems

Andrew S. H. Lai and Ferdinand S. K. Chu

28.1 Deranged Renal Function

28.1.1 *Ultrasound*

Ultrasound is the most common and noninvasive investigation used for patients with deranged renal function. It is useful in detecting parenchymal changes, especially for reversible pathologies such as obstruction and hydronephrosis.

Ultrasound can be used to guide the nephrologist in determining which site to biopsy and to avoid lesions such as renal cyst or angiomyolipoma (AML). Common indications of renal biopsy include glomerulonephritis, interstitial nephritis, and unexplained deranged renal function. Absolute contraindications for renal biopsy include bleeding diathesis, uncooperative patient, uncontrolled hypertension, and solitary kidney. Relative contraindications include large cyst or tumor, hydronephrosis, contracted kidney, acute pyelonephritis, and pregnancy.

28.1.2 *Nuclear Medicine*

Radiopharmaceuticals used for evaluating anatomy and renal function fall into three categories:

- Excretion by glomerular filtration
- Excretion by tubular secretion
- Renal cortical assessment — those bound in renal tubules to assess cortical anatomic imaging

28.1.2.1 *Excretion by Glomerular Filtration*

- ^{99m}Tc-DTPA is used in the evaluation of glomerular filtration. DTPA is cleared by the renal glomeruli, and measurement of its excretion can provide an accurate estimate of the glomerular filtration rate (GFR).
- In patients who are allergic to radiographic contrast, it provides information that can be shown by intravenous urography (IVU).
- DTPA makes an excellent, inexpensive agent for routine renal imaging.

28.1.2.2 *Tubular Secretion Agents*

- ^{99m}Tc-MAG3 is used in clinical practice to assess tubular function. MAG3 is predominately cleared by proximal tubules (95%) with minimal filtration (<5%).

28.1.2.3 *Renal Cortical Agent*

- DMSA is the most commonly used agent, with about 40% of the injected dose concentrated in the renal cortex at 6 h and the remainder being excreted slowly. DMSA provides an image of the renal cortex with high resolution and is useful in assessing renal mass or scarring.

28.2 Urinary Tract Infection (UTI)

- Urinary tract infection is a clinical, biochemical, and microbiological diagnosis. Diagnosis is made by a routine urine culture.
- Imaging is not usually relevant in the microscopy and diagnosis of UTI.
- Radiological investigations are indicated in complicated cases of UTI and male patients, and are sometimes useful in identifying the source of infection.
- Ultrasound is quick and noninvasive. Pathologies such as hydronephrosis, renal stones, dilated upper ureter, and other renal or perinephric inflammation can be detected on ultrasound. It is also the imaging modality of choice for patients with impaired renal function and pregnancy.
- Non-contrast computerized tomography (NCCT) and, when necessary, contrast CT is useful in providing information on the site and cause of obstruction. Contrast CT is the modality

of choice for complicated/resistant cases of UTI. Renal or per-inephric abscesses, collections, and even congenital anomaly can be detected.

28.3 Stone Disease and Renal Colic

Renal stone affects approximately 1 in every 500 individuals in the USA each year. Over a lifetime, approximately 3%–5% of the population experience symptoms. Men are three times more likely than women to develop this disease. Asians, African-Americans, and individuals of American-Indian descent are relatively less likely to develop renal stones than Caucasians. Commons symptoms include renal colic, flank pain, and hematuria. Renal calculi may give rise to obstruction and acute renal failure, especially in patients with impaired renal function or a single nonfunctioning kidney.

28.3.1 *Intravenous Urography*

- IVU is the historical gold standard of investigation for renal stones. It gives a good overview of the entire urinary tract.
- IVU is also useful in the assessment of renal size, renal position, renal calcifications, distorting mass lesion, abnormalities of cortical contour, dilation or blunting of calyces, courses of ureters, congenital abnormalities, bladder morphology, and bladder emptying.
- The main disadvantage is that it requires the use of contrast and reliance on reasonably good excretory function to obtain images of good quality.

28.3.2 *Non-contrast Computed Tomography*

- CT has superseded IVU as the investigation of choice for diagnosis of renal stone. NCCT can visualize up to 99% of all renal stones. Other advantages include short examination time, avoidance of intravenous contrast, and detection of extra-urinary cause of flank pain.

28.3.3 *Ultrasound*

- Ultrasound is used in detecting acute hydronephrosis and in identifying renal calyceal stones, but small stones and masses may be missed. With the aid of ultrasound, procedures such as percutaneous nephrostomy (PCN) can be performed to relieve acute obstruction.

28.3.4 *Magnetic Resonance (MR) Urography*

- MR urography is clinically useful in the evaluation of suspected urinary tract obstruction, hematuria, congenital anomalies, and surgically altered anatomy. It can be performed as a non-contrast or contrast examination with no radiation. It is useful in pediatric patients, but sedation is often required. It has no known untoward effect on pregnant patients, but the long-term effects are yet to be determined.
- MR urographic techniques for displaying the urinary tract can be divided into two categories:

  (i) Single-shot fast spin-echo MR urography — makes use of heavily T2-weighted sequences to image the urinary tract as a static collection of fluid. This can be repeated sequentially to better demonstrate the ureters and to confirm the presence of fixed stenoses. It is most successful in patients with dilated or obstructed collecting systems.
  (ii) Excretory MR urography — performed during the excretory phase after intravenous administration of gadolinium-based contrast agent. The examination requires patients to have sufficient renal function.

- Single-shot fast spin-echo and excretory MR urography can be combined with conventional MR imaging for comprehensive evaluation of the urinary tract.

28.4 Hematuria

- Hematuria results from bleeding from any site of the urinary tract. Hematuria can be broadly classified into medical and surgical causes.
- Common medical causes of hematuria include glomerulonephritis, UTI, and coagulopathy. The glomerular origin of hematuria is suggested by urine microscopy of dysmorphic red blood cells and red cell cast (refer to Chapter 1).
- Common surgical causes include calculous disease, nephrocalcinosis, neoplasms, cystitis (postchemotherapy or postradiation), and trauma.

- Ultrasound is the first-line investigation in most renal diseases, and is especially useful in differentiating between a cystic and a solid mass lesion. Ultrasound also plays a role in screening for polycystic disease, nephrocalcinosis, and renal calculi.
- IVU gives a good overview of the entire urinary system. IVU can also assess calcifications, distorting mass lesion, and uroepithelial tumors.
- CT is the modality of choice for upper urinary tract lesions such as tumor mass, renal stones, fluid collection, and abscess. CT urography can be performed with unenhanced, nephrographic-phase, and excretory-phase imaging. The unenhanced images are ideal for detecting calculi. Renal masses can also be detected and characterized with a combination of unenhanced and nephrographic-phase imaging. The excretory-phase images provide evaluation of the collecting system and screening for uroepithelial lesions.
- Radiological examination for different etiologies of hematuria is summarized in Table 28.1.

28.5 Hypertension

The most important and potentially treatable cause of renal hypertension is renal artery stenosis (RAS). RAS accounts for 1%–4% of hypertensive individuals. Atherosclerosis is the most common cause of RAS, followed by fibromuscular dysplasia (FMD) for Caucasians and Takayasu's arteritis for Asians.

Indications of screening test for RAS include:

- abrupt-onset or severe hypertension
- resistant hypertension (not responding to triple drug therapy)
- abdominal bruits
- unexplained renal failure in the elderly with hypertension
- worsening of renal function during antihypertensive therapy (especially with angiotensin-converting enzyme inhibitors or angiotensin II receptor blockers)
- onset of hypertension at <30 years or >55 years of age
- hypertension in children.

28.5.1 *Renal Artery Stenosis*

- Visualization of renal artery on ultrasound is operator- and patient-dependent. In obese patients, those who cannot hold their

Table 28.1　Radiological examination for different etiologies of hematuria.

Location	Condition	Suggested investigation
Glomerular	Different types of glomerulonephritis (IgA nephropathy, thin basement membrane disease, Alport's syndrome, lupus nephritis, etc.)	Urinalysis for RBC cast followed by ultrasound and/or biopsy
Upper urinary tract	Renal stone	IVU/USG/NCCT
	Renal tumor (RCC or TCC)	CT/USG/MRI
	Renal trauma	CT
	Renal tuberculosis	IVU/CT
	Pyelonephritis	Clinical history/CT
	Polycystic kidney	USG/CT/MRI
	Angiomyolipoma	USG/CT/MRI
Lower urinary tract		
Bladder	Bladder cancer	USG/CT/MRI
	Cystitis/Prostatitis or urethritis	Clinical history, cystoscopy
Prostate	Prostate cancer	MRI/TRUS
	Prostatitis	Clinical history
Other	Over-anticoagulation	History and blood test
	Drug toxicity e.g. cyclophosphamide	Clinical history

Note: RBC: red blood cell; RCC: renal cell carcinoma; TCC: transitional cell carcinoma; IVU: intravenous urography; USG: ultrasonography; NCCT: non-contrast computerized tomography; CT: computerized tomography; MRI: magnetic resonance imaging; TRUS: transrectal ultrasound.

breath properly, and those whose renal artery is atherosclerotic, visualization of renal artery would be difficult. Very often, the renal artery is only partially visualized.

- Direct diagnostic signs of RAS on Doppler ultrasound are a flow velocity of ≥1.8–2 m/s, a renal artery: aortic velocity ratio of ≥3.5, or poststenotic spectral broadening (i.e. turbulence). Indirect sign of RAS is through examination of intrarenal lobar or interlobar arteries. Dampened Doppler waveforms in lobar, arcuate, or interlobar arteries, with slow acceleration to peak systole of >0.07 s, would be suggestive.

28.5.2 MR Angiography (MRA)

- MR angiography is increasingly used as a tool for the evaluation of renal arteries. Recent studies of renal MRA performed with high-dose gadolinium contrast report sensitivities and specificities of more than 90% for the detection of RAS (>50% stenosis) when compared with conventional angiography as the standard of reference.
- MRA, with its higher cost and lesser availability, should be reserved for patients with indeterminate functional imaging results or for patients with normal functional imaging results but high clinical suspicion of renal hypertension.

28.5.3 Digital Subtraction Angiography (DSA)

- DSA has long been the standard of reference for quantifying arterial stenosis. Despite the emergence of other less invasive modalities that provide high-quality images, DSA is still used as a diagnostic tool for several reasons.
- DSA findings are easy to interpret and can depict the whole target artery with a higher spatial resolution than CT angiography or MR angiography. In addition, DSA allows easier, more accurate lumen evaluation in calcified vessels and in vessels containing stents compared to CT angiography and MR angiography, owing to fewer artifacts from calcification and metal structures.
- However, DSA has other shortcomings. As DSA yields two-dimensional images, multiple views are obtained at different angles for evaluating the stenosis; even with multiple views, however, eccentric stenosis or stenosis of a tortuous vessel may be underestimated. Overlapping vessels may also interfere with the assessment of stenosis. Rotational DSA (if available) will depict stenosis better than the combination of two or three DSA projections.

28.5.4 Angioplasty/Stenting

- It is usually performed as an extension to the procedure of DSA.
- Renal angioplasty/stenting is undertaken for hypertension or ischemic renal failure. The majority of renal stenoses are secondary to atherosclerotic lesions that tend to involve the proximal renal artery or its ostium (Fig. 28.1).

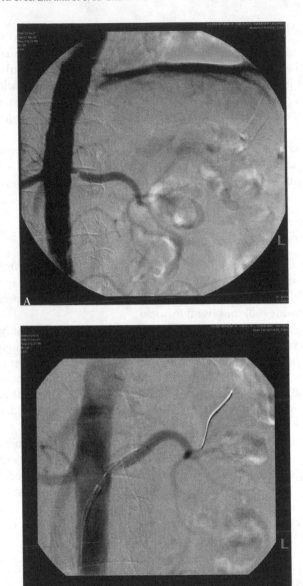

Fig. 28.1 Arteriography showing proximal renal artery stenosis (arrow) (A) before and (B) after stenting.

- Fibromuscular dysplasia can affect any part of the renal artery and has a characteristic beaded appearance on angiography. The success rate of lone angioplasty is highest with FMD, moderate with non-ostial atherosclerotic stenosis, and poorest with ostial lesion. Ostial lesions are prone to elastic recoil, and many radiologists opt for a primary stent placement.

28.6 Renal Osteodystrophy

Renal osteodystrophy is a multifactorial disorder of bone remodeling comprising high-turnover hyperparathyroid bone disease; low-turnover bone disease, including osteomalacia and adynamic bone disease (ABD); and mixed uremic osteodystrophy. Histological abnormalities can be detected early during the course of renal failure, and are present in over half of the patients with a GFR < 50% of normal. Bone disease is not a static phenomenon; evolution from one form to another can occur and may reflect the effects of treatment. Radiological examination may help to predict bone histology in selected situations. One must be aware that radiological changes of renal bone disease often appear late, as patients can have severe histological changes and normal radiographs.

28.6.1 *Plain Radiograph*

As radiographic findings are less sensitive than parathyroid hormone, many dialysis centers have abandoned routine radiographic screening, reserving radiographs for symptomatic patients. Subperiosteal erosions of hyperparathyroidism are first noted in the phalanges (Fig. 28.2), and so the hand radiograph probably remains the most commonly requested radiograph. It is important to optimize the quality of radiographs by using fine-grained, single-sided emulsion film and a fine focal spot (0.6 mm or less). Looser's zones are rarely seen nowadays, although metastatic calcification remains common.

28.6.2 *Bone Densitometry*

The most widely available technique to determine bone mass is dual-energy X-ray absorptiometry (DEXA). Other techniques include single-energy X-ray absorptiometry, quantitative CT, and quantitative

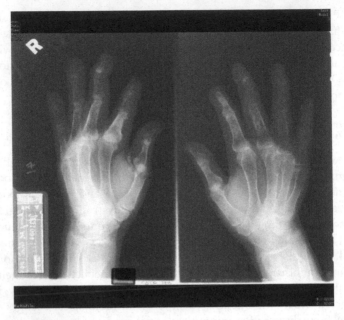

Fig. 28.2 Plain X-ray of the phalanges showing subperiosteal erosions of secondary hyperparathyroidism.

ultrasound (QUS). DEXA is regarded as the gold standard because of its high precision and accuracy, short acquisition time, and low radiation dose.

Patients with end-state renal disease (ESRD) are likely to be at risk of reduced bone mineral density (BMD) and osteoporosis because of hyperparathyroidism, increasing age, immobility, gonadal dysfunction, and corticosteroid exposure. The interpretation of bone densitometry scans in patients with renal osteodystrophy is complex. Isolated measurements of BMD are unlikely to be helpful in the diagnosis of renal osteodystrophy due to poor correlation between bone density measurements and histology.

Taken as a whole, studies do show a higher prevalence of osteopenia and osteoporosis in patients with ESRD compared with age-matched and sex-matched control individuals. Osteoporosis is also more common than expected in predialysis patients, and BMD decreases in relation to a decrease in GFR. Rapid bone loss of the order of 3%–9% at the lumbar spine occurs during the immediate period after renal transplantation, and steroid therapy could be a contributory factor. However, prospective data linking BMD to fracture risk are lacking in patients with ESRD.

28.6.3 *Quantitative Ultrasound*

Quantitative ultrasound (QUS) of peripheral sites offers a portable, quick, relatively inexpensive, and radiation-free method of bone mass assessment. In postmenopausal and elderly females with a hip fracture, ultrasound-measured parameters produce a comparable prediction as DEXA. Ultrasound techniques are now being used in dialysis patients showing lower measurements at the phalanges and heel than in matched controls. Some investigators have suggested that QUS could be used as a screening test to exclude those patients who are unlikely to have BMD in the osteoporotic range.

28.7 Hyperparathyroidism

Decreased serum calcium and increased phosphate are common in patients with chronic renal failure. This would lead to an increase in parathyroid hormone secretion, termed "secondary hyperthyroidism". Management of secondary hyperparathyroidism does not usually require any imaging.

Prolonged secondary hyperparathyroidism may lead to autonomous hyperfunction of parathyroid glands, with an increase in both serum calcium and phosphate. Previously, this was termed "tertiary hyperparathyroidism". The treatment relies on surgical excision of the hyperfunctioning gland. Though disputed by some, preoperative imaging has the theoretical advantage of a more focused operation/limited neck dissection and a higher cure rate. About 13% of patients have a parathyroid gland in the mediastinum. Approximately 3% of patients have less than four parathyroid glands.

Ultrasonography, scintigraphy, and a combination of both ultrasonography and scintigraphy are the most common imaging modalities used. Operative success can be confirmed by intraoperative quick parathyroid hormone assay.

28.7.1 *Ultrasound*

- High-resolution ultrasound using a linear transducer can produce high-quality images of the lower neck.

- Sensitivity in detecting a hyperplastic parathyroid gland is 60%–79%.
- Ultrasound is difficult to detect ectopic parathyroid glands and in patients who have had previous neck dissection.

28.7.2 *Scintigraphy*

- Most parathyroid scintigraphy is performed using single-tracer dual-phase imaging by technetium-99m sestamibi.
- Uptake in the parathyroid is based on the same mechanism as uptake in the thyroid, and it includes mitochondrial activity. The thyroid, however, releases the tracer earlier than the parathyroid. Therefore, delayed scanning 1.5–2 h after injection of the tracer may localize the hyperfunctioning parathyroid gland.
- Sometimes, faster wash-out of the tracer is noted in parathyroid hyperplasia, and that tracer can accumulate in the thyroid nodule. These explain why the sensitivity is only 77%–88%.

28.7.3 *Combination of Sonography and Scintigraphy*

Sensitivity is reported to be up to 89%–98%. It is especially advantageous in ectopic parathyroids.

28.7.4 *Other Imaging and Interventional Techniques*

28.7.4.1 *Percutaneous Ablation*

Ultrasound-guided percutaneous ablation using 100% alcohol can achieve long-term remission in 66%–80% of cases. Complications include vocal cord palsy and paraglandular fibrosis.

28.7.4.2 *Contrast CT and Contrast MR*

Contrast CT and contrast MR have a sensitivity of 46%–87% and 80%, respectively. In view of renal impairment, both iodine contrast (CT) and gadolinium contrast (MR) should only be used with great caution.

28.8 Complications of Contrast Imaging in Renal Patients

28.8.1 *Iodinated Contrast-Induced Nephropathy*

Refer to Chapter 9.

28.8.2 *Prophylactic Treatment for Subjects at Risk*

Premedication with corticosteroids and antihistamines is recommended for patients who are at risk, including those with an allergic-like reaction to contrast media, asthma, and other allergies. A prophylactic regimen is highly recommended.

For elective procedures:

- Prednisolone 50 mg orally 13, 7, and 1 h before the examination and diphenhydramine 50 mg orally 1 h before the examination
- Patients should be advised not to drive or perform potentially dangerous tasks.

For emergent situations:

- Hydrocortisone 200 mg intravenously given immediately and repeated every 4 h until the examination is complete; diphenhydramine 50 mg intravenously 1 h before the examination.

28.8.3 *Gadolinium Contrast — Nephrogenic Systemic Fibrosis*

- It is a commonly held myth among the very junior clinicians that if the patient's function is too poor to undergo contrast CT, then contrast MRI is the way to go.
- Nephrogenic systemic fibrosis (NSF) is also known as nephrogenic fibrosing dermopathy. It is a multisystem fibrosing disorder and is a potentially fatal disease. It could confine an affected patient to a wheelchair and may lead to contractures.
- It occurs only in patients with renal disease.
- It has never been known to occur before 1997. It occurs in 3%–5% of renal-impaired patients receiving gadolinium-based contrast within the preceding 3–6 months.
- About 90% of cases occur with gadodiamide (Omniscan®).
- There is no evidence that prompt dialysis can reduce the risk of NSF.

For patients with GFR < 15 mL/min:

- Use gadolinium only if it is absolutely necessary and there is no alternative.

For patients with GFR < 30 mL/min but > 15mL/min:

- Consider alternative imaging or no imaging.
- Inform the patient of specific risks and benefits.
- Use the lowest dose possible, but no more than half a dose.
- Add nonenhanced sequences if necessary.
- If gadolinium has to be used, adopt one of the following different strategies:

    o For patients already on dialysis — dialysis within 3 h, and the second dialysis within 24 h.
    o For patients on peritoneal dialysis — ensure there is no period with dry abdomen and more frequent exchanges in the next 48 h.
    o For patients not on dialysis — since dialysis also incurs risks, one-off hemodialysis or peritoneal dialysis can be spared.

- Refrain from gadolinium in the presence of a relatively protected space that allows accumulation of gadolinium (e.g. amniotic space, loculated ascites, pleural effusion).

Suggested Reading

Bakker J, Beek FJ, Beutler JJ, *et al.* (1998) Renal artery stenosis and accessory renal arteries: accuracy of detection and visualization with gadolinium-enhanced breath-hold MR angiography. *Radiology* 207:497–504.

De Cobelli F, Vanzulli A, Sironi S, *et al.* (1997) Renal artery stenosis: evaluation with breath-hold, three-dimensional, dynamic, gadolinium-enhanced versus three-dimensional, phase-contrast MR angiography. *Radiology* 205:689–695.

Deo A, Fogel M, Cowper SE. (2007) Nephrogenic systemic fibrosis: a population study examining the relationship of disease development to gadolinium exposure. *Clin J Am Soc Nephrol* 2:264–267.

Dong Q, Schoenberg SO, Carlos RC, *et al.* (1999) Diagnosis of renal vascular disease with MR angiography. *Radiographics* 19:1535–1554.

Hany TF, Debatin JF, Leung DA, Pfammatter T. (1997) Evaluation of the aor-toiliac and renal arteries: comparison of breath-hold, contrast-enhanced, three-dimensional MR angiography with conventional catheter angiography. *Radiology* 204:357–362.

Kawashima A, Vrtiska TJ, LeRoy AJ, *et al.* (2004) CT urography. *Radiographics* 24:S35–S54.

Lavely WC, Goetze S, Friedman KP, *et al.* (2007) Comparison of SPECT/CT, SPECT, and planar imaging with single- and dual-phase ^{99m}Tc-sestamibi parathyroid scintigraphy. *J Nucl Med* 48:1084–1089.

Leyendecker JR, Barnes CE, Zagoria RJ. (2008) MR urography: techniques and clinical applications. *Radiographics* 28:23–46.

Ota H, Takase K, Rikimaru H, *et al.* (2005) Quantitative vascular measurements in arterial occlusive disease. *Radiographics* 25:1141–1158.

Roe S, Cassidy MJ. (2000) Diagnosis and monitoring of renal dystrophy. *Curr Opin Nephrol Hypertens* 9:675–681.

Soulez G, Oliva VL, Turpin S, *et al.* (2000) Imaging of renovascular hypertension: respective values of renal scintigraphy, renal Doppler US, and MR angiography. *Radiographics* 20:1355–1368.

29

Imaging and Interventional Treatment of Dialysis-Related Problems

Andrew S. H. Lai and Ferdinand S. K. Chu

29.1 Temporary and Tunneled Catheter Access

29.1.1 *Simple/Straightforward Cases*

- Venous puncture guided by anatomical landmark is a practice of the past.
- The initial puncture is to be performed under ultrasound guidance.
- The catheter tip position is to be confirmed by fluoroscopy.
- The vein of first choice is the right internal jugular vein.
- Other choices include right external jugular vein, left internal and external jugular veins, subclavian vein, femoral vein, and translumbar/transhepatic access to inferior vena cava.
- Note that subclavian and brachiocephalic (continuation of subclavian vein) veins are prone to stenosis (Fig. 29.1), and that femoral veins are prone to infection.

29.1.2 *Difficult Cases*

29.1.2.1 *Ultrasound and Doppler Ultrasound*

- Ultrasound or Doppler ultrasound should be used in all cases to ascertain the presence or absence of the vein to be punctured.
- Routinely, bilateral internal jugular and subclavian veins are examined.
- The patency of the venous lumen is first assessed.
- The waveform of jugular and subclavian veins is usually very pulsatile due to phasic changes. When the waveform is dampened, it signifies problems (Fig. 29.2).

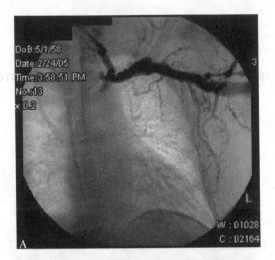

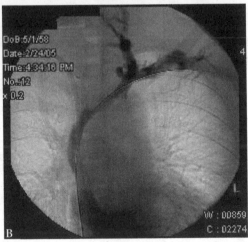

Fig. 29.1   Brachiocephalic vein stenosis, (A) pre- and (B) post-angioplasty.

- Brachiocephalic veins and superior vena cava are hidden behind bones, so they cannot be directly examined by ultrasound methods.
- When brachiocephalic or superior vena cava stenosis is clinically suspected, the collective findings on the bilateral subclavian and jugular veins can infer the likely site of obstruction.

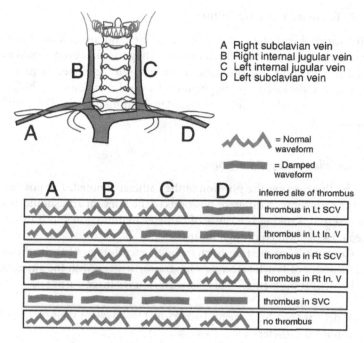

A Right subclavian vein
B Right internal jugular vein
C Left internal jugular vein
D Left subclavian vein

⋀⋁⋀ = Normal waveform

▬▬▬ = Damped waveform

A	B	C	D	inferred site of thrombus
⋀⋀	⋀⋀	⋀⋀	▬▬	thrombus in Lt SCV
⋀⋀	⋀⋀	▬▬	▬▬	thrombus in Lt In. V
▬▬	⋀⋀	⋀⋀	⋀⋀	thrombus in Rt SCV
▬▬	▬▬	⋀⋀	⋀⋀	thrombus in Rt In. V
▬▬	▬▬	▬▬	▬▬	thrombus in SVC
⋀⋀	⋀⋀	⋀⋀	⋀⋀	no thrombus

Fig. 29.2 The schematic depicts the way the site of thrombosis is inferred by the location of abnormal signs. In. V: innominate (brachiocephalic) vein; Lt: Left; Rt: right; SCV: subclavian vein; SVC: superior vena cava. [Adopted from Patel MC *et al. Radiology* 1999; 211: 579–583, used with permission].

29.1.2.2 *Venogram*

- Venogram is indicated when spectral Doppler suggests the presence of central vein obstruction.
- Venogram helps to map out the exact anatomy and configuration of the venous structure, which could be very complicated in a renal patient.
- The radiologist can then assess whether angioplasty or stent placement is feasible or necessary, prior to the insertion of the hemodialysis catheter.
- Note that when cannulating a peripheral vein is proved to be difficult by the bedside method, ultrasound with a linear high-frequency (7–12 Hz) probe should be used to locate a suitable vein for injection of contrast.

29.2 Tunneled Catheter Failure

All tunneled catheters eventually fail. Their failure can be due to various causes, some of which could be diagnosed or even solved by medical imaging. By the time a patient with catheter failure is sent to a radiologist, the nephrologist would have done all he/she could at the bedside, such as catheter flushing and dwelling with uirokinase.

29.2.1 *Fluoroscopy/Venogram*

Under fluoroscopy, the position of the catheter is noted. The position of the catheter with different positions of the relevant arm should also be assessed. Kinking is a cause of catheter malfunction and it can be treated using interventional means.

Contrast is injected, in turn, through each lumen of the catheter, and a series of fast-frame-rate venograms (usually with the superior vena cava) is performed. This maneuver serves three purposes:

- It detects the fibrin sheath (occurs in 13%–57% of malfunctioned tunneled catheters).
- It detects any downstream venous stenosis/obstruction.
- It detects whether the catheter is apposed to a vessel wall, thereby causing malfunction.

29.2.2 *Stripping of Tunneled Catheter*

A snare is passed to the site of the catheter tip via a femoral venous access. The snare is then tightened around the catheter, and a series of downward movements strips the fibrin sheath (if any) away from the catheter. The fibrin sheath is so common that empirical stripping of the catheter can be done sometimes even without actual visualization of the fibrin sheath.

29.2.3 *Alternatives to Fibrin Sheath Stripping*

A new catheter can be exchanged by the over-guidewire technique. A balloon catheter can be used as an adjunct to mechanically disrupt the fibrin sheath. Studies showed that there is no significant difference in patency rate between stripping, replacement of catheter, and replacement of catheter with balloon disruption of fibrin sheath.

29.3 Pre-arteriovenous Fistula Workup

Surgically created arteriovenous fistula (AVF) is the most reliable access for hemodialysis. Unfortunately, primary failure is not uncommon (approx. 25%). One quarter of newly created fistulas never reach maturity to be clinically useful.

Many studies have demonstrated that preoperative vascular mapping may help to revise the operative plan formulated following preoperative assessment by physical examination alone. In patients deemed to be "fit" as per assessment by preoperative ultrasound mapping for AVF creation, the primary failure is much lower. Assessment may reveal that the patient has small-caliber veins in the forearm, and hence it would only be suitable for the AV graft to be placed more proximally. Assessment may reveal central vein stenosis, which might require interventional treatment before hemodialysis could even be considered.

29.3.1 *Venous Anatomy*

Veins in the upper limbs could be assessed by ultrasound for:

- caliber
- patency.

The venous diameter tends to taper, as it runs distally. The cut-off diameter is between 2.5 mm and 3 mm (after application of tourniquet).

The central veins, i.e. those which are usually hidden behind bony structures and not amenable to direct visualization by ultrasound, can be indirectly assessed by performing spectral Doppler analysis of the bilateral jugular and subclavian veins. Any deviation from the normal pulsatile and phasic waveform is noted. The site of any possible central vein stenosis or obstruction could then be inferred. In case of any suspicion of stenosis or obstruction, findings could be confirmed by venogram with preoperative dilatation or stenting as appropriate.

29.3.2 *Arterial Anatomy*

Ulnar and radial arteries are assessed for:

- caliber
- atherosclerotic changes

- direction of flow
- flow velocity.

The cut-off diameter is about 2 mm.

29.4 Poor Flow in Arteriovenous Fistula or Polytetrafluoroethylene (PTFE) Graft

In patients with poor flow without upper limb swelling, thrombosis or focal stenosis must be considered.

29.4.1 *Acute Thrombosis (Fresh Clot)*

- Thrombosis can occur acutely with no clinically palpable thrill.
- Diagnosis can be made with Doppler ultrasound — acute/fresh thrombus tends to be hypoechogenic.
- The thrombus may be dissolved by catheter-directed thrombolysis, but this is a high-risk procedure that requires strong radiological support and intensive care unit (ICU)/high-dependency inpatient care.
- Thrombolysis can be achieved by the infusion or pulse-spray administration of a thrombolytic agent. Repeated fistulogram is needed for assessment.
- Once the thrombus is dissolved, fistulogram and venogram are required to identify the presence of any predisposing stenosis, which should then be treated (as per the section below) in order to eliminate the culprit of recurrent thrombosis.

29.4.2 *Focal Stenosis*

- Focal stenosis of AVF, most common along the venous limb, can be diagnosed using ultrasound by visualizing a focal area of turbulence.
- Fistulogram under fluoroscopy will confirm the diagnosis and guide the interventional treatment.
- Balloon dilatation is most often used to reopen the stenotic segment; often, a high-pressure balloon or even a cutting balloon is required for stenosis of AVF.
- Pain is often experienced by the patient; therefore, adequate sedation and/or local anesthetic infiltration around the stenotic segment is required.

- Recurrence of stenosis can be treated by repeated balloon dilatation.
- Metallic stenting is technically possible, but is usually not recommended since the location of the fistula is subject to trauma.

29.4.3 *Chronic Thrombosis*

- Chronic thrombosis is easily diagnosed by ultrasound, but is not amenable to interventional treatment.

In patients with poor flow accompanied with upper limb swelling, central venous obstruction or stenosis must be considered. Swelling is suggestive of a proximal vascular problem. Patients with a distal AVF may have a history of previous venous injury of the central veins due to repeated jugular or subclavian puncture/catheter insertion. Indirect assessment of the central veins using ultrasound may point to the culprit. It could be further assessed by venogram and treated by interventional means such as balloon dilatation or venous metallic stenting. A metallic stent, once deployed, is not retrievable and carries a risk of stent migration. Therefore, the decision to place a metallic stent in a central vein is not to be taken lightly. An oversized stent should be chosen to minimize the chance of stent migration, if necessary.

29.5 Complications Related to Continuous Ambulatory Peritoneal Dialysis (CAPD)

29.5.1 *Fluoroscopy*

Fluoroscopy is useful for the detection of catheter migration, breakage, or malposition (Fig. 29.3).

29.5.2 *Ultrasound*

- Ultrasound is useful in evaluating catheter exit-site infection.
- In appropriate cases, it can also guide ultrasound-guided aspiration of exit-site collection.

29.5.3 *Peritoneogram*

Peritoneogram can identify:

- loculated fluid collection
- adhesion

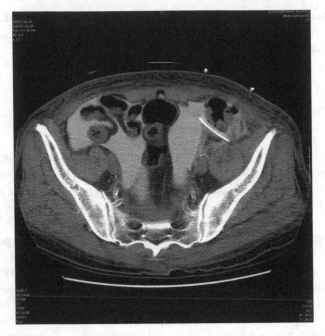

Fig. 29.3 Malposition of peritoneal dialysis catheter (arrow), as shown by computerized tomography (CT) scan of the abdomen.

- tunnel leak
- catheter migration, breakage, malposition
- catheter kink
- hernia
- retroperitoneal leakage
- leakage into other spaces such as pleural cavity and subcutaneous tissue.

After instillation of iodinated contrast into the peritoneal cavity via the CAPD catheter under aseptic precaution, CT peritoneogram is performed after thorough mixing with the peritoneal fluid (Fig. 29.4). It has been reported that instillation of gadolinium-based contrast would facilitate magnetic resonance (MR) peritoneogram; however, radiologists are hesitant to use this type of contrast agent in an enclosed space such as the peritoneal cavity, given the recent reports of nephrogenic systemic fibrosis. Making use of the contrast between the dialysate and adjacent tissue, one can perform MR peritoneogram without gadolinium contrast. This is a useful modality, but sometimes

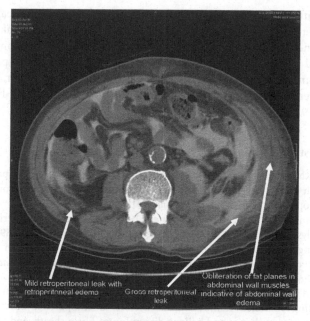

Fig. 29.4 CT peritoneogram showing retroperitoneal leakage.

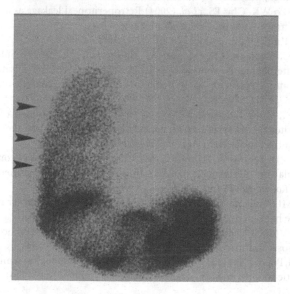

Fig. 29.5 ^{99m}Tc peritoneal scintigraphic peritoneogram showing increased radioactivity (arrowheads) in the right pleural cavity 60 min after intraperitoneal injection, suggesting a peritoneopleural leakage.

it is difficult to differentiate between a genuine retroperitoneal leak and a retroperitoneal edema or resolving retroperitoneal leak. MR peritoneogram with gadolinium cannot differentiate concomitant pleural effusion from diaphragmatic leakage. Scintigraphic peritoneogram lacks the anatomic details required for surgical repair, but is very sensitive in diagnosing leakage into pleural space and hernia (Fig. 29.5).

Suggested Reading

Berri RN, Lloyd LR. (2006) Detection of parathyroid adenoma in patients with primary hyperparathyroidism: the use of office-based ultrasound in preoperative localization. *Am J Surg* 191:311–314.

Cochran ST, Do HM, Ronaghi A, *et al.* (1997) Complications of peritoneal dialysis: evaluation with CT peritoneography. *Radiographics* 17:869–878.

Gooding GA, Hightower DR, Moore EH, *et al.* (1986) Obstruction of the superior vena cava or subclavian veins: sonographic diagnosis. *Radiology* 159:663–665.

Janne d'Othée B, Tham JC, Sheiman RG. (2006) Restoration of patency in failing tunneled hemodialysis catheters: a comparison of catheter exchange, exchange and balloon disruption of fibrin sheath, and femoral stripping. *J Vasc Interv Radiol* 17:1011–1015.

Lam MF, Lo WK, Chu FS, *et al.* (2004) Retroperitoneal leakage as a cause of ultrafiltration failure. *Perit Dial Int* 24:466–470.

National Kidney Foundation. (2006) *K/DOQI Guidelines 2006.*

Patel MC, Berman LH, Moss HA, McPherson SJ. (1999) Subclavian and internal jugular veins at Doppler US: abnormal cardiac pulsatility and respiratory phasicity as a predictor of complete central occlusion. *Radiology* 211:579–583.

Prischl FC, Muhr T, Seiringer EM, *et al.* (2002) Magnetic resonance imaging of peritoneal cavity among peritoneal dialysis patients, using the dialysate as "contrast medium". *J Am Soc Nephrol* 13:197–203.

Prokesch PW, Schima W, Schober E, *et al.* (2000) Complications of continuous ambulatory peritoneal dialysis: findings on MR peritoneography. *Am J Roentgenol* 174:987–991.

Robbin ML, Gallichio MH, Deierhoi MH, *et al.* (2000) US vascular mapping before hemodialysis access placement. *Radiology* 217:83–88.

Santilli J. (2002) Fibrin sheaths and central venous catheter occlusions: diagnosis and management. *Tech Vasc Interv Radiol* 5:89–94.

Surlan M, Popovic P. (2003) The role of interventional radiology in management of patients with end-stage renal disease. *Eur J Radiol* 46:96–114.

30

Imaging and Interventional Treatment of Renal Transplant-Related Problems

Ferdinand S. K. Chu and Andrew S. H. Lai

30.1 Imaging of the Donor

Prior to kidney donation, we have to ascertain that:

- the donor has two kidneys
- there is no anatomical abnormality in the kidneys

Usually, a gray-scale ultrasonic examination of the donor's kidneys would suffice. In case any significant abnormality is found, the usual line of investigation for kidney disorder should be followed.

In addition, the surgeon wishes to know detailed information about the vascular anatomy of donor kidneys, particularly:

- the number of main renal arteries
- any early branching
- any accessory branches

The traditional gold standard is digital subtraction angiography (DSA). Computerized tomography angiography (CTA) also provides good details of the vascular anatomy. It also provides additional anatomic information of the renal parenchyma, such as scarring, masses, or cysts. Moreover, if delayed scanning is performed, the structure of the pelvicalyceal system and ureters can be shown. Magnetic resonance angiography (MRA) has also been recently studied; however, it remains controversial whether the detailed vascular anatomy shown is as good as that by CTA.

30.2 Imaging of the Recipient

The recipient does not need imaging under normal circumstances. In patients who are suspected to have distorted vascular anatomy in or around the intended transplant site, imaging may be required. Doppler ultrasound should provide some useful information; but if it is not adequate, then a venogram/arteriogram would be the next step.

30.3 Graft Dysfunction and Other Graft Problems

Any pathology that affects the native kidney can inflict upon the graft. Examples are renal stone, tumor, and glomerulopathy. The line of investigations to follow is usually similar to that for disease of the native kidney; however, there are conditions that only affect the graft, but not the native kidney. Ultrasound is usually the first imaging modality to use for any problem with the graft kidney. It can usually differentiate between nephrological, surgical, and vascular problems.

30.3.1 Complications Related to Graft Renal Parenchyma

Often, sonographic appearance is nonspecific. Ultrasound is nevertheless mandatory for localization, if renal biopsy is contemplated.

30.3.1.1 Hyperacute Rejection

- Hyperacute rejection is a rare condition with accurate tissue typing.
- Doppler examination may reveal total absence of perfusion.
- DSA examination or scintigraphy shows no perfusion.

30.3.1.2 Acute Rejection

- The ultrasonic appearance of the graft is often normal on gray-scale ultrasound.
- Doppler examination of the intrarenal arteries often reveals an elevated resistivity index >0.8; this is, however, a nonspecific finding.
- A resistivity index of >0.9 is usually suggestive of acute rejection.
- The diagnosis is confirmed by renal biopsy under ultrasound guidance.

30.3.1.3 *Chronic Rejection*

- Radiological findings are nonspecific.
- Ultrasound shows a generalized increase in parenchymal echogenicity, akin to chronic renal parenchymal disease in native kidneys.

30.3.2 *Acute Tubular Necrosis*

- No diagnostic sonographic feature is visible.
- The perfusion is normal in scintigraphy, but later phases of ^{99m}Tc-DTPA or Hippuran/^{99m}Tc-MAG3 show slow wash-out and persistent isotope accumulation (Fig. 30.1).

30.3.3 *Cyclosporine Nephrotoxicity*

- No diagnostic sonographic feature is visible.
- Scintigraphy shows prolonged clearance of Hippuran/^{99m}Tc-MAG3.
- Cyclosporine level in blood and renal biopsy are the confirmatory tests.

30.4 Surgical Complications of Graft Kidneys

30.4.1 *Obstructive Uropathy*

- Different from native kidney, stone is a rare cause of obstructive uropathy. The usual cause is blood clot, anastomotic site edema, or anastomotic stricture.
- Ultrasound is extremely useful in diagnosing obstructive uropathy by visualizing a dilated pelvicalyceal system or even part of the ureter (Fig. 30.2).
- The resistivity index determined by Doppler ultrasound is usually high in obstructive uropathy.
- Ultrasound combined with fluoroscopy is useful in performing a percutaneous nephrostomy (PCN) in order to relieve the obstruction.
- An antegrade pyelogram can identify the site and possible nature of the obstruction with the PCN *in situ* (Fig. 30.3).
- It is possible that a patient could have a dilated ureter/pelvicalyceal system without having obstruction. In the case of genuine obstruction, scintigraphy with ^{99m}Tc-DTPA scan shows a normal perfusion

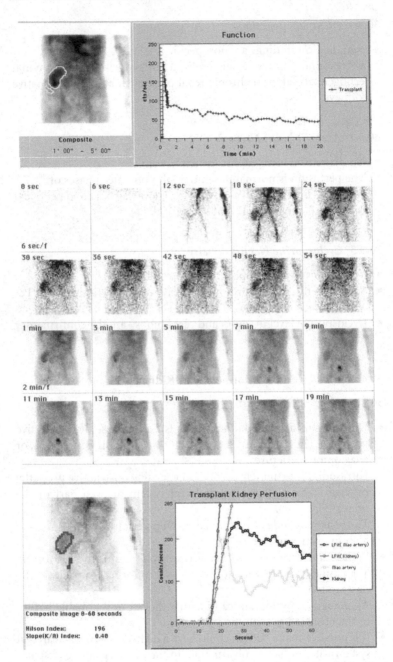

Fig. 30.1 Radionuclide scintigraphy in a renal transplant patient with acute tubular necrosis.

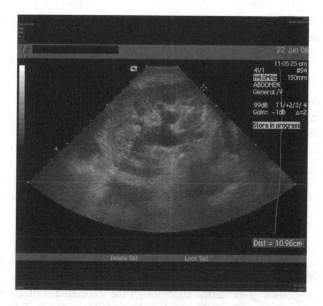

Fig. 30.2 Ultrasound showing a dilated pelvicalyceal system of the transplanted kidney.

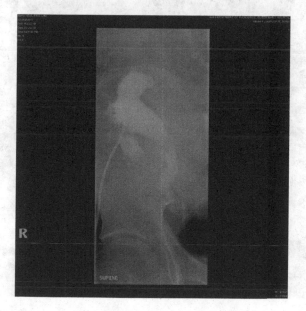

Fig. 30.3 An antegrade pyelogram identifying the site of obstruction with the PCN *in situ.*

phase yet prolongation of the excretory phase, with an ascending slope of the renogram curve.

30.4.2 Perinephric Collection

- Nonspecific sonographic features are visible.
- Lymphocele is the most common posttransplant perinephric collection (Fig. 30.4).
- Abscess or hematoma can sometimes be distinguished by its complex content.
- The diagnosis of abscess or hematoma is usually clinical, and sometimes is combined with ultrasound-guided aspiration or drainage.

30.4.3 Vascular Complications of Graft Kidney

Vascular complications are diverse. They have different etiologies and presentations. Doppler ultrasound gives excellent information. DSA is the diagnostic gold standard, although the iodinated contrast poses a risk of nephrotoxicity. DSA also has the added benefit of a follow-on

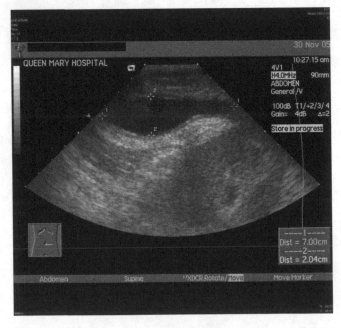

Fig. 30.4 Ultrasound of a transplanted kidney showing a lymphocele.

intervention procedure. DSA could be performed using CO_2 and has been shown to give similar information. Similarly, computed tomography (CT) is associated with a risk of contrast nephropathy. Magnetic resonance imaging (MRI) is also associated with contrast risk, especially in patients with a poor glomerular filtration rate (GFR).

30.4.3.1 Renal Arterial Occlusion

- It is often accompanied by acute rejection.
- Doppler ultrasound shows an absence of flow.
- DSA would be confirmatory, but there is an associated contrast risk.
- CT/MRI is supposed to show an absence of or decreased perfusion, but is generally not advisable.

30.4.3.2 Renal Arterial Stenosis

- The principle of diagnosis is the same as for renal artery stenosis in the native kidney.
- However, the graft renal artery does not arise from the aorta; therefore, the reno-aortic ratio measured in Doppler ultrasound does not play a part.
- Doppler features of graft renal artery stenosis include a high systolic velocity of >2.5–3 m/s with delayed upstroke of intrarenal arteries.
- Beware of kinks in the arterial anastomosis, which can simulate stenosis.
- DSA is the diagnostic gold standard. It can then be followed by appropriate intervention such as balloon dilatation or stenting. It should be noted that these should be proceeded with very cautiously in the immediate posttransplant period (Fig. 30.5).

30.4.3.3 Renal Vein Stenosis and Thrombosis

- These are rare in posttransplant kidneys.
- In renal vein stenosis, a focal narrowing might be visualized, often with turbulence, by Doppler ultrasound.
- In renal vein thrombosis, Doppler ultrasound shows an absence of flow in the veins with high-resistance flow in the renal arteries.

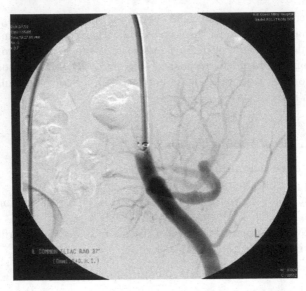

Fig. 30.5   DSA showing renal artery stenosis (arrow) of the transplant kidney.

30.5 Arteriovenous Fistula (AVF) and Pseudoaneurysm

- These usually occur as complications of interventional procedures such as biopsy and percutaneous nephrostomy.
- These can occur in native as well as graft kidneys.
- AVF is depicted as an abnormal communication between the arterial and venous sides by Doppler ultrasound, with low-resistance arterial inflow.
- Pseudoaneurysm is depicted as a rounded vascular structure with flow by Doppler ultrasound.
- AVF fistulae can be self-limiting; if not, both AVF and pseudoaneurysm should be treated by angiographic embolization.
- DSA is the gold standard in diagnosis, and is essential if intervention is indicated.

Suggested Reading

Diaz JM, Guirado L, Facundo C, *et al.* (2006) Assessment of the arteries in living kidney donors: correlation of magnetic resonance angiography with intraoperative findings. *Transplant Proc* 38:2376–2377.

Janoff DM, Davol P, Hazzard J, *et al.* (2004) Computerized tomography with 3-dimensional reconstruction for the evaluation of renal size and arterial anatomy in the living kidney donor. *J Urol* 171:27–30.

Kim JC, Kim CD, Jang MH, *et al.* (2007) Can magnetic resonance angiogram be a reliable alternative for donor evaluation for laparoscopic nephrectomy? *Clin Transplant* 21:126–135.

Rajiah P, Lim YY, Taylor P. (2006) Renal transplant imaging and complications. *Abdom Imaging* 31:735–746.

Part VI
Drug Use in Renal Patients

31

Drug Doses in Patients with Renal Impairment

Siu-Kim Chan and Laurence K. Chan

The kidney is the major regulator of the internal environment and also an important organ involved in the elimination of drugs. Changes in the absorption, distribution, metabolism, and excretion of drugs and their active metabolites are common in patients with impaired renal function. If a drug or its metabolites are primarily excreted through the kidneys and increased drug levels are associated with adverse effects, drug dosages must be reduced in patients with renal impairment to avoid toxicity. It is therefore important to understand the basic principles of pharmacokinetic properties and various processes controlling the clearance of drugs from the body in patients with renal impairment. Furthermore, the optimal therapeutic regimen for a patient with renal impairment requires knowledge of the degree and type of pharmacokinetic alterations of a given drug, which are associated with the patient's degree of renal impairment.

31.1 Influence of Renal Impairment on Drug Absorption and Bioavailability

Before drugs have systemic effects, they must be absorbed into the body and metabolized into their active form. Bioavailability can be affected in patients with renal failure. Vomiting and impaired peristalsis due to uremic enteropathy may reduce the drug absorption rate. Drugs commonly used in renal failure, including phosphate binders and proton pump inhibitors, reduce acidic drug absorption; while phosphate binders also form a complex with certain antibiotics and iron tablets. Renal failure frequently causes gastrointestinal tract

Table 31.1 Bioavailability of drugs in patients with renal impairment.

Decreased bioavailability	Increased bioavailability
Furosemide	Dihydrocodein
Pindolol	Erythromycin
	Propanaolol
	Tacrolimus

edema, which further affects drug absorption. Examples of altered bioavailability with renal impairment are listed in Table 31.1.

31.2 Influence of Renal Impairment on Volume of Distribution and Protein Binding

The volume of distribution (V_d) of drugs extensively bound to plasma proteins, but not to tissue components, approaches the plasma volume. For example, in a typical 70-kg human, the plasma volume is ~3 L and extracellular water outside the vasculature is ~42 L; the V_d for warfarin is close to 3 L. By contrast, for drugs highly bound to tissues, the V_d of digoxin and tricyclic antidepressants approximates hundreds of liters. Such drugs are not readily removed by dialysis.

A number of factors can also affect the V_d of an individual drug. These include body size, age, gender, renal function, protein binding, and presence of other drugs. A decrease in protein binding causes an increase in V_d. Renal impairment induces a decrease in the ability of plasma proteins to bind certain drugs, especially for acidic drugs existing as anions in blood. The possible mechanisms include a reduction in binding protein concentration, competitive displacement from normal binding sites in tissue, or synthesis of a protein with reduced binding sites.

For drugs that are normally highly protein-bound to plasma proteins, small changes in the extent of binding due to renal impairment produce a large change in the amount of unbound drugs, and hence susceptibility to toxicity for a drug with a narrow therapeutic ratio. Hypoalbuminemia, commonly seen in renal failure, may increase the free fraction of drugs appearing in the plasma. So, drug efficacy and toxicity are enhanced if total (free + bound) drug concentration is used to monitor therapy. Conversely, an increased binding can lead to reduced pharmacologic effects on the therapeutic concentration

Table 31.2   Effect of renal impairment on the distribution of selected drugs.

Drug	Normal (L/kg)	ESRD (L/kg)
Increased distribution		
Amikacin	0.20	0.29
Cefazolin	0.13	0.16
Cefuroxime	0.20	0.26
Cloxacillin	0.14	0.26
Erythromycin	0.57	1.09
Furosemide	0.11	0.18
Gentamicin	0.20	0.29
Isoniazid	0.60	0.80
Minoxidil	2.60	4.90
Phenytoin	0.64	1.40
Trimethoprim	1.36	1.83
Vancomycin	0.64	0.85
Decreased distribution		
Digoxin	7.30	4.10
Ethambutol	3.70	1.60
Pindolol	2.10	1.10

ESRD: end-stage renal disease.

of a total drug. Examples of drug distribution affected by renal impairment are shown in Table 31.2.

31.3 Influence of Renal Impairment on Drug Elimination

Most drugs undergo biotransformation to metabolites, which are then excreted. The usual pathways of drug metabolism include oxidation, reduction, and hydrolysis. The renal component of drug clearance will be reduced in renal failure patients, while hepatic metabolism may be increased as a compensatory mechanism. Hepatic metabolism of some drugs, however, will be slower in renal failure patients (e.g. propranolol oxidation, hydrocortisone reduction, cephalosporin hydrolysis).

The renal elimination of drugs depends on the glomerular filtration, tubular secretion and reabsorption, and renal epithelial cell metabolism. Glomerular filtration is obviously affected in renal failure, while tubular secretion and reabsorption could be influenced by decreased renal blood flow. Organic acids accumulated in renal failure compete with the acidic drugs like diuretics for tubular secretion.

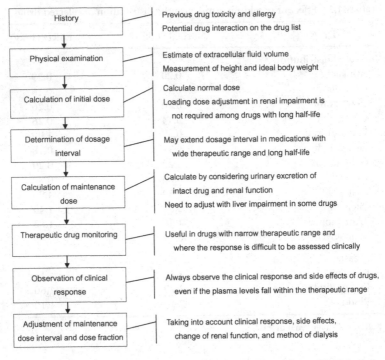

Fig. 31.1 Approach to dosage determination in patients with renal impairment.

Insulin catabolism relies on renal parenchymal enzymes, and will be declined in the uremic state.

31.4 Dosing of Drugs in the Presence of Renal Impairment

31.4.1 *Calculation of Initial Dose*

$$\text{Loading dose} = V_d \text{ (L/kg)} \times \text{IBW (kg)} \times C_p \text{ (mg/L)},$$

Where V_d = volume of distribution of the drug
 IBW = patient's ideal body weight
 C_p = desired plasma drug concentration.

31.4.2 *Calculation of Dose Fraction of Maintenance Dose*

$$\text{Dose fraction} = F[(\text{CrCl}/120) - 1] + 1,$$

where   F = fraction of the drug excreted unchanged in the urine
       CrCl = creatinine clearance.

31.4.3 The Cockcroft–Gault Equation for Estimating Creatinine Clearance

$$CrCl = \frac{(140 - age) \times IBW}{72 \times Scr} \times (0.85 \text{ if female}),$$

where   CrCl = creatinine clearance (mL/min)
           Scr = serum creatinine (mg/dL)
  IBW(kg) of men = 50 kg + 2.3 kg per 2.54 cm over 150 cm
IBW(kg) of women = 45.5 kg + 2.3 kg per 2.54 cm over 150 cm.

31.5 Drug Removal During Hemodialysis and Peritoneal Dialysis

Several factors affect the efficiency of drug removal by hemodialysis. The most crucial factor is the molecular weight of the drug: drugs larger than 500 Da are mainly removed by convection. Drugs with high lipid solubility tend to accumulate in the lipophilic tissue and have large V_d, while high protein binding of drugs limits the availability of free drugs for dialysis. The pore size of the dialysis filter obviously affects the clearing of drugs; other dialysis parameters like blood flow, dialysate flow, and ultrafiltration rate also determine the drug clearance.

Peritoneal dialysis has low drug clearance. Those dialyzable drugs should be small in size and have low V_d. Due to protein loss during peritoneal dialysis, drugs with high protein binding may be removed more substantially.

31.6 Drug Removal During Continuous Renal Replacement Therapy (CRRT)

Drugs are cleared in CRRT by convection. Their efficiency can be expressed by the sieving coefficient (SC). SC is the ratio of the solute concentration in the ultrafiltrate (UF) to the concentration in the arterial blood (A):

$$SC = [UF]/[A].$$

Drug clearance can be calculated as:

$$SC \times UF \text{ rate.}$$

Factors affecting the SC include the drug-membrane binding and the charge of the molecules. Protein binding also limits the portion of free drugs for filtration.

31.7 Therapeutic Drug Monitoring

Monitoring of drug levels is most useful for drugs with a narrow therapeutic range and where the drug response is difficult to be assessed clinically. The peak level should be obtained 30 min after intravenous dose when the steady state is achieved. The trough level is drawn just prior to the next dose.

Suggested Reading

Aronoff GR, Bennett WM, Berns JS, *et al.* (2007) *Drug Prescribing in Renal Failure: Dosing Guidelines for Adults and Children*, 5th ed. American College of Physicians, Philadelphia, PA, pp. 73, 97–100, 170, 171.

Burton ME, Shaw LM, Schentag JJ, Evans WB. (2006) *Applied Pharmacokinetics and Pharmacodynamics*, 4th ed. Lippincott Williams & Wilkins, Baltimore, pp. 187–212.

Schrier RW (ed.). (2007) *Diseases of the Kidney and Urinary Tract*, 8th ed. Lippincott Williams & Wilkins, Philadelphia, pp. 2765–2802.

32

Recommended Maintenance Drug Doses in Patients with Renal Impairment and in HD/CAPD/CVVH

Laurence K. Chan and Siu-Kim Chan

This chapter summarizes the dosage of common medication for subjects with normal or impaired renal function. In the latter, the dose is adjusted according to the renal function defined by the glomerular filtration rate (GFR). The medication regime of frequently used drugs for patients undergoing dialytic renal replacement therapy — herit hemodialysis (HD), continuous ambulatory peritoneal dialysis (CAPD), or continuous venovenous hemofiltration (CVVH) — is also outlined.

The kidney may be the site for degradation of certain compounds such as insulin. Electrolyte disturbance and renal impairment may confound drug effects (e.g. hypokalemia and digitalis toxicity). Concurrent drug use may also interfere with the metabolism and excretion of individual compounds (e.g. reduced renal excretion of penicillin by probenecid). The dialytic clearance of drugs should be taken into consideration in patients on dialysis. Hemodialysis is very efficient in clearing small molecules with low protein binding. Scheduled or supplementary doses after dialysis should be given. The peritoneal clearance of drugs can be estimated from the molecular weight of the compound:

$$\frac{\text{Peritoneal clearance of the drug}}{\text{Peritoneal clearance of creatinine}}$$

$$= \sqrt{\frac{\text{molecular weight of creatinine}}{\text{molecular weight of the drug}}}.$$

Strong electrostatic charge and protein binding decrease the peritoneal clearance of a drug, while lipid solubility results in an increase.

32.1 Antibiotics[a]

32.1.1 Aminoglycoside Antibiotics

Drugs	Normal dosage	Dosage adjustment in renal failure			HD	CAPD	CVVH
		GFR > 50	GFR 10–50	GFR < 10			
Gentamicin	1.7 mg/kg q8h	q12–24h	q24–48h	q48–72h	1/2 full dose after HD	3–4 mg/L/d	dose for GFR 10–50
Tobramycin	1.7 mg/kg q8h	q12–24h	q24–48h	q48–72h	1/2 full dose after HD	3–4 mg/L/d	dose for GFR 10–50
Netilmicin	2 mg/kg q8h	q12–24h	q24–48h	q48–72h	1/2 full dose after HD	3–4 mg/L/d	dose for GFR 10–50
Amikacin	7.5 mg/kg q12h	q12–24h	q24–48h	q48–72h	1/2 full dose after HD	15–20 mg/L/d	dose for GFR 10–50
Streptomycin	7.5 mg/kg q12h	q24h	q24–72h	q72–96h	1/2 normal dose after HD	20–40 mg/L/d	dose for GFR 10–50

(Continued)

Drugs	Normal dosage	Dosage adjustment in renal failure			HD	CAPD	CVVH
		GFR > 50	GFR 10–50	GFR < 10			
32.1.2 Cephalosporin							
Ceftibuten	400 mg q12h	normal dose	normal dose	50% dose	300 mg after HD	dose for GFR < 10	dose for GFR 10–50
Cefuroxime	250–500 mg bid	normal dose	normal dose	normal dose	dose after HD	dose for GFR < 10	no data
Cefuroxime (IV)	0.75–1.5g q8h	q8h	q8–12h	q12–24h	dose after dialysis	dose for GFR < 10	1 g q12h
Cefazolin	1–2 g q8h	q8h	q12h	q12–24h	0.5–1 g after HD	0.5 g q12h	dose for GFR 10–50
Cefepime	1–2 g q8h	q8–12h	q12h	q24h	1 g after HD	dose for GFR < 10	dose for GFR 10–50
Cefoperazone/ Sulbactam	1–2 g q12h	normal dose	1 g q12h	500 mg q12h	1 g after HD	dose for GFR < 10	no data
Ceftazidime	1–2 g q8h	q8h	q12h	q24h	1 g after HD	0.5 g/d	dose for GFR 10–50
Cefotaxime	1–2 g q6–q8h	q8h	q12h	q12–24h	1 g after HD	1 g/d	1 g q12h
Ceftriaxone	1–2 g q12–24h	normal dose	normal dose	normal dose	dose after HD	750 mg q12h	dose for GFR 10–50
Cephalexin	250–500 mg tid	normal dose	normal dose	normal dose	dose after HD	dose for GFR < 10	no data

(Continued)

(Continued)

Drugs	Normal dosage	Dosage adjustment in renal failure			HD	CAPD	CVVH
		GFR > 50	GFR 10–50	GFR < 10			
32.1.3 Penicillin (Oral)							
Amoxicillin	500 mg tid	normal dose	normal dose	50–75%	dose after HD	250 mg q12h	dose for GFR 10–50
Amoxicillin/ Clavulanate	250–500 mg q8h	normal dose	q8–12h	q24h	dose during and after HD	q12h	q12h
Ampicillin	500 mg q6h	normal dose	normal dose	50–75%	dose after HD	250 mg q12h	dose for GFR 10–50
Cloxacillin	250–500 mg q6h	normal dose	normal dose	normal dose	no adjustment	no adjustment	no adjustment
32.1.4 Penicillin (IV)							
Ampicillin	1–2 g q6h	q6h	q8h	q12h	dose after HD	250 mg q12h	dose for GFR 10–50
Ampicillin/ Sulbactam	1.5–3 g q6–8h	normal dose	q8–12h	q24h	dose after HD	q24h	dose for GFR 10–50
Penicillin G	2–3 MU q4h	q4–q6h	q6h	q8h	dose after HD	dose for GFR < 10	dose for GFR 10–50
Piperacillin	3–4 g q4–6h	normal dose	normal dose	normal dose	dose after HD	dose for GFR < 10	dose for GFR 10–50

(Continued)

(Continued)

Drugs	Normal dosage	Dosage adjustment in renal failure			HD	CAPD	CVVH
		GFR > 50	GFR 10–50	GFR < 10			
Piperacillin/ Tazobactam	4.5/3.375 g q6–8h	normal dose	3.375/2.25 g q6h	2.25 g q6–8h	dose after HD	dose for GFR < 10	dose for GFR 10–50
Ticarcillin/ Clavulanate	3.1 g q4–6h	q8h	q8–12h	q12h	suppl dose after HD	dose for GFR < 10	dose for GFR 10–50
32.1.5 Quinolones							
Ciprofloxacin	200–400 mg q12h	normal dose	q12–24h	q24h	200 mg q24h	200 mg q24h	200 mg q12h
Levofloxacin	500 mg daily	normal dose	250 mg q24–48h	250 mg q48h	dose for GFR < 10	dose for GFR < 10	dose for GFR 10–50
Moxifloxacin	400 mg daily	normal dose	normal dose	normal dose	no adjustment	no adjustment	no adjustment
Nalidixic acid	1 g q6h	normal dose	avoid use	avoid use	avoid use	avoid use	no data
Norfloxacin	400 mg q12h	q12h	q12–24h	q24h	dose for GFR < 10	dose for GFR < 10	no data
Ofloxacin	200–400 mg q12h	q12h	q12–24h	q24h	100–200 mg after HD	dose for GFR < 10	300 mg/d

(Continued)

(Continued)

Drugs	Normal dosage	Dosage adjustment in renal failure			HD	CAPD	CVVH
		GFR > 50	GFR 10–50	GFR < 10			
32.1.6 Macrolides							
Azithromycin	250–500 mg bid	normal dose	normal dose	normal dose	no adjustment	no adjustment	no adjustment
Clarithromycin	500 mg bid	normal dose	normal dose	normal dose	no adjustment	no adjustment	no adjustment
Clindamycin	150–450 mg tid	normal dose	normal dose	normal dose	no adjustment	no adjustment	no adjustment
Erythromycin	250–500 mg qid	normal dose	normal dose	normal dose	no adjustment	no adjustment	no adjustment
32.1.7 Carbapenem							
Aztreonam	0.5–2 g q8–12h	normal dose	50–100% dose	25% dose	suppl 12.5% dose	dose for GFR < 10	q12h
Ertapenem	1 g q24h	normal dose	0.5–1 g q24h	500 mg q24h	suppl 150 mg if last dose given within 6 h of HD	no data	no data

(Continued)

(Continued)

Drugs	Normal dosage	Dosage adjustment in renal failure			HD	CAPD	CVVH
		GFR > 50	GFR 10–50	GFR < 10			
Imipenem/ Cilastatin	250–500 mg q6h	500 mg q8h	250–500 mg q8–12h	250 mg q12h	dose after HD	dose for GFR < 10	dose for GFR 10–50
Meropenem	1 g q8h	1 g q8h	0.5–1g q12h	0.5–1 g q24h	dose after HD	dose for GFR < 10	dose for GFR 10–50
32.1.8 *Other Antibiotics*							
Doxycycline	100–200 mg/d qd to bid dose	normal dose	normal dose	normal dose	no adjustment	no adjustment	no adjustment
Metronidazole	500 mg q6–8h	normal dose	normal dose	normal dose	dose after HD	dose for GFR < 10	dose for GFR 10–50
Pentamidine	4 mg/kg/d	q24h	q24–36h	q48h	no adjustment	no adjustment	no adjustment q18h
Trimethoprim/ Sulfamethoxazole	960 mg bid q12h	q18h	q12h (50%)	q24h (50%)	dose after HD	q24h	
Vancomycin	1 g q12h	q12h	q24–48h	q48–72h	suppl 0.5–1 g after HD	q48–72h	500 mg q12h

(Continued)

(Continued)

Drugs	Normal dosage	Dosage adjustment in renal failure			HD	CAPD	CVVH
		GFR > 50	GFR 10–50	GFR < 10			
32.2 Antituberculosis Antibiotics							
Ethambutol	15–25 mg/kg/d	normal dose	q24–36h	q48h	dose after HD	dose for GFR < 10	dose for GFR 10–50
Isoniazid	300 mg daily	normal dose	normal dose	may reduce (50% in slow acetylator)	dose after HD	dose for GFR < 10	dose for GFR < 10
Rifampicin	300–600 mg daily	normal dose	normal dose	normal dose	no adjustment	no adjustment	no adjustment
Pyrazinamide	15–30 mg/kg/d	normal dose	reduce dose to 12–20 mg/ kg/d or usual dose 3 times per week	avoid use	avoid use	avoid use	avoid use

(Continued)

(Continued)

Drugs	Normal dosage	Dosage adjustment in renal failure			HD	CAPD	CVVH
		GFR > 50	GFR 10–50	GFR < 10			
32.3 Antifungal Agents							
Amphotericin B (lipid)	0.5–1.5 mg/kg/d	normal dose	normal dose	q24–36h	no adjustment	no adjustment	no adjustment
Fluconazole	200–800 mg/d	normal dose	normal dose	50% dose	200 mg after HD	dose for GFR < 10	dose for GFR 10–50
Flucytosine	25–37.5 mg/kg q6h	q12h	q12–24h	q24h	dose after HD	0.5–1 g/d	dose for GFR 10–50
Griseofulvin	125–250 mg q6h	normal dose	normal dose	normal dose	no adjustment	no adjustment	no adjustment
Itroconazole	200 mg q12h	normal dose	normal dose	50% dose	100 mg q12–24h	100 mg q12–24h	100 mg q12–24h
Ketoconazole	200–400 mg daily	normal dose	normal dose	normal dose	no adjustment	no adjustment	no adjustment
Terbinafine	250 mg daily	normal dose	use half-normal dose if CrCl < 50	normal dose	no adjustment	no adjustment	no adjustment

(Continued)

(Continued)

Drugs	Normal dosage	Dosage adjustment in renal failure			HD	CAPD	CVVH
		GFR > 50	GFR 10–50	GFR < 10			
32.4 Antiviral Agents							
Acyclovir (oral)	200–800 mg 5x/d	normal dose	q8h	q12h	dose after HD	dose for GFR < 10	3.5 mg/kg/d
Acyclovir (IV)	5–10 mg/kg q8h	normal dose	q12–24h	50% q24h	dose after HD	50% daily	5–7.5 mg/kg/d
Adefovir	10 mg daily	normal dose	q48–72h	q1wk	dose after HD	no data	no data
Amantadine	100–200 mg q12h	normal dose	50% dose	25% dose	no adjustment	no adjustment	dose for GFR 10–50
Cidofovir	5 mg/kg qwk × 2 (induction), 5 mg/kg q2wk (maintenance)	50–100%	avoid use	avoid use	avoid use	avoid use	no data
Entecavir	0.5–1 mg daily	normal dose	q48–72h	q1wk	dose after HD	dose for GFR < 10	no data
Famciclovir	250–500 mg bid/tid	q8h	q12h	q24h	dose after HD	no data	dose for GFR 10–50

(Continued)

(Continued)

Drugs	Normal dosage	Dosage adjustment in renal failure			HD	CAPD	CVVH
		GFR > 50	GFR 10–50	GFR < 10			
Foscarnet	40–80 mg/kg q8h	20–40 mg/kg q8–24h according to CrCl (see package insert)			dose after HD	dose for GFR < 10	dose for GFR 10–50
Ganciclovir (IV)	5 mg/kg q12h	q12h	q24h	2.5 mg/kg qd	dose after HD	dose for GFR < 10	2.5 mg/kg q24h
Ganciclovir (PO)	1000 mg tid	1000 mg tid	1000 mg bid	1000 mg qd	dose after HD	dose for GFR < 10	no data
Lamivudine	150 mg bid (HIV)	100%	q24h	50 mg q24h	dose after HD	dose for GFR < 10	dose for GFR 10–50
	100 mg qd (HBV)	100%	50 mg q24h	25 mg q24h	dose after HD	dose for GFR < 10	dose for GFR 10–50
Ribavirin	500–600 mg q12h	normal dose	normal dose	normal dose	dose after HD	dose for GFR < 10	dose for GFR 10–50
Ritonavir	600 mg q12h	normal dose	normal dose	normal dose	no adjustment	dose for GFR < 10	dose for GFR 10–50
Telbivudine	600 mg daily	normal dose	q48–72h	q96h	dose after HD	no data	no data

(Continued)

(Continued)

Drugs	Normal dosage	Dosage adjustment in renal failure			HD	CAPD	CVVH
		GFR > 50	GFR 10–50	GFR < 10			
Valacyclovir	500–1000 mg q8h	normal dose	50% dose	25% dose	dose after HD	dose for GFR < 10	dose for GFR 10–50
Zidovudine	300 mg q12h	normal dose	normal dose	100 mg q8h	dose after HD	dose for GFR < 10	100 mg q8h
32.5 Analgesics							
Acetaminophen	500 mg q4h	normal dose	normal dose	normal dose	no adjustment	no adjustment	dose for GFR 10–50
Acetylsalicylic acid	650 mg q4h	q4h	q4–6h	avoid	dose after HD	no adjustment	dose for GFR 10–50
Codeine	30–60 mg q4–6h	normal dose	75% dose	50% dose	no data	no data	dose for GFR 10–50
Fentanyl	individualized	normal dose	75% dose	50% dose	not applicable	not applicable	not applicable
Methadone	2.5–5 mg q6–8h	normal dose	normal dose	50–70% dose	no adjustment	no adjustment	no data
Morphine	20–25 mg q4h	normal dose	75% dose	50% dose	no adjustment	no data	dose for GFR 10–50
Naloxone	0.4–2 mg	normal dose	normal dose	normal dose	not applicable	not applicable	dose for GFR 10–50

(Continued)

(Continued)

32.6 Antihypertensive Drugs and Diuretics

32.6.1 ACE Inhibitors

Drugs	Normal dosage	Dosage adjustment in renal failure			HD	CAPD	CVVH
		GFR > 50	GFR 10–50	GFR < 10			
Benazepril	10–80 mg daily	normal dose	75% dose	25–50% dose	no adjustment	no adjustment	dose for GFR 10–50
Captopril	6.25–100 mg tid	normal dose	75% dose	50% dose	suppl 25–30% dose	no adjustment	dose for GFR 10–50
Enalapril	5 mg qd–20 mg bd	normal dose	75% dose	50% dose	suppl 20–25% dose	no adjustment	dose for GFR 10–50
Fosinopril	10 mg qd–20 mg bd	normal dose	normal dose	75% dose	no adjustment	no adjustment	dose for GFR 10–50
Lisinopril	2.5 mg qd–20 mg bd	normal dose	50–75% dose	25–50% dose	suppl 20% dose	no adjustment	dose for GFR 10–50
Perindopril	2–16 mg qd	normal dose	75% dose	25% dose	suppl 25–50% dose	no data	dose for GFR 10–50
Quinapril	10–20 mg qd	normal dose	75–100% dose	75% dose	suppl 25% dose	no adjustment	dose for GFR 10–50
Ramipril	2.5 mg qd–10 mg bd	normal dose	50–75% dose	25–50% dose	suppl 20% dose	no adjustment	dose for GFR 10–50

(Continued)

(Continued)

Drugs	Normal dosage	Dosage adjustment in renal failure			HD	CAPD	CVVH
		GFR > 50	GFR 10–50	GFR < 10			
32.6.2 Angiotensin II Receptor Blockers							
Candesartan	16–32 mg qd	normal dose	normal dose	50% dose	no adjustment	no adjustment	no adjustment
Eprosartan	400–800 mg qd	normal dose	normal dose	normal dose	no adjustment	no adjustment	no adjustment
Irbesartan	150–300 mg qd	normal dose	normal dose	normal dose	no adjustment	no adjustment	no adjustment
Losartan	50–100 mg qd	normal dose	normal dose	normal dose	no data	no data	dose for GFR 10–50
Telmisartan	20–80 mg qd	normal dose	normal dose	normal dose	no adjustment	no adjustment	no adjustment
Valsartan	80–160 mg qd	normal dose	normal dose	normal dose	no adjustment	no adjustment	no adjustment
32.6.3 Beta Blockers							
Atenolol	25–100 mg qd	normal dose	75% dose	50% dose	suppl 25–50 mg	no adjustment	dose for GFR 10–50
Carvedilol	3.125 mg bd– 25 mg tid	normal dose	normal dose	normal dose	no adjustment	no adjustment	dose for GFR 10–50

(Continued)

(Continued)

Drugs	Normal dosage	Dosage adjustment in renal failure			HD	CAPD	CVVH
		GFR > 50	GFR 10–50	GFR < 10			
Esmolol (IV)	50–300 mcg/kg/min	normal dose	normal dose	normal dose	no adjustment	no adjustment	no data
Labetalol	50–400 mg bid	normal dose	normal dose	normal dose	no adjustment	no adjustment	dose for GFR 10–50
Metoprolol	50–100 mg bid	normal dose	normal dose	normal dose	no adjustment	no adjustment	no adjustment
Nadolol	80 mg qd–160 mg bid	normal dose	50% dose	25% dose	suppl 40 mg	no adjustment	dose for GFR 10–50
Pindolol	10–40 mg bid	normal dose	normal dose	normal dose	no adjustment	no adjustment	dose for GFR 10–50
Propranolol	10–80 mg tid	normal dose	normal dose	normal dose	no adjustment	no adjustment	dose for GFR 10–50
Sotalol	80–160 mg bid	normal dose	50% dose	25–50% dose	suppl 80 mg	no adjustment	dose for GFR 10–50
Timolol	10–20 mg bid	normal dose	normal dose	normal dose	no adjustment	no adjustment	dose for GFR 10–50

(Continued)

(Continued)

Drugs	Normal dosage	Dosage adjustment in renal failure			HD	CAPD	CVVH
		GFR > 50	GFR 10–50	GFR < 10			
32.6.4 Calcium Channel Blockers							
Amlodipine	2.5–10 mg qd	normal dose	normal dose	normal dose	no adjustment	no adjustment	dose for GFR 10–50
Diltiazem	30–90 mg tid	normal dose	normal dose	normal dose	no adjustment	no adjustment	dose for GFR 10–50
Felodipine	2.5–20 mg qd	normal dose	normal dose	normal dose	no adjustment	no adjustment	dose for GFR 10–50
Nicardipine	20–30 mg tid	normal dose	normal dose	normal dose	no adjustment	no adjustment	no adjustment
Nifedipine SR	20–40 mg bid	normal dose	normal dose	normal dose	no adjustment	no adjustment	no adjustment
Nimodipine	60 mg q4h	normal dose	normal dose	normal dose	no adjustment	no adjustment	dose for GFR 10–50
Verapamil	40–80 mg tid	normal dose	normal dose	normal dose	no adjustment	no adjustment	dose for GFR 10–50

(Continued)

(*Continued*)

Drugs	Normal dosage	Dosage adjustment in renal failure			HD	CAPD	CVVH
		GFR > 50	GFR 10–50	GFR < 10			
32.6.5 *Diuretics*							
Acetazolamide	125–500 mg tid	normal dose	50% dose	avoid	no data	no data	no data
Amiloride	5–10 mg qd	normal dose	normal dose	avoid	avoid	avoid	avoid
Bemetanide	1–4 mg qd	normal dose	normal dose	normal dose	no adjustment	no adjustment	not applicable
Furosemide	20 mg qd–120 mg tid	normal dose	normal dose	normal dose	no adjustment	no adjustment	not applicable
Hydrochlorothiazide	12.5–200 mg qd	normal dose	normal dose	avoid	not applicable	not applicable	not applicable
Indapamide	2.5 mg qd	normal dose	avoid	ineffective	no adjustment	not applicable	no adjustment
Metolazone	2.5 mg qd–10 mg tid	normal dose	normal dose	normal dose	no adjustment	no adjustment	no adjustment
Spironolactone	100–300 mg qd	normal dose	normal dose	avoid	not applicable	not applicable	avoid
Triamterene	25–50 mg bid	normal dose	normal dose	avoid	avoid	avoid	avoid

(*Continued*)

(Continued)

Drugs	Normal dosage	Dosage adjustment in renal failure			HD	CAPD	CVVH
		GFR > 50	GFR 10–50	GFR < 10			
32.6.6 Alpha Blockers							
Doxazosin	1–16 mg/d	normal dose	normal dose	normal dose	no adjustment	no adjustment	dose for GFR 10–50
Prazosin	1–15 mg/d	normal dose	normal dose	normal dose	no adjustment	no adjustment	dose for GFR 10–50
Terazosin	1–10 mg bid	normal dose	normal dose	normal dose	no adjustment	no adjustment	dose for GFR 10–50
32.6.7 Other Antihypertensive Drugs							
Clonidine	0.1–1.2 mg bid	normal dose	normal dose	normal dose	no adjustment	no adjustment	dose for GFR 10–50
Hydralazine	10–100 mg qid	normal dose	normal dose	normal dose	no adjustment	no adjustment	dose for GFR 10–50
Minoxidil	2.5–10 mg bid	normal dose	normal dose	normal dose	no adjustment	no adjustment	dose for GFR 10–50
Nitroprusside	1–10 mcg/kg/min	normal dose	normal dose	normal dose	no adjustment	no adjustment	dose for GFR 10–50

(Continued)

(Continued)

32.7 Antiarrhythmic Agents

Drugs	Normal dosage	Dosage adjustment in renal failure			HD	CAPD	CVVH
		GFR > 50	GFR 10–50	GFR < 10			
Amiodarone	200–600 mg/d	normal dose	normal dose	normal dose	no adjustment	no adjustment	dose for GFR 10–50
Disopyramide	150 mg q6h	q8h	q12h	100 mg q24h	no adjustment	no adjustment	dose for GFR 10–50
Digoxin	0.125–0.25 mg qd	normal dose	25–75% dose	25% dose	no adjustment	no adjustment	dose for GFR 10–50
Flecainide	40 mg bid–100 mg tid	normal dose	normal dose	50–75%	no adjustment	no adjustment	dose for GFR 10–50
Lidocaine	1–1.5 mg/kg	normal dose	normal dose	normal dose	no adjustment	no adjustment	dose for GFR 10–50
Magnesium	start 1–2 g IV, then 0.5–1 g/h prn	normal dose	normal dose	max 20 g/48h	no data	no data	dose for GFR 10–50 no data
Procainamide	0.5–1 g q6h	normal dose	q6–12h	q8–24h	suppl 200 mg	no adjustment	dose for GFR 10–50
Propafenon	150 mg q8h	normal dose	normal dose	normal dose	no adjustment	no adjustment	dose for GFR 10–50
Quinidine ER	300–600 mg q8–12h	normal dose	normal dose	75% dose	suppl 100–200 mg	no adjustment	dose for GFR 10–50

(Continued)

(Continued)

32.8 Oral Hypoglycemic Agents

Drugs	Normal dosage	Dosage adjustment in renal failure			HD	CAPD	CVVH
		GFR > 50	GFR 10–50	GFR < 10			
Acarbose	25–100 mg tid	normal dose	50% dose	avoid	no data	no data	avoid
Chlorpropamide	100–500 mg q24h	50% dose	avoid	avoid	no data	no adjustment	avoid
Gliclazide	40 mg qd–160 mg bid	50–100% dose	avoid	avoid	no data	no data	avoid
Glipizide	5 mg qd–20 mg bid	normal dose	50% dose	50% dose	no data	no data	avoid
Metformin	500 mg bid–750 mg tid	normal dose	avoid	avoid	no data	no data	avoid
Tolbutamide	0.5–1 g bid	normal dose	normal dose	normal dose	no adjustment	no adjustment	avoid
Pioglitazone	15–45 mg qd	normal dose	normal dose	normal dose	no adjustment	no data	no data
Rosiglitazone	4–8 mg/d, qd to bid	normal dose	normal dose	normal dose	no adjustment	no data	no data
Sitagliptin	100 mg qd	normal dose	25–50 mg qd	25 mg qd	no adjustment	no adjustment	no data

(Continued)

(Continued)

Drugs	Normal dosage	Dosage adjustment in renal failure			HD	CAPD	CVVH
		GFR > 50	GFR 10–50	GFR < 10			
32.9 Lipid-Lowering Agents							
Atorvastatin	10–80 mg qd	normal dose	normal dose	normal dose	no data	no data	no data
Cholestyramine	2–8 mg bid	normal dose	normal dose	normal dose	no data	no data	no data
Clofibrate	500–1000 mg bid	normal dose	normal dose	normal dose	no data	no data	no data
Rosuvastatin	5–20 mg qd	normal dose	max 10 mg for CrCl < 30		no data	no data	no data
Fluvastatin	20–80 mg qd	normal dose	normal dose	normal dose	no data	no data	no data
Gemfibrozil	600 mg bid	normal dose	normal dose	normal dose	no data	no data	no data
Lovastatin	5–20 mg qd	normal dose	normal dose	normal dose	no data	no data	no data
Nicotinic acid	1–2 g tid	normal dose	50% dose	25% dose	no data	no data	no data
Parvastatin	10–80 mg qd	normal dose	normal dose	normal dose	no data	no data	no data
Simvastatin	5–80 mg qd	normal dose	normal dose	normal dose	no data	no data	no data
Ezetimibe	10 mg qd	normal dose	normal dose	normal dose	no data	no data	no data
32.10 Gastrointestinal Agents							
Cimetidine	400–800 mg bid	normal dose	75% dose	25% dose	no adjustment	no adjustment	dose for GFR 10–50
Cisapride	10 mg tid–20 mg qid	normal dose	normal dose	50–75% dose	no data	no data	50–100% dose

(Continued)

(Continued)

Drugs	Normal dosage	Dosage adjustment in renal failure			HD	CAPD	CVVH
		GFR > 50	GFR 10–50	GFR < 10			
Famotidine	20–40 mg bid	normal dose	75% dose	25% dose	no adjustment	no adjustment	dose for GFR 10–50
Lansoprazole	15 mg qd–30 mg bid	normal dose	normal dose	normal dose	no data	no data	no data
Metoclopramide	10 mg tid	normal dose	normal dose	50–75% dose	no adjustment	no data	50–75% dose
Misoprostol	100 mcg bid–200 mcg qid	normal dose	normal dose	normal dose	no data	no data	no data
Omeprazole	20 mg qd–40 mg bid	normal dose	normal dose	normal dose	no data	no data	no data
Rabeprazole	10 mg qd–40 mg bid	normal dose	normal dose	normal dose	no data	no data	no data
Ranitidine	150–300 mg bid	normal dose	75% dose	25% dose	suppl 1/2 dose	no adjustment	dose for GFR 10–50
Pantoprazole	40 mg qd–80 mg bid	normal dose	normal dose	normal dose	no data	no data	no data
Sucralfate	1 g qid	normal dose	normal dose	normal dose	no data	no data	no data

(Continued)

(Continued)

Drugs	Normal dosage	Dosage adjustment in renal failure			HD	CAPD	CVVH
		GFR > 50	GFR 10–50	GFR < 10			
32.11 Neurological Agents/Anticonvulsants							
Carbamazepine	2–8 mg/kg/d	normal dose	normal dose	normal dose	no adjustment	no adjustment	no adjustment
Clonazepam	0.5–2 mg tid	normal dose	normal dose	normal dose	no adjustment	no data	not applicable
Ethosuximide	5 mg/kg/d	normal dose	normal dose	normal dose	no adjustment	no data	no data
Gabapentin	150–900 mg tid	normal dose	50% dose	25% dose	suppl 200–300 mg	300 mg qod	dose for GFR 10–50
Lamotrigine	25–150 mg/d	normal dose	normal dose	normal dose	no data	no data	dose for GFR 10–50
Levetiracetam	500–1500 mg bid	normal dose	50% dose	50% dose	250–500 mg after HD	dose for GFR < 10	dose for GFR 10–50
Phenobarbital	loading 15–20 mg/kg, maintenance 60 mg bid/tid	q8–12h	q8–12h	q12–16h	dose after HD	1/2 normal dose	dose for GFR 10–50
Phenytoin	300–400 mg/d	normal dose	normal dcse	normal dose	no adjustment	no adjustment	no adjustment
Primidone	750–1500 mg/d	q8h	q8–12h	q12–24h	suppl 1/3 dose	no data	no data
Sodium valproate	7.5–15 mg/kg/d	normal dose	normal dose	normal dose	no adjustment	no adjustment	no adjustment

(Continued)

(Continued)

Drugs	Normal dosage	Dosage adjustment in renal failure			HD	CAPD	CVVH
		GFR > 50	GFR 10–50	GFR < 10			
Topiramate	50 mg qd–200 mg bid	normal dose	50% dose	avoid	no data	no data	dose for GFR 10–50
Trimethadione	300–600 mg tid/qid	q8h	q8–12h	q12–24h	no data	no data	dose for GFR 10–50
Vigabatrin	1–2 g bid	normal dose	50% dose	25% dose	no data	no data	dose for GFR 10–50
Carbidopa/Levodopa	1 tablet tid to 6 tablets qd (according to preparation)	normal dose	normal dose	50–100% dose	no adjustment	50–100% dose	dose for GFR 10–50
Selegiline	1.25–2.5 mg qd	normal dose	normal dose	normal dose	no data	no data	no data
32.12 Arthritis and Gout							
Allopurinol	300 mg qd	75% dose	50% dose	25% dose	1/2 dose after HD	no data	dose for GFR 10–50
Auranofin	6 mg qd	50% dose	avoid	avoid	no adjustment	no adjustment	no adjustment
Colchicine	Acute: 0.5 mg q6h Chronic: 0.5–1 mg qd	normal dose	50% dose	25% dose	no adjustment	no data	dose for GFR 10–50

(Continued)

(*Continued*)

Drugs	Normal dosage	Dosage adjustment in renal failure			HD	CAPD	CVVH
		GFR > 50	GFR 10–50	GFR < 10			
Gold sodium	25–50 mg/wk	50% dose	avoid	avoid	no adjustment	no adjustment	avoid
Penicillamine	250–1000 mg qd	normal dose	avoid	avoid	suppl 1/3 dose	no data	dose for GFR 10–50
Probenecid	500 mg bid	normal dose	avoid	avoid	avoid	no data	avoid
Sulfasalazine	1–2 g/d, bid to qid	normal dose	q12h	q24h	no data	no data	no data
Methotrexate	7.5–25 mg qwk	75% dose	25–50% dose	avoid	suppl 50% dose	no adjustment	50% dose
32.13 NSAIDs[b]							
Diclofenac	25–75 mg bid	normal dose	normal dose	normal dose	no adjustment	no adjustment	dose for GFR 10–50
Ibuprofen	300–800 mg tid	normal dose	normal dose	normal dose	no adjustment	no adjustment	dose for GFR 10–50
Indomethacin	25–50 mg tid	normal dose	normal dose	normal dose	no adjustment	no adjustment	dose for GFR 10–50
Ketoprofen	25–75 mg tid	normal dose	normal dose	normal dose	no adjustment	no adjustment	dose for GFR 10–50
Mefenamic acid	250 mg qid	normal dose	normal dose	normal dose	no adjustment	no adjustment	dose for GFR 10–50

(*Continued*)

(Continued)

Drugs	Normal dosage	Dosage adjustment in renal failure			HD	CAPD	CVVH
		GFR > 50	GFR 10–50	GFR < 10			
Naproxen	500 mg bid	normal dose	normal dose	normal dose	no adjustment	no adjustment	dose for GFR 10–50
Piroxicam	20 mg qd	normal dose	normal dose	normal dose	no adjustment	no adjustment	dose for GFR 10–50
Sulindac	200 mg bid	normal dose	normal dose	normal dose	no adjustment	no adjustment	dose for GFR 10–50
32.14 Sedatives							
32.14.1 Barbiturates							
Pentobarbital	30 mg q6–8h	normal dose	normal dose	normal dose	no adjustment	no adjustment	dose for GFR 10–50
Phenobarbital	50–100 mg q8–12h	q8–12h	q8–12h	q12–16h	dose after HD	1/2 normal dose	dose for GFR 10–50
Thiopental	individualized	normal dose	normal dose	normal dose	no data	no data	no data

(Continued)

(Continued)

Drugs	Normal dosage	Dosage adjustment in renal failure			HD	CAPD	CVVH
		GFR > 50	GFR 10–50	GFR < 10			
32.14.2 Benzodiazepines							
Alprazolam	0.25–0.5 mg q8h	normal dose	normal dose	normal dose	no adjustment	no data	no data
Clorazepate	15–60 mg q24h	normal dose	normal dose	normal dose	no data	no data	no data
Chlordiazepoxide	5–25 mg tid–qid	normal dose	normal dose	50% dose	no adjustment	no data	dose for GFR 10–50
Clonazepam	0.5 mg tid	normal dose	normal dose	normal dose	no adjustment	no data	no data
Diazepam	2–10 mg tid–qid	normal dose	normal dose	normal dose	no adjustment	no data	no adjustment
Lorazepam	1–2 mg q8–12h	normal dose	normal dose	normal dose	no adjustment	no data	dose for GFR 10–50
Midazolam	individualized	normal dose	normal dose	50% dose	no data	no data	no data
Temazepam	7.5–30 mg bedtime	normal dose	normal dose	normal dose	no adjustment	no adjustment	no data
Triazolam	0.25–0.5 mg bedtime	normal dose	normal dose	normal dose	no adjustment	no adjustment	no data
32.14.3 Benzodiazepine Antagonist							
Flumazenil	0.2 mg IV	normal dose	normal dose	normal dose	no adjustment	no data	no data

(Continued)

(Continued)

Drugs	Normal dosage	Dosage adjustment in renal failure			HD	CAPD	CVVH
		GFR > 50	GFR 10–50	GFR < 10			
32.14.4 Lithium							
Lithium	300 mg tid–qid	normal dose	50–75% dose	25–50% dose	dose after HD	no adjustment	dose for GFR 10–50
32.15 Antipsychotics							
Chlorpromazine	300–800 mg/d	normal dose	normal dose	normal dose	no adjustment	no adjustment	dose for GFR 10–50
Clozapine	300–450 mg/d	normal dose	normal dose	normal dose	no data	no data	no data
Haloperidol	0.5–5 mg bid/tid	normal dose	normal dose	normal dose	no adjustment	no adjustment	dose for GFR 10–50
Olanzapine	5–10 mg qd	normal dose	normal dose	normal dose	no adjustment	no data	no data
Promethazine	20–100 mg/d	normal dose	normal dose	normal dose	no data	no data	dose for GFR 10–50
Quetiapine	150–750 mg/d	normal dose	normal dose	normal dose	no data	no data	no data
Risperidone	1–3 mg bid	normal dose	start at lower dose	normal dose	no data	no data	no data
Thioridazine	50–100 mg tid	normal dose	normal dose	normal dose	no adjustment	no data	no data
Trifluoperazine	1–2 mg bid	normal dose	normal dose	normal dose	no adjustment	no data	no data

(Continued)

(Continued)

Drugs	Normal dosage	Dosage adjustment in renal failure			HD	CAPD	CVVH
		GFR > 50	GFR 10–50	GFR < 10			
32.16 Antidepressants							
Citalopram	20–60 mg qd	normal dose	normal dose	avoid	no data	no data	no data
Escitalopram	10 mg qd	normal dose	normal dose	use with caution	no data	no data	no data
Fluoxetine	20–60 mg qd	normal dose	normal dose	normal dose	no adjustment	no adjustment	no data
Mirtazapine	15–45 mg bedtime	normal dose	70% clearance	50% clearance	no data	no data	no data
Paroxetine	20–50 mg qd	normal dose	50% dose	25% dose	no data	no data	no data
Sertraline	50–200 mg qd	normal dose	normal dose	normal dose	no adjustment	no data	no data
Venlafaxine	37.5–75 mg bid to tid	75% dose	75% dose	50% dose	dose after HD	no data	no data
32.17 Anticoagulants							
Alteplase	60 mg over 1 h, then 20 mg/h for 2 h	normal dose in renal failure			no data	no data	dose for GFR 10–50
Aspirin	80–300 mg/d	normal dose	normal dose	normal dose	dose after HD	no adjustment	dose for GFR 10–50

(Continued)

(Continued)

Drugs	Normal dosage	Dosage adjustment in renal failure			HD	CAPD	CVVH
		GFR > 50	GFR 10–50	GFR < 10			
Clopidogrel	75 mg qd	normal dose	normal dose	normal dose	no data	no data	no data
Nadroparin	171 IU/kg/d	normal dose	dosage reduction recommended		no data	no data	no data
Dipyridamole	50 mg tid	normal dose	normal dose	normal dose	no data	no data	no data
Enoxaparin	1 mg/kg q12h	normal dose	75–50% dose	50% dose	no data	no data	no data
Heparin	75 mg/kg loading, then 15 mg/kg/h	normal dose in renal failure			no adjustment	no adjustment	dose for GFR 10–50
Streptokinase	1.5 MU over 1 h	normal dose	normal dose	normal dose	no data	no data	dose for GFR 10–50
Ticlopidine	250 mg bid	normal dose	normal dose	normal dose	no data	no data	dose for GFR 10–50
Urokinase	4400 U/kg/h × 12 h	no data	no data	no data	no data	no data	no data
Warfarin	adjust with INR	normal dose	normal dose	normal dose	no adjustment	no adjustment	no data
32.18 Antihemophilic Agent							
Tranexamic acid	25 mg/kg/dose tid to qid	50% dose	25% dose	10% dose	no data	no data	no data

(Continued)

(*Continued*)

Drugs	Normal dosage	Dosage adjustment in renal failure			HD	CAPD	CVVH
		GFR > 50	GFR 10–50	GFR < 10			
32.19 Chemotherapy							
Bleomycin	individual protocol	normal dose	45–70% dose	40% dose	no adjustment	no data	75% dose
Busulfan	individual protocol	normal dose	normal dose	normal dose	no data	no data	no data
Capecitabine	individual protocol	normal dose	75% dose	CrCl < 30 contraindicated	no data	no data	no data
Chlorambucil	individual protocol	normal dose	75% dose	50% dose	no data	50% dose	no data
Cyclophosphamide	individual protocol	normal dose	normal dose	75% dose	50% dose after HD	75% dose	100% dose
Cytarabine	low dose (100–200 mg/m²)	no adjustment	no adjustment	no adjustment	no data	no data	no data
	high dose (1–3 g/m²)	60% dose	50% dose	avoid use if CrCl < 30	avoid	avoid	no data
Doxorubicin	individual protocol	normal dose	normal dose	normal dose	no adjustment	no data	no data

(*Continued*)

(Continued)

Drugs	Normal dosage	Dosage adjustment in renal failure			HD	CAPD	CVVH
		GFR > 50	GFR 10–50	GFR < 10			
Etoposide	individual protocol	normal dose	75% dose	50% dose	no adjustment	no adjustment	75% dose
Fluorouracil	individual protocol	normal dose	normal dose	normal dose	suppl 50% dose	no data	no data
Imatinib	400–800 mg qd	no data, urinary excretion: 5% intact drug			no data	no data	no data
Melphalan	individual protocol	normal dose	75% dose	50% dose	dose after HD	50% dose	75% dose
Mitomycin	individual protocol	Cr > 1.7 mg/dL (150 μmol/L) contraindicated			no data	no data	no data
Thalidomide	100–400 mg qd	no data, urinary excretion: <1% intact drug			no data	no data	no data
Tretinoin	45 mg/m^2/d bid-tid	no data, urinary excretion: 63%			no data	no data	no data
Vinblastine	0.1–0.5 mg/kg/wk individual protocol	normal dose	normal dose	normal dose	no data	no data	no data
Vincristine	individual protocol	normal dose	normal dose	normal dose	no data	no data	no data
32.20 Iron-Chelating Agent							
Deferoxamine	20–40 mg/kg/d over 8 h	normal dose	normal dose	50% dose	no data	no data	no data

(Continued)

(Continued)

Drugs	Normal dosage[a]	Dosage adjustment in renal failure			HD	CAPD	CVVH
		GFR > 50	GFR 10–50	GFR < 10			
32.21 Immunosuppressants							
Azathioprine	1–3 mg/kg/d	normal dose	75% dose	50% dose	suppl	no adjustment	no data
Cyclosporin	7–9 mg/kg/d bid (tapered down to achieve desirable drug level)	normal dose	normal dose	normal dose	0.25 mg/kg no adjustment	no adjustment	normal dose
Sirolimus	loading 4–6 mg/d, maintenance 1–2 mg/d, adjust according to drug level	normal dose	normal dose	normal dose	no adjustment	no adjustment	no data
Everolimus	0.75 mg bid	normal dose	normal dose	normal dose	no adjustment	suggested	no data
Tacrolimus	0.075–0.2 mg/kg/d	lowest dose of recommended range			no adjustment	no adjustment	no data
Mycophenolic acid	720 mg bid	normal dose	normal dose	normal dose	no adjustment	no adjustment	no data
Mycophenolic mofetil	1 g bid	normal dose	normal dose	normal dose	no adjustment	no adjustment	no data

[a] Drug-level monitoring is crucial in determining the dosage interval.
[b] In general, NSAIDs are not recommended in patients with significant renal impairment.

33

Drug Interactions with Commonly Used Immunosuppressants

Laurence K. Chan and Siu-Kim Chan

Knowledge of the pharmacology and drug interactions of immunosuppressants is crucial in the prescription of immunosuppressive therapy for solid organ transplant. Any changes in plasma drug level due to the addition of interacting drugs can potentially cause devastating consequences, as most of the commonly used immunosuppressants have a narrow therapeutic range. An inadequate level is associated with acute rejection, while a high level can result in toxicity. Besides interaction with medications competing in their metabolic pathway, immunosuppressive agents are usually prescribed in combination with the components that interact with each other. There are potential interactions throughout the metabolic pathway, from absorption to elimination of the drugs. Furthermore, variations of pharmacokinetics or pharmacodynamics are commonly observed in individuals as a result of varying degrees of gene expression, and they are dealt with in pharmacogenetics. Therefore, it is important to understand the pharmacokinetics and pharmacodynamics of individual immunosuppressive agents, and to have therapeutic drug monitoring.

Immunosuppressants can be classified on the basis of their primary site of action, as inhibitors of transcription (cyclosporine and tacrolimus), as inhibitors of nucleotide synthesis (azathioprine, mycophenolate mofetil, and enteric-coated mycophenolic acid), or as inhibitors of growth factor signal transduction (sirolimus and everolimus). The current standard practice for chronic immunosuppression includes a calcineurin inhibitor, an antiproliferative agent, and steroids. The calcineurin inhibitor is either cyclosporine (CsA) or tacrolimus; the antiproliferative agent is typically mycophenolate mofetil (MMF)/mycophenolic acid (MPA) or sirolimus/everolimus; and low-dose prednisone is used as a basic immunosuppressive drug for induction and maintenance immunosuppressive therapy.

The commonly used regimens to be discussed include cyclosporine, tacrolimus, mycophenolic acid, and sirolimus/everolimus. The pharmacology of these regimens will be discussed, and focus will be put on the metabolic site where potential drug interactions take place.

33.1 Cyclosporine

The microemulsion form of cyclosporine (Neoral) significantly improves the absorption and bioavailability of the drug when compared with a preparation developed earlier. The generic form of cyclosporine is now available in different preparations. Subtle differences in pharmacokinetics exist among the different formulations, and caution should be made in switching between them. Cyclosporine exerts its immunosuppressive effect by binding to the intracellular FK-binding protein and the complex formed inhibits calcinuerin, an important phosphatase in the cellular signal transduction pathway, leading to inhibition of T-cell proliferation.

The metabolism of cyclosporine is mainly performed by the liver cytochrome P450 3A4 (CYP3A4) enzyme system. It is both a substrate and an inhibitor of this well-described enzyme system, which metabolizes more than 50% of commonly used drugs. Besides drugs, grapefruit juice, St. John's wort, and red wine also interact with cyclosporine through their modulating effect on CYP3A4. Clinically significant drug interactions of cyclosporine are summarized in Table 33.1.

33.2 Tacrolimus

Tacrolimus behaves similarly to cyclosporine in its pharmacodynamics, metabolism, and drug interaction. Its oral bioavailability is poor, reaching around 25%, and is decreased extensively by the activity of intestinal cytochrome P450 3A and P-glycoprotein. P-glycoprotein is a membrane-bound transporter protein involved in the transport of tacrolimus out of intestinal epithelial cells. The trough level of tacrolimus is inversely proportional to the expression of P-glycoprotein in the mucosa of the upper jejunum.

Table 33.1   Clinically significant drug interactions of cyclosporine.

Drugs that increase blood cyclosporine level
  Antifungal agents — ketoconazole, fluconazole, itraconazole
  Macrolides — clarithromycin, erythromycin
  Antivirals (HIV) — ritonavir, tipranavir, fosamprenavir
  Calcium channel blockers — verapamil, nicardipine, diltiazem
  Others — methylprednisolone, allopurinol, bromocriptine, danazol,
    metoclopramide, cimetidine

Drugs that decrease blood cyclosporine level
  Antiepileptics — phenytoin, phenobarbital, carbamazepine
  Antibiotics — co-trimoxazole, rifampicin, nafcillin
  Others — ticlopidine, octreotide

Drugs that increase risk of hyperkalemia when given with cyclosporine
  Angiotensin-converting enzyme inhibitors (ACEIs) and angiotensin II
    antagonists, potassium-sparing diuretics

Drugs that increase risk of nephrotoxicity when given with cyclosporine
  Aminoglycosides, vancomycin, co-trimoxazole, amphotericin B,
    melphalan, non-steroidal anti-inflammatory drugs (NSAIDs)

Tacrolimus is metabolized by the hepatic enzyme system CYP3A; therefore, many drug interactions are expected. Similar to cyclosporine, grapefruit juice and St. John's wort also exert an inhibitory effect on CYP3A and P-glycoprotein, and thus increase the exposure of tacrolimus. A summary of drug interactions of tacrolimus can be seen in Table 33.2. The CYP3A subfamily exhibits significant pharmacogenetic variability. One of its isoforms, CYP3A4, which is the most abundantly expressed, shows a 10–100-fold difference in hepatic expression and up to a 30-fold difference in intestinal expression. Liver and intestinal disease could possibly affect the exposure of tacrolimus if the CYP3A system and P-glycoprotein expression are significantly affected during the disease course. These pharmacokinetic interactions and pharmacogenetic variability contribute to the interindividual and intraindividual variability of tacrolimus exposure, making therapeutic drug monitoring crucial in maintaining immunosuppression.

33.3 Mycophenolic Acid (MMF or Myfortic)

Mycophenolic mofetil (MMF), a prodrug of mycophenolic acid (MPA), was developed to improve the bioavailability of MPA. MMF is rapidly

Table 33.2   Clinically significant drug interactions of tacrolimus.

Drugs that increase blood tacrolimus level
Bromocriptine, chloramphenicol, cimetidine, cisapride, clarithromycin,
clotrimazole, cyclosporine, danazol, diltiazem, erythromycin, ethinyl
estradiol, fosamprenavir, itraconazole, ketoconazole, methylprednisolone, metoclopramide, nicardipine, omeprazole, ritonavir,
theophylline, tipranavir, verapamil, voriconazole

Drugs that decrease blood tacrolimus level
Carbamezepine, phenobarbitol, phenytoin, rifabutin, rifampicin

Drugs that increase risk of nephrotoxicity when given with tacrolimus
Aminoglycosides, amphotericine B, cisplatin, cyclosporine, NSAIDs

hydrolyzed to form MPA in various tissues after absorption. MPA is then metabolized in the liver and gastrointestinal tract to form 7-O-MPA-β-glucuronide (MPAG), which undergoes enterohepatic recirculation to enter the blood stream. MPAG is excreted in the bile and converted to MPA by the β-glucuronidase of the microorganism in the gut. The subsequent reabsorption of MPA contributes significantly to its area under the time–concentration curve (AUC).

Myfortic is an enteric-coated formulation of mycophenolate sodium that delivers the active moiety MPA. It is enteric-coated and is primarily absorbed in the intestine. Similar to CellCept, it is an uncompetitive and reversible inhibitor of inosine monophosphate dehydrogenase and therefore inhibits the *de novo* pathway of guanosine nucleotide synthesis without incorporation to DNA. The recommended dose of Myfortic is 720 mg administered twice daily 1 h before or 2 h after food intake. The side effects between Myfortic and MMF are similar in both *de novo* and maintenance patients.

MPA (from CellCept or Myfortic) is an antimetabolite that decreases the synthesis of guanosine nucleotides by inhibiting the rate-limiting enzyme inosine monophosphate dehydrogenase. It exerts the pharmacodynamic action mainly by inhibiting lymphocyte proliferation and antibody formation.

The potential drug interactions with MPA are mainly through its absorption and enterohepatic recirculation (Table 33.3). Combination therapy commonly used (like cyclosporine) inhibits the MPAG excretion in the bile, thus limiting the enterohepatic recycling of MPA.

Table 33.3   Clinically significant drug interactions of mycophenolic acid (MPA).

Drugs that increase blood MPA level
   Tacrolimus[a]

Drugs that decrease blood MPA level
   Iron salts, calcium polycarbophil, cyclosporine, aluminum and magnesium
   antacids, cholestyramine, corticosteroids

---

[a] Controversial evidence regarding the effect of tacrolimus on blood MPA level.

In contrast, tacrolimus was found to have a controversial effect on the metabolism of MPA, and therefore further studies are required to confirm its effect. Corticosteroids may decrease the MPA AUC, as evidenced by the comparison between standard triple therapy and steroid-withdrawn therapy. Other medications like antacids inhibit MMF/MPAG absorption during the initial and enterohepatic recirculation phases. Calcium salt in the form of calcium polycarbophil and iron salts can inhibit MMF absorption, and therefore significantly decrease the MPA AUC.

33.4 The TOR Inhibitors: Sirolimus and Everolimus

Target of rapamycin (TOR) is a key regulatory kinase in the process of cell division. Both sirolimus and everolimus are TOR inhibitors or proliferation signal inhibitors (PSI) that block growth-factor-dependent cellular proliferation through a calcium-independent signal. Sirolimus resembles tacrolimus in its structure. It binds to cytoplasmic FK-binding protein 12 and the complex formed inhibits the enzymatic activity of mammalian target of rapamycin (mTOR), thus limiting its catalytic effect on multiple intracellular cascades after T- or B-cell stimulation. This results in indirectly inhibiting the function of T helper cell and cytotoxic T cell, while B-cell proliferation and differentiation are also affected.

Absorption of sirolimus or everolimus is significantly impaired by the metabolism of intestinal cytochrome P450 enzyme systems and possibly by the epithelial P-glycoprotein transport system. The variable expression of these enzymes results in significant interpatient variation in sirolimus exposure. The concomitant use of cyclosporine shows a marked increase in the sirolimus AUC but not vice versa, as a much higher dose of cyclosporine than sirolimus is usually used clinically. The trough level of sirolimus can increase up to 50% when sirolimus is administered together with cyclosporine. Tacrolimus–sirolimus interaction is mainly on antagonistic competition for the T-cell binding site (FK-binding protein), eventually leading to their antiproliferative action. However, in clinical use, their therapeutic concentrations are usually too low to cause a significant antagonistic effect, although their additive side effects should not be overlooked.

Sirolimus is mainly metabolized by the liver CYP3A4 enzyme system, and therefore drugs modulating this enzyme system can potentially affect its AUC. The possible interacting drugs are listed in Table 33.4.

33.5 Potential Drug Interactions Among Commonly Used Immunosuppressants

Knowledge of the drug absorption, metabolism, and elimination is essential in investigating the possible drug interactions on the various immunosuppressants. There are also clinically significant interactions among these immunosuppressants, as summarized in Fig. 33.1. Those drugs that are highly probable in generating interactions through different mechanisms are summarized in Table 33.5.

It is important for the clinician to be aware of drug interactions in transplant patients when initiating new therapies or witnessing unexpected toxicities. The interactions can result from changes in absorption, metabolism, or excretion, or through additive or synergistic toxicity with agents that have similar side effects. Simple medications such as antacids, cholestyramine, promotility agents, and even food can affect the absorption of immunosuppressive agents.

Table 33.4   Clinically significant drug interactions of sirolimus.

Drugs that increase blood sirolimus level
  Clarithromycin, erythromycin, clotrimazole, fluconazole, itraconazole, ketoconazole, voriconazole, bromocriptine, cimetidine, danazole, cisapride, metoclopramide, diltiazem, nicardipine, verapamil, ritonavir, cyclosporine

Drugs that decrease blood sirolimus level
  Carbamazepine, phenobarbital, phenytoin, rifabutin, rifampicin

Drugs that increase risk of toxicity when given with sirolimus
  Tacrolimus (e.g. development of hyperlipidemia), statins (e.g. development of rhabdomyolysis)

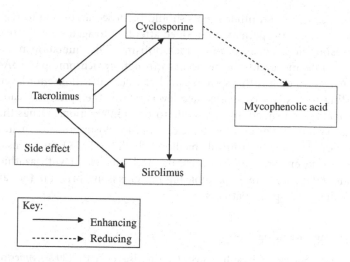

Fig. 33.1 Potential drug interactions among commonly used immuno-suppressants.

Table 33.5 Drugs of high risk in generating interactions through different mechanisms.

Mechanism	High-risk drugs	Affected drugs
Inhibitor of CYP3A (increase concentration of interacting drugs)	Verapamil, diltiazem, erythromycin, clarithromycin, ketoconazole, itraconazole, St. John's wort, ritonavir	Cyclosporin, tacrolimus, sirolimus, everolimus
Induction of hepatic enzymes (decrease concentration of interacting drugs)	Carbamazipine, rifampicin, phenytoin, phenobarbitone	Cyclosporine, tacrolimus, sirolimus, warfarin, oral contraception
Xanthine oxidase inhibitor	Allopurinol	Azathioprine
P-glycoprotein inhibition (increase exposure of drugs)	Cyclosporine, erythromycin, quinidine, itraconazole	Tacrolimus, digoxin, sirolimus
Interfere with gut absorption	Antacids, cholestyramine	Mycophenolic mofetil

Antimicrobials and other agents should be dosed according to renal function as in any patient, with added attention to agents which affect cyclosporine or tacrolimus metabolism. The metabolism of tacrolimus and cyclosporine occurs through cytochrome p450 3A4, so agents that affect this system can alter calcineurin-inhibitor levels, leading to toxicity or inadequate levels. Statin therapies may cause myopathy and rhabdomyolysis due to p450 interactions. Drugs that cause synergistic or additive toxicities and myelosuppression include allopurinol, trimethoprim/sulfamethoxazole (TMP/SMX), angiotensin-converting enzyme (ACE) inhibitors, and ganciclovir with azathioprine. Attention to these possible interactions is important in the care of kidney transplant patients.

Suggested Reading

American Society of Health-System Pharmacists (ASHP). (2008) *American Hospital Formulary Service (AHFS) Drug Information* 2008. ASHP, Bethesda, MD.

Augustine JJ, Bodziak KA, Hricik DE. (2007) Use of sirolimus in solid organ transplantation. *Drugs* 67:369–391.

Christians U, Jacobsen W, Benet LZ, Lampen A. (2002) Mechanisms of clinically relevant drug interactions associated with tacrolimus. *Clin Pharmacokinet* 41:813–851.

Christians U, Pokaiyavanichkul T, Chan L. (2006) *Tacrolimus. Applied Pharmacokinetics and Pharmacodynamics: Principles of Therapeutic Drug Monitoring*, 4th ed. Lippincott Williams & Wilkins, Baltimore, pp. 529–563.

Dahan A, Altman H. (2004) Food–drug interaction: grapefruit juice augments drug bioavailability — mechanism, extent and relevance. *Eur J Clin Nutr* 58:1–9.

Iwasaki K. (2007) Metabolism of tacrolimus (FK506) and recent topics in clinical pharmacokinetics. *Drug Metab Pharmacokinet* 22:328–335.

Izzo AA. (2004) Drug interactions with St. John's wort (*Hypericum perforatum*): a review of the clinical evidence. *Int J Clin Pharmacol Ther* 42: 139–148.

Kato R, Ooi K, Ikura-Mori M, *et al.* (2002) Impairment of mycophenolate mofetil absorption by calcium polycarbophil. *J Clin Pharmacol* 42:1275–1280.

Picard N, Prémaud A, Rousseau A, *et al.* (2006) A comparison of the effect of ciclosporin and sirolimus on the pharmokinetics of mycophenolate in renal transplant patients. *Br J Clin Pharmacol* 62:477–484.

Ting LS, Partovi N, Levy RD, *et al.* (2008) No pharmacokinetic interactions between mycophenolic acid and tacrolimus in renal transplant recipients. *J Clin Pharm Ther* 33:193–201.

Zwerner J, Fiorentino D. (2007) Mycophenolic mofetil. *Dermatol Ther* 20:229–238.

Index